FUNDAMENTALS OF
Psychopharmacology

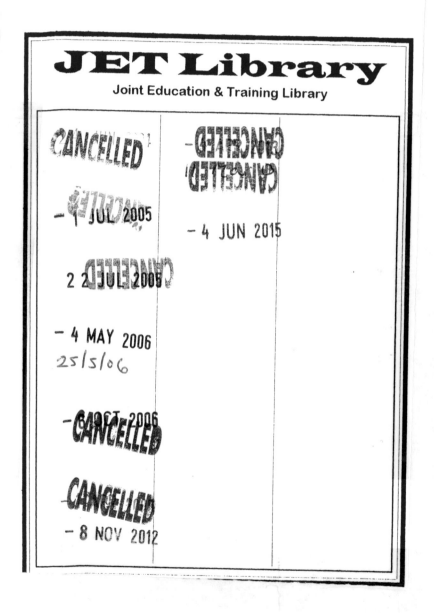

32.50

FUNDAMENTALS OF
Psychopharmacology

Third Edition

BRIAN E. LEONARD

Emeritus Professor of Pharmacology
National University of Ireland, Galway

WILEY

Other Wiley Editorial Offices

John Wiley & Sons Inc., 111 River Street, Hoboken, NJ 07030, USA

Jossey-Bass, 989 Market Street, San Francisco, CA 94103-1741, USA

Wiley-VCH Verlag GmbH, Boschstr. 12, D-69469 Weinheim, Germany

John Wiley & Sons Australia Ltd, 33 Park Road, Milton, Queensland 4064, Australia

John Wiley & Sons (Asia) Pte Ltd, 2 Clementi Loop #02-01, Jin Xing Distripark,
Singapore 129809

John Wiley & Sons Canada Ltd, 22 Worcester Road, Etobicoke, Ontario, Canada M9W 1L1

Wiley also publishes its books in a variety of electronic formats. Some content that appears
in print may not be available in electronic books.

All CNSforum figures are reprinted with permission from www.cnsforum.com. Original
colour images, with and without text, can be found on CNSforum. Reuse of the images
is permitted, as long as the copyright notice on the images is not hidden or removed.

Library of Congress Cataloging-in-Publication Data

Leonard, B. E.
  Fundamentals of psychopharmacology / Brian E. Leonard. – 3rd ed.
    p. cm.
  Includes bibliographical references and index.
  ISBN 0-471-52178-7 (alk. paper)
    1. Psychopharmacology. 2. Psychotropic drugs. I. Title.

RM315.L42 2003
615'.78–dc22

                                                    2003057597

British Library Cataloguing in Publication Data

A catalogue record for this book is available from the British Library

ISBN 0 471 52178 7

Typeset in 10/12pt Palatino by Dobbie Typesetting Ltd, Tavistock, Devon
Printed and bound in Great Britain by TJ International, Padstow, Cornwall
This book is printed on acid-free paper responsibly manufactured from sustainable forestation,
for which at least two trees are planted for each one used for paper production.

This book is dedicated to

HELGA

INGRID HEIDE

SAMUEL BENJAMIN

Contents

Preface to Third Edition ix

Preface to Second Edition xi

Preface to First Edition xiii

Introduction xv

1 Functional Neuroanatomy of the Brain 1

2 Basic Aspects of Neurotransmitter Function 15

3 Pharmacokinetic Aspects of Psychopharmacology 79

4 Clinical Trials and their Importance in Assessing the Efficacy and Safety of Psychotropic Drugs 101

5 Molecular Genetics and Psychopharmacology 113

6 Psychotropic Drugs that Modify the Serotonergic System 133

7 Drug Treatment of Depression 153

8 Drug Treatment of Mania 193

9 Anxiolytics and the Treatment of Anxiety Disorders 211

10 Drug Treatment of Insomnia 241

11 Drug Treatment of Schizophrenia and the Psychoses 255

12 Drug Treatment of the Epilepsies 295

13 Drug Treatment of Parkinson's Disease 319

14 Alzheimer's Disease and Stroke: Possible Biochemical Causes and Treatment Strategies 341

15 Psychopharmacology of Drugs of Abuse 375

16 Paediatric Psychopharmacology 417

17 Geriatric Psychopharmacology 425

18 The Inter-relationship Between Psychopharmacology and
     Psychoneuroimmunology   431

19 Endocoids and their Importance in Psychopharmacology   445

Appendix 1 Some Important Psychotropic Drug Interactions   459

Appendix 2 Glossary of some Common Terms Used
             in Psychopharmacology   463

Appendix 3 Generic and Proprietary Names of Some
             Common Psychotropic Drugs   483

Appendix 4 Key References for Further Reading   489

Index   499

Preface to Third Edition

The second edition of *Fundamentals of Psychopharmacology* was published in 1996 and therefore a thorough revision of the text became essential. This revision has taken me much longer than originally anticipated because I soon came to realize that every chapter would require a thorough reassessment. Retrospectively it would have been easier to have written a completely new book, but hopefully this edition will be a compromise between the style of the previous editions and the requirement to include increasingly complex concepts with the inclusion of molecular neurobiology and molecular genetics. In attempting to make such areas accessible to the non-specialist neuroscientist and clinical psychiatrist, I hope I have managed to accurately interpret the areas in which I have no specialist knowledge.

Besides thoroughly revising every chapter contained in the second edition, I have added a new short chapter on clinical trials of psychotropic drugs. The methods used to determine the efficacy and safety of new psychotropic drugs are becoming of major importance and now have an impact on all areas of medicine. I hope that this chapter will help to fill the gap that occurred in the earlier editions of the text. I have also broadened the final chapter to discuss the role of endogenous factors (the endocoids) that might play a crucial role in psychiatric disorders. Besides the endogenous opioids, it is now apparent that cannabinoids, benzodiazepine ligands and various neuropeptides (such as the sleep factor) may play a fundamental role not only in the psychopathology of the various disorders but also in the mechanisms whereby psychotropic drugs act.

As in the previous editions, I have been guided by the need to integrate the various areas of psychopharmacology. It is my belief that the neurosciences, like most branches of medicine, have become too fragmented into their specialist areas so that their important impact in our understanding of the whole organism (whether animal or man) is lost. The brain is not just a collection of cells that function in a tissue culture and genes are not independent, deterministic entities that function independently of their environment. Neither is it sufficient to classify psychiatric disorders by diagnostic criteria, quantified by esoteric rating scales, without seriously considering the biological components that contribute to the nature of the behavioural disorder. Perhaps it is time to return to a more integrated and dialectical approach to the basic and clinical neurosciences.

The revision of the third edition largely occurred between January 2002 and January 2003. Despite my early retirement as Head of the Pharmacology Department in 1999, I have found even less time to devote to writing a textbook than I did during my years as a full-time academic. Nevertheless, I am eternally grateful to the numerous students and colleagues who, over the past 4 years, have continued to stimulate my interest and excitement in the neurosciences and helped me to expand, and hopefully improve, this textbook. Special thanks must go to CNS forum (which has been supported by the Lundbeck Foundation, Skodsborg, Denmark), for permission to use several of the figures used to illustrate this edition.

I wish to give thanks in particular to Dr Brian O'Shea of Newcastle Hospital, Co. Wicklow, for the care and attention he gave in pointing out some of the errors in the second edition of the text. My thanks are also due to Charlotte Brabants of John Wiley and Sons Ltd, for her encouragement and regular e-mails to ensure that, though overdue, the third edition did materialize. Lastly, I again thank my wife for her support and understanding of my obsession with the brain, behaviour and the psychopathology of mental illness.

Brian E. Leonard
Emeritus Professor of Pharmacology
National University of Ireland, Galway

February 2003

Preface to Second Edition

The first edition of *Fundamentals of Psychopharmacology* was completed five years ago and, due to the major advances which have been made in the subject in the intervening years, a thorough revision of the text was necessary. Unfortunately, I did not have the privilege of a sabbatical leave on this occasion to rewrite all the chapters that would ideally be necessary. However, I have tried to compromise by adding several new chapters (on molecular genetics and functional neuroanatomy for example) and to revise intensively those areas (such as the antidepressants, antipsychotics and the importance of serotonin in psychiatric illness) that have undergone major advances in the intervening five years. In addition, I have added two chapters that hopefully will give a flavour to the development of psychopharmacology in the 21st century. One of these deals with the growing area of psychoimmunology and its importance in integrating the immune, endocrine and neurotransmitter systems with behaviour. The second area concerns the role of the enigmatic sigma receptors that appear to play a role in modulating the immune, endocrine and neurotransmitter systems.

Despite my best intentions, I am aware of the deficiencies and limitations that still exist in this volume. I have tried to correct the numerous minor errors in the first edition which undoubtedly reflected my lax proof reading. In this respect I wish to express my sincere thanks to the numerous friends and colleagues who took the time to comment on the strengths and deficiencies of the first edition. Hopefully, the second edition has remedied the more glaring errors and omissions. In producing the second edition, my intention has been to keep the volume as concise as possible without compromising on the accuracy of the contents.

The last five years have seen the publication of numerous excellent texts and monographs in psychopharmacology, many of which are mentioned in the bibliography. Hopefully, the second edition of *Fundamentals of Psychopharmacology* will generate sufficient enthusiasm for the reader to be encouraged to delve more deeply into the subject.

The revision of the second edition largely occurred between April and October 1996. As with the first edition, I am particularly indebted to the staff and postgraduate students of the Department of Pharmacology for their help and encouragement for this venture. In particular, I wish to express sincere thanks to my secretary Marie Morrissey for her help in

processing some of the new text, to Ambrose O'Halloran for his assistance
with all the technical aspects of my word processing, diagrams, etc. and to
Dr John Kelly who enabled me to dedicate time and energy to writing by
taking over the organization of the research group and many of my
departmental activities. Several of the post-doctoral students from the
department have also indirectly contributed to the ideas which have been
incorporated into the second edition. In particular I wish to thank Maeve
Caldwell, Bernadette Earley, Mairead McNamara, Anna Redmond, Cai
Song, Alan O'Connell and Michael O'Neill. Michael Davis and Hilary Rowe
of John Wiley and Sons have been a constant source of encouragement and
monthly faxes to ensure that the second edition materialized. Lastly, I thank
my long-suffering wife for having endured yet another period of physical
and mental absence from our domestic life while I remained obsessed with
the fascination of receptors, ion channels and the biochemistry of the brain.

B. E. Leonard
Department of Pharmacology
University College Galway
October 1996   Ireland

Preface to First Edition

This textbook started life some ten years ago as a collection of lecture notes in neuro- and psychopharmacology. These notes were produced in response to the needs of the undergraduate medical students and postgraduates studying for membership examinations at University College Galway and at the Muhibili Medical Centre, University of Dar es Salaam, where I was involved for several years in teaching under the auspices of an Irish Development Aid programme. Clearly the time had come to completely rewrite the lecture notes or to produce a proper textbook.

The problem was partly solved by my election as a visiting Fellow at Magdalen College, Oxford, during my sabbatical year 1990–1991, and I am particularly grateful to the Fellows of Magdalen College for having given me this opportunity. The access to the Radcliffe Science Library and the tranquillity of life in Magdalen College provided the ideal setting for this undertaking. Whether the pleasure I achieved in writing this text is reflected in the quality of its content is for the reader to judge. One thing is certain, without the support of Dr Jim O'Donnell and the postgraduates and staff of my department in Galway, who undertook many of the vital teaching and administrative duties during my year of absence, the completion of the textbook would have been impossible.

I am particularly grateful to my secretary, Marie Morrissey, for her dedication and determination to ensure that my appallingly bad word-processing was made intelligible to the reader. Ambrose O'Halloran not only taught me what little I know about word-processing but also had the patience and creativity to convert my illiterate sketches of chemical formulae and anatomical drawings into comprehensible figures. Without his enthusiastic support for this project, I am certain that the text would have been even more mediocre!

My colleagues Drs Ted Dinan and Veronica O'Keane of the Department of Psychiatry, Trinity College, Dublin, kindly offered to read critically the penultimate draft of the text. Their contribution was crucial in highlighting the errors, inconsistencies and lack of clarity in the draft. Their time and energy in helping to improve the text is gratefully acknowledged. Any errors and omissions that remain are, of course, entirely the responsibility of the author!

Michael Davis of John Wiley and Sons has also given invaluable support during the gestation of the text and made many useful suggestions regarding its content.

Finally I express my thanks to my long-suffering wife for having endured my obsessional preoccupation with this enterprise and with my physical and mental absence from our domestic life for the past year.

My sincere wish is that you, the reader, will look upon this modest contribution as merely an introduction to the exciting world of psychopharmacology. Your comments and criticisms will be particularly welcome.

B. E. Leonard
Department of Pharmacology
University College Galway
Ireland

September 1991

Introduction

The pain and suffering of those with major psychiatric illness has been appreciated since the dawn of civilization. For over 5000 years, drugs have been used in an attempt to alleviate the suffering of such patients. There is evidence that the Sumerians in the Tigris–Euphrates valley were aware of the mood-elevating effects of the juice of the opium poppy and cultivated these plants for that purpose. The potent analgesic effect of opium was well known to the inhabitants of Asia Minor, Cyprus, Mycenae and Egypt 2000 years BC. Indeed it should not be forgotten that opiates were still being used in the 19th century to relieve depression.

Other plants known to contain psychoactive compounds include hellebore, which was used for centuries in Europe to treat mania, violent temper, mental retardation and epilepsy. However, a drug of major importance in modern psychopharmacology arose from the discovery by medicinal chemists of the alkaloids of *Rauwolfia serpentina*, a root which had been used in the Indian subcontinent for centuries, not only for the treatment of snake bite but also for alleviating "insanity". Understandably, the mechanism of action of reserpine, the alkaloid purified from *Rauwolfia serpentina*, helped to lay the basis to psychopharmacology by demonstrating how the depletion of central and peripheral stores of biogenic amines was correlated with a reduction in blood pressure and tranquillization.

An unexpected discovery also arose during the therapeutic use of reserpine in the treatment of hypotension when it was found that approximately 15% of patients became clinically depressed. As it has been shown that reserpine depletes both the central and peripheral nervous system of noradrenaline, it was postulated that depression would be a consequence of the defective synthesis of noradrenaline and possibly serotonin. This helped to form the basis of the amine therapy of depression.

It is interesting to note that one of the founders of modern psychiatry, Kraepelin, listed only nine substances that were available for the treatment of psychiatric illness in the 1890s. These were: opium, morphine, scopolamine, hashish, chloral hydrate, a barbiturate, alcohol, chloroform and various bromides. Later Bleuler, another founder of modern psychiatry, added paraldehyde and sodium barbitone to the list. Thus psychopharmacology is a very recent area of medicine which largely arose from the chance discovery of chlorpromazine by Delay and Deniker in France in 1952, and of imipramine by Kuhn in Switzerland in 1957.

Although the chemical structure of the benzodiazepines was first described by Sternbach in the 1930s, the clinical efficacy of these anxiolytics was only fully realized following a clinical trial of chlordiazepoxide by Harris in the USA in 1960.

The purpose of this book is to give the basic neuroscientist and the psychiatrist an overview of psychopharmacology, that branch of pharmacology which is concerned with the study of drugs used to treat mental illness. The scope of the subject also covers the use of drugs and other chemical agents as tools that enable the researcher to investigate how the brain functions. This is one of the most rapidly advancing fields of medicine and therefore any short textbook on the subject is bound to omit many aspects which are fundamentally important.

Nevertheless, based on several years of experience teaching psychopharmacology to undergraduates and to postgraduate clinicians studying for their membership examination for the Royal College of Psychiatrists, I have tried to emphasize the practical advantages of understanding how psychotropic drugs work, not only because this may lead to an improvement in their therapeutic use but also that their side effects may be predicted. A brief glance through this book will persuade the reader that this is not a "cook-book" containing proprietary drug names, doses and a list of side effects. Neither have I attempted to give anything but a brief synopsis of the clinical features of the psychiatric illnesses for which the psychotropic drugs are used. There are many good texts available that cover clinical aspects of psychiatry and most countries have produced excellent formularies to provide practising clinicians with a summary of the therapeutic uses and side effects of the psychotropic drugs in common use. I hope that the reader will not only gain some insight into psychopharmacology as a result of this text but, more importantly, that it will enable the basic and clinical neuroscientist to better understand how the brain works in health and disease.

1 Functional Neuroanatomy of the Brain

Understanding the relationship between brain structure and function, and particularly how this relationship becomes disturbed in the mentally ill, is one of the major challenges to clinical and experimental neuroscientists. The brain may be described in terms of its general structure and key anatomical areas. It may also be described in terms of the cellular or subcellular structure of the different types of cells that constitute the brain. Finally it may be considered in terms of its functional importance in memory, consciousness and control of bodily functions. However the brain is described, each level of organization is essentially linked to another level of organization. Conventionally, neuroscientists have concentrated on the structural aspects of the brain and its cellular components while psychologists and psychiatrists have concentrated on the more functional aspects such as consciousness, thought processing and emotion. With the advent of sophisticated imaging methods and the introduction of novel drugs that combine therapeutic efficacy with subcellular specificity of action, it is now possible to show how all the levels of brain structure and function are interlinked. This will be illustrated by presenting an overview of brain structure and function and the reader is referred to the key references for further details of neuroanatomy. The principal regions of the human brain which are important in psychiatry and neurology are shown in Figure 1.1.

Structural and functional subdivision of the brain

Figure 1.2 presents a coronal section through the human brain. In brief, the brain may be divided into the brainstem (consisting of the medulla, pons and midbrain) that is linked to the diencephalon which is composed of the thalamus and the hypothalamus. The two cerebral hemispheres are linked by the corpus callosum, a large tract of nerve fibres that enables the two

Fundamentals of Psychopharmacology. Third Edition. By Brian E. Leonard
© 2003 John Wiley & Sons, Ltd. ISBN 0 471 52178 7

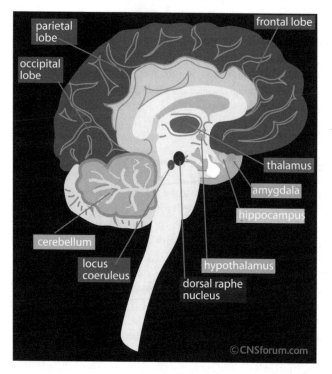

Figure 1.1. Main function of brain areas shown:

Amygdala – An anatomically coherent subsystem within the basal forebrain. Verbal and non-verbal expressions of fear and anger are interpreted by the amygdala.

Cerebellum – One of the seven parts of the brain that is responsible for muscle co-ordination and modulation of the force and range of movement. It is involved in the learning of motor skills.

Cortex – The most highly developed area in humans and divided into four main regions, namely frontal, parietal, temporal and occipital. The cortex mediates and integrates higher motor, sensory and association functions.

Dorsal raphé – Main serotonin (5-HT)-containing neurons that project through the brain. Other raphé neurons project down the spinal cord where they act as a gating mechanism for pain perception from the periphery. Main activity is in the regulation of mood, anxiety, sexual behaviour, sleep.

Hippocampus – Region primarily concerned with learning and short-term memory.

Hypothalamus – Part of the diencephalon comprising several nuclei where hormones such as oxytocin and antidiuretic hormone are synthesized and pass to the pituitary gland. Involved in the regulation of the peripheral autonomic system and pituitary hormones such as prolactin, growth hormone and adrenocorticotrophic hormone.

Locus coeruleus – Collection of cell bodies containing about 50% of the noradrenergic neurons. Main activity is in the regulation of mood, anxiety and attention. Noradrenergic tracts innervate most regions of the brain.

Thalamus – This acts as a relay station for pain, temperature and other bodily sensations.

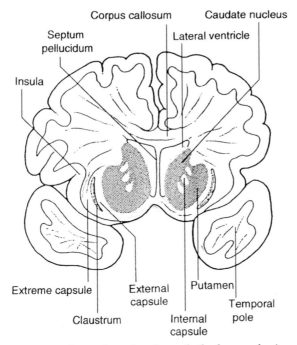

Figure 1.2.   Coronal section through the human brain.

halves of the brain to communicate. The brain is permeated by four ventricles, the two largest of which occur beneath the cerebral cortex.

More details of brain structure become evident in the coronal section through the brain (see Figure 1.2). From this figure it is evident that the _basal ganglia_ occupies a prominent role. The basal ganglia consists of the corpus striatum (consisting of the caudate nucleus, globus pallidus and putamen) and the substantia nigra. This region is concerned primarily with the control of movement and is malfunctional in Parkinson's disease and Huntington's disease. Figure 1.2 also illustrates the highly indented features of the cerebral cortex which can be visually differentiated into the surface grey matter, consisting of the cell bodies, and the much larger area of white matter which contains the myelinated axons connecting the cells of the cortex to the subcortical regions. The cerebrum contains the largest area of the brain, namely the two cerebral hemispheres.

From this brief description, it is apparent that the brain is really an assembly of organs all of which are structurally and functionally interconnected. Undoubtedly one of the most important areas for the psychopharmacologist is the so-called _limbic system_ which is concerned with emotion. This region consists of the hippocampus (concerned with memory

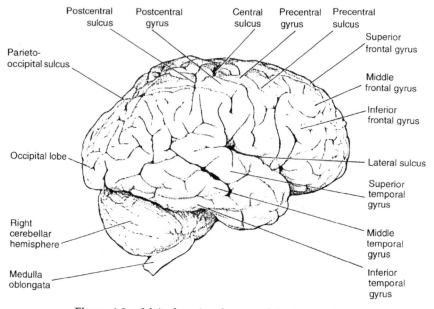

Figure 1.3. Main functional areas of the human brain.

processing), the thalamus and hypothalamus (concerned with the control of the endocrine system, temperature regulation, feeding, etc.), the amygdala and septum (the emotional centres of the subcortex), the fornix and the cingulate gyrus of the cortex.

The cerebral cortex is conventionally subdivided into four main regions that may be delineated by the sulci, or large clefts, termed the frontal, temporal, parietal and occipital lobes. These names are derived from the bones of the skull which overlay them. Each lobe may be further subdivided according to its cellular structure and composition. Thus Brodmann has divided the cortex into approximately 50 discrete areas according to the specific cellular structure and function. For example, electrical stimulation of the strip of cerebral cortex in front of the central sulcus (see Figure 1.3) is responsible for motor commands to the muscles. This is termed the *primary motor cortex* and can be further subdivided according to which muscles are controlled in different parts of the body.

Similar maps exist in other parts of the brain; for example, the areas concerned with sensory input such as the *primary somatosensory cortex* (see Figure 1.3). Such brain maps of the body are important because information from various organs converge on the brain in a highly organized fashion and can therefore be reflected at all levels of information processing. Such

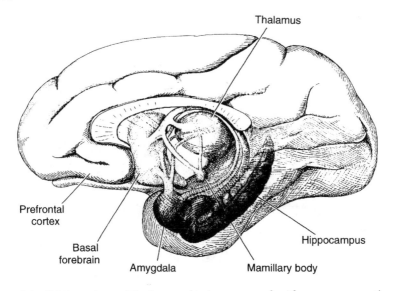

Figure 1.4. Main regions of the human brain concerned with memory, emotion and intellect.

integration also allows the brain to obtain a true representation of the external environment as projected by the sensory organs.

The functional importance of specific cortical and subcortical regions of the brain may also be elucidated by studying the consequences of specific neurological lesions. For example, it has been shown by imaging methods that blood flow to the hippocampus of patients with Alzheimer's disease is dramatically reduced, the reduction paralleling the degree of short-term memory impairment. In addition, blood flow to the parietotemporal association cortex is also greatly reduced. Such changes in the functional activity of these brain areas may account for the memory and cognitive deficits that are symptomatic of the disease, the main function of the parietotemporal association cortex being the integration of sensory and cognitive processes in the brain.

Figures 1.4 and 1.5 show the main structures of the human brain and the areas of the brain which are primarily affected in different types of neurological disease.

In SUMMARY, areas of the cerebral cortex can be identified according to the bodily functions which they control. For example, the motor cortex for muscle control, somatosensory cortex for sensory input, visual cortex for visual input, an area concerned with speech, etc. In addition to these specific areas, the cortex also contains highly developed association areas which are probably involved in the complex synthesis of information.

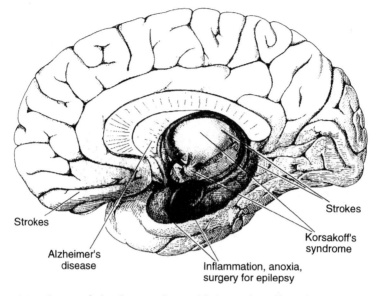

Figure 1.5. Areas of the human brain likely to be affected in some types of neurological dementing diseases.

Blood supply to the brain and the role of the blood–brain barrier

Although the brain constitutes only 2% of body weight, it receives approximately 15% of the blood supply and consumes nearly 20% of the total oxygen and glucose available to the body. In order to supply these essential nutrients for brain function, there must be a consistent and rapid blood supply to the brain in order that the brain cells may function. This is supplied by the cerebral arteries derived from the internal carotid arteries which branch over the surface of the brain and send smaller branches into the deeper subcortical structures. The capillaries are highly branched and it has been calculated that every nerve cell is no more than 40–50 μm from a capillary.

Because of the unique dependence of the brain on oxygen and glucose to enable the extensive oxidative metabolism to take place within the nerve cells, it is essential that the composition of nutrients, electrolytes, etc. in the fluid surrounding the brain cells is controlled. The composition of the blood varies to some extent according to the composition of the diet and therefore a mechanism has evolved to ensure that the composition of the extracellular fluid surrounding the brain cells is constant. The extracellular fluid is in equilibrium with the cerebrospinal fluid which fills the four ventricles of the brain, and covers the surface of the brain and the spinal cord.

Cerebrospinal fluid is formed from the blood and may be considered as an ultra filtrate of plasma. Thus cerebrospinal fluid contains most of the electrolytes and low molecular weight nutrients but is low in protein. It is formed from a network of capillaries in the ventricles termed the *choroid plexus* but the cerebral capillaries also contribute to the production of cerebrospinal fluid. The extracellular fluid and the cerebrospinal fluid compartment is separated from the blood by the *blood–brain barrier*. This is a barrier formed by tight junctions that exist between the endothelial cells lining the capillaries and the epithelial cells at the choroid plexus. Such a barrier prevents the influx of large molecular weight molecules but enables small molecular weight substances such as glucose, amino acids, fatty acids, electrolytes, etc., which are essential for normal brain function, to enter. In addition to the structural nature of the blood–brain barrier, there also exist specific transport sites that assist the transport of glucose and essential amino acids into the extracellular fluid. Thus the blood–brain barrier has both a structural and a metabolic role to play in maintaining homeostasis.

Cellular structure of the brain

It has been calculated that the human brain contains approximately 10^{-12} neurons of which the cortex probably contains 10^{-10}. Such complexity is further magnified by the neuronal interconnections. Structurally the neuronal cell body contains a number of organelles that are characteristic of all cell types (see Figure 1.6). The most important features are the *nucleus*, which contains the deoxyribonucleic acid (DNA) together with specific proteins that form chromosomes, and which functions to control the synthesis of all molecules within the neuron, and the *nucleolus* which is involved in ribosome synthesis and in the transfer of ribonucleic acid (RNA) to the cytosol. There is now evidence that the messenger RNA forming specific proteins is targeted to specific parts of the nerve cell. For example, the messenger RNA for microtubule associated protein-2 (MAP-2) targets the dendrites. This provides a mechanism for maintaining the structural integrity and differentiation of the neuron. The mitochondria, as in all types of cells, provides energy to the nerve cell in the form of adenosine triphosphate (ATP). The *smooth endoplasmic reticulum* is involved in lipid synthesis and in protein glycosylation whereas the *rough endoplasmic reticulum* is formed from the attachment of ribosomes to the smooth endoplasmic reticulum. These ribosomes are the main sites of membrane protein synthesis.

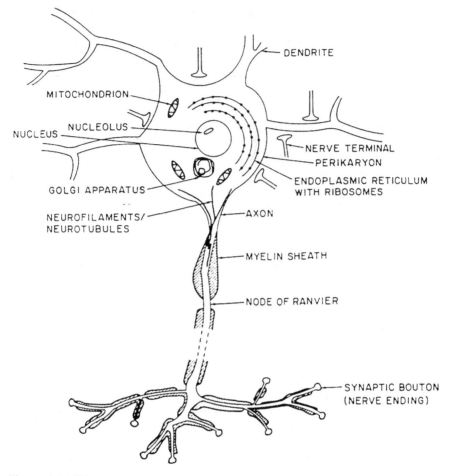

Figure 1.6. Diagrammatic representation of a nerve cell and nerve ending from mammalian brain.

The *Golgi apparatus* is situated near the nucleus and is responsible for protein glycosylation, membrane assembly and protein sorting. *Lysosomes* are responsible for the degradation of all types of cellular debris. The *plasma membrane* surrounds the neuron and consists of a phospholipid bilayer, inserted into which are intrinsic and extrinsic membrane proteins and cholesterol. The plasma membrane provides an impermeable barrier for many large molecular weight and charged molecules. The plasma membrane is transversed by different types of proteins that act as neurotransmitter receptors and voltage-sensitive ion channels.

The *cytosol* is the fluid compartment of the cell and contains the enzymes responsible for cellular metabolism together with free ribosomes concerned with local protein synthesis. In addition to these structures which are common to all cell types, the neuron also contains specific organelles which are unique to the nervous system. For example, the *neuronal skeleton* is responsible for monitoring the shape of the neuron. This is composed of several fibrous proteins that strengthen the axonal process and provide a structure for the location of specific membrane proteins. The axonal cytoskeleton has been divided into the internal cytoskeleton, which consists of microtubules linked to filaments along the length of the axon, which provides a track for the movement of vesicular material by fast axonal transport, and the cortical cytoskeleton.

The cytoskeleton is found near the axonal membrane and consists of microfilaments linked internally to microtubules and the plasma membrane by a network of filamentous protein that includes the brain-specific protein fodrin. This protein forms attachment sites for integral membrane proteins either by means of the neuronal cell adhesion molecule (N-CAM) or indirectly by means of a specific protein called ankyrin in the case of the sodium channels. This may provide a means whereby the sodium channels are concentrated in the region of the nodes of Ranvier. Thus the cortical cytoskeleton plays a vital role in neuronal function by acting as an attachment site for various receptors and ion channels, but also for synaptic vesicles at nerve terminals, thereby providing a mechanism for concentrating the vesicles prior to the release of the neurotransmitter.

There is also interest in the involvement of the cytoskeleton in such degenerative diseases as Alzheimer's disease (see Chapter 14) which is characterized by tangles (paired helical filaments). It seems likely that one of the microtubule-associated proteins (tau protein) is an important component of the tangles found in Alzheimer's disease.

Another unique feature of the neuron is the presence of synaptic and coated vesicles. The former are small smooth-coated vesicles 30–100 nm in diameter and containing the neurotransmitters. The latter are rough-coated vesicles that contain the protein clathrin. These are thought to be involved in the retrieval and recycling of membrane components including the synaptic vesicles once they have liberated their neurotransmitter into the synaptic cleft.

Some types of cell that are important to brain function

The neurons are surrounded by *neuroglia* (or glia) cells. These differ from the neurons in that they do not have electrically excitable membranes. They comprise nearly half the brain volume and function to separate and support the neurons. There are two main types of neuroglial cells, termed the *macroglia* and *microglia*. The macroglia are divided into the astrocytes, oligodendrocytes and ependymal cells. The astrocytes are characterized by long narrow cellular processes which give them a star-like structure; through their feet-like endings they can make contact with both the capillaries and neurons. It has been suggested that the astrocytes play a role in conducting nutrients from the blood to the neurons. Other roles include the removal by active transport of released neurotransmitters (particularly the inhibitory transmitter gamma-aminobutyric acid – GABA), the provision of precursors for transmitter synthesis (e.g. glutamine for the synthesis of GABA) and the buffering of the neuron against excessive concentrations of potassium ions formed following depolarization. Thus the astrocytes appear to play a critical role both in terms of physical protection of the neurons and in providing a metabolic buffer to ensure homeostasis. The *oligodendrocytes* occur in both grey and white matter. In white matter they form the insulating myelin sheath around the axon, whereas in grey matter they probably provide myelin for axons coursing through the grey matter. In the peripheral nervous system, these functions are fulfilled by the Schwann cells. The myelin is formed by the outgrowth of the plasma membrane of the oligodendrocyte which is wrapped several times around the axon, thereby excluding extracellular fluid from between the layers of the plasma membrane and thereby generating a highly insulating coat. This insulating coat, which is interrupted at the nodes of Ranvier, is important for the efficient transmission of the electrical impulses down the axon.

The *ependymal* cells line the inner surfaces of the ventricles and, together with the neuroglial cells, appear to be involved in the exchange of material with the surrounding cerebrospinal fluid. The *microglia* can be considered as the macrophage cells of the brain whose function is to remove cell debris by a process of phagocytosis following neuronal damage. There is also evidence that the macroglia are involved in localized inflammatory processes within the brain and may play an important role in the cause of neurodegenerative diseases such as Alzheimer's disease (see Chapter 14). Damage to brain tissue is associated with the proliferation of neuroglia. This is termed *gliosis* and is associated with an increase in the number of macroglia and microglia. Scar tissue is frequently associated with gliosis.

Structure and function of nerve cells

Nerve cells have two distinct properties that distinguish them from all other types of cells in the body. First, they conduct bioelectrical signals for relatively long distances without any loss of signal strength. Second, they possess specific, intracellular connections with other cells and with tissues that they innervate such as muscles and glands. These connections determine the type of information a neuron can receive and also the nature of the responses it can yield.

It is not within the scope of this text to give a detailed account of the anatomical structure of the central nervous system; this has been very adequately covered in a number of excellent textbooks, some of which are listed in the Appendix. However, to understand the physiological mechanisms which form the basis of psychopharmacology, a brief outline of the subject will be given.

Essentially all nerve cells have one or more projections termed *dendrites* whose primary function is to receive information from other cells in their vicinity and pass this information on to the cell body. Following the analysis of this information by the nerve cell, bioelectrical changes occur in the nerve membrane that result in the information being passed to the nerve terminal situated at the end of the *axon*. The change in membrane permeability at the nerve terminal then triggers the release of the *neurotransmitter*.

There is now evidence that the mammalian central nervous system contains several dozen neurotransmitters such as acetylcholine, noradrenaline, dopamine and 5-hydroxytryptamine (5-HT), together with many more co-transmitters, which are mainly small peptides such as met-enkephalin and neuromodulators such as the prostaglandins. It is well established that any one nerve cell may be influenced by more than one of these transmitters at any time. If, for example, the inhibitory amino acids (GABA or glycine) activate a cell membrane then the activity of the membrane will be depressed, whereas if the excitatory amino acid glutamate activates the nerve membrane, activity will be increased. The final response of the nerve cell that receives all this information will thus depend on the balance between the various stimuli that impinge upon it.

The structure of the nerve cell and nerve terminal is shown in Figure 1.6. Although different neurotransmitters can be produced at different synapses within the brain, the individual neuron seems capable of releasing only one major neurotransmitter from its axonal terminal, for example noradrenaline or acetylcholine. This view was originally postulated by Sir Henry Dale in 1935 and was subsequently called *Dale's Law*, not incidentally by Dale himself! It is now known that, in addition to such "classical transmitters", peptides and/or prostaglandins may also be co-released, and Dale's Law has been modified in the light of such evidence. The nature of the physiological response to any transmitter will depend on the function of the target *receptor* upon which it acts. For example, acetylcholine released from a motor neuron will stimulate the nicotinic receptor on a muscle end-plate and cause muscle contraction. When the same neurotransmitter is released from the vagus nerve innervating the heart, however, it acts on muscarinic receptors and slows the heart.

Recently it has become apparent that neurotransmitters can also be released from dendrites as well as axons. For example, in dendrites found on the cells of the substantia nigra dopamine may be released which then diffuses over considerable distances to act on receptors situated on the axons and dendrites of GABAergic and dopaminergic neurons in other regions of the basal ganglia. Another means of communication between nerve cells involves dendrodendritic contacts, where the dendrites from one cell communicate directly with those of an adjacent cell. In the olfactory bulb, for example, such synapses appear to utilize GABA as the main transmitter. Thus any neuron responding to inputs that may converge from several sources may inhibit, activate or otherwise modulate the cells to which it projects and, because many axons are branched, the target cells may be widely separated and varied in function. In this way, one one neuron may project to an inhibitory or excitatory cell which may then excite, inhibit or otherwise modulate the activity of the original cell. As most neurons are interlinked in an intricate network the complexity of such transmitter interactions becomes phenomenal! In brief, neurons can be conceived as complex gates which integrate the data they receive and, via their specific collection of transmitters and modulators, have a large repertoire of effects which they impose upon their target cells.

Neuronal plasticity

Neuronal plasticity is an essential component of neuronal adaptability and there is increasing evidence that this is primarily a biochemical rather than a morphological process. The neuron is not a fixed entity in terms of the quantity of transmitter it releases, and transmitters which are co-localized in a nerve terminal may be differentially secreted under different conditions. This, together with the repeated firing of some neurons that appear to have "leaky" membranes, may underlie the rhythmicity of neuronal activity within the brain.

Plasticity is also evident at the level of the neurotransmitter receptors. These are fluid structures that can be internalized into the membrane so that their density, and affinity for a transmitter, on the outer surface of the nerve membrane may change according to functional need.

Perhaps it is not surprising to find that our knowledge of how the brain works and where defects that lead to abnormal behaviour can arise is so deficient. The approach to understanding the biochemical basis of psychiatric disease is largely based on the assumption that the brain is chemically homogeneous, which is improbable! Nevertheless, there has been some success in recent years in probing the changes that may be causally related to schizophrenia, depression and anxiety. It should be apparent to anyone interested in the neurosciences that the brain is more than a sophisticated computer that follows a complicated programme, and any dogmatic approach to unravelling the complexities of this dynamic, plastic collection of organs which we call "brain" is doomed to failure.

In CONCLUSION, it can be seen that the adaptability of the organism to external and internal environmental changes is largely dependent on the functional flexibility of the cellular structure of the different brain areas. It is too often assumed that the brain is structurally homogeneous and that, like the heart or liver, once a drug penetrates the blood–brain barrier, it has access to most central compartments. Clearly this is not the case and the pharmacokinetic properties of a psychotropic drug (lipophilicity, molecular size, etc.), as well as the relative blood perfusion rate of a specific brain region which will depend on the metabolic activity at the time of day the drug is administered, could profoundly affect its concentration in a part of the brain. In support of this view, it is known that following its parenteral administration, the concentration of chlorpromazine in the left hemisphere is higher than in the right hemisphere, which presumably reflects the increased functional activity of the left hemisphere. Hopefully this chapter will provide a basis for understanding the physical substrate upon which psychotropic drugs act to produce their effects on the brain.

2 Basic Aspects of Neurotransmitter Function

Introduction

The concept of chemical transmission in the nervous system arose in the early years of the century when it was discovered that the functioning of the autonomic nervous system was largely dependent on the secretion of acetylcholine and noradrenaline from the parasympathetic and sympathetic nerves respectively. The physiologist Sherrington proposed that nerve cells communicated with one another, and with any other type of adjacent cell, by liberating the neurotransmitter into the space, or *synapse*, in the immediate vicinity of the nerve ending. He believed that transmission across the synaptic cleft was unidirectional and, unlike conduction down the nerve fibre, was delayed by some milliseconds because of the time it took the transmitter to diffuse across the synapse and activate a specific neurotransmitter receptor on the cell membrane.

While it was generally assumed that the brain also contained acetylcholine and noradrenaline as transmitters, it was only in the early 1950s that experimental evidence accumulated that there were also many other types of transmitter in the brain. The indoleamine neurotransmitter 5-hydroxytryptamine (5-HT), or serotonin, which is now recognized as an important component of mental function, was first studied by Erspamer in Italy and by Page in the United States in enterochromaffin tissue and platelets, respectively. It was left to Gaddum and colleagues in Edinburgh to show that 5-HT was present in the mammalian brain where it may have neurotransmitter properties. The potential importance of 5-HT to psychopharmacology arose when Woolley and Shaw in the United States suggested that lysergic acid diethylamide (LSD) owed its potent hallucinogenic properties to its ability to interfere in some way with brain 5-HT, the similarity in chemical structure of these molecules suggesting that they might compete for a common receptor site on the neuronal membrane.

Fundamentals of Psychopharmacology. Third Edition. By Brian E. Leonard
2003 John Wiley & Sons, Ltd. ISBN 0 471 52178 7

The neuron

It has been estimated that there are several billion neurons that comprise the mammalian brain which, together with their surrounding glial cells, form a unique network of connections which are ultimately responsible for all thoughts and actions. While the glial cells may play a critical role in brain development, their main function in the mature brain is to maintain the structure and metabolic homeostasis of the neurons which they surround.

A typical neuron consists of a cell body and an axonal projection through which information in the form of an action potential passes from the cell body to the axonal terminal. Information is received by the cell body via a complex array of dendrites which make contact with adjacent neurons. The structural complexity and the number of dendritic processes vary according to the type of nerve cell and its physiological function. For example, the granule cells in the dentate gyrus of the hippocampus (a region of the brain which plays a role in short-term memory) receives and integrates information from up to 10 000 other cells in the vicinity.

The majority of the inputs to the granule cells are excitatory, each of which provides a small depolarizing current to the membrane of the cell body. The point of contact between the axonal projection from the neuron and an adjacent cell is termed the synapse which under the electron microscope appears as a swelling at the end of the axon. Most synapses are excitatory and are usually located along the dendritic branches of the neuron. The contributions of the individual excitatory synapses are additive and, as a result, when an excitatory stimulus occurs a wave of depolarizing current travels down the axon to stimulate the adjacent cell body. However, some synapses are inhibitory, usually fewer in number and strategically located near the cell body. These synapses, when activated, inhibit the effects of any excitatory currents which may travel down the dendritic processes and thereby block their actions on the neuron (Figure 2.1).

The nerve impulse

Action potentials are the means whereby information is passed from one neuron to an adjacent neuron. The balance between the excitatory and inhibitory impulses determines how many action potentials will reach the axonal terminal and, by releasing a specific type of neurotransmitter from the terminal, influence the adjacent neuron. Thus, in summary, chemical information in the form of small neurotransmitter molecules released from axonal terminals is responsible for changing the membrane potential at the synaptic junctions which may occur on the dendrites or directly on the cell body. The action potential then passes down the axon to initiate the release

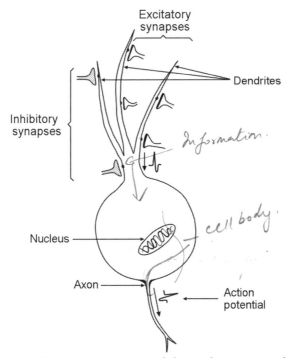

Figure 2.1. A single neuron, represented by a dentate granule cell, receives numerous synaptic contacts which are either of excitatory or inhibitory type.

of the neurotransmitter from the axonal terminal and thereby pass information on to any adjacent neurons.

A summary of the neurotransmitters and neuromodulators that have been identified in the mammalian brain is given in Table 2.1. The term *neuromodulator* is applied to those substances that may be released with a transmitter but which do not produce a direct effect on a receptor; a neuromodulator seems to work by modifying the responsiveness of the receptor to the action of the transmitter.

The metabolic unity of the neuron requires that the same transmitter is released at all its synapses. This is known as Dale's Law (or principle) which Sir Henry Dale proposed in 1935. Dale's Law only applies to the presynaptic portion of the neuron, not the postsynaptic effects which the transmitter may have on other target neurons. For example, acetylcholine released at motor neuron terminals has an excitatory action at the motor neuron junction, whereas the same transmitter released at vagal nerve terminals has an inhibitory action on the heart.

In addition to the diversity of action of a single transmitter released from a neuron, it has become well established that among invertebrates up to

Table 2.1. Some of the neurotransmitters and neuromodulators that have been identified in the mammalian brain

Transmitter	Distribution in brain	Physiological	Involvement in CNS disease
Noradrenaline	Most regions: long axons project from pons and brainstem	α_1 receptors – inhibitory β_1 receptors – inhibitory β_2 receptors – excitatory?	Depression Mania
Dopamine	Most regions: short, medium and long axonal projections	D_1/D_5 receptors – stimulatory D_2 receptors – inhibitory D_3/D_4 receptors – ?	Schizophrenia ?Mania
5-Hydroxytryptamine	Most regions: project from pons and brainstem	$5\text{-}HT_{1A}$ receptors – inhibitory $5\text{-}HT_2$ receptors – ? $5\text{-}HT_3$ receptors – ?	Depression ?Schizophrenia Anxiety
Acetylcholine	Most regions: long and short axonal projections from basal forebrain	M_1 receptors – excitatory M_2 receptors – inhibitory N receptors – excitatory	Dementias ?Mania
Adrenaline	Midbrain and brainstem	Possibly same as for noradrenaline	?Depression
GABA	Supraspinal interneurons	A receptors – hyperpolarize membranes (inhibitory) B receptors – inhibitory	Anxiety Seizures, epilepsy
Glycine	Spinal interneurons; modulates NMDA amino acid receptors in brain	Hyperpolarize membranes Strych-sensitive receptors – inhibitory Strych-insensitive receptors – excitatory	?Seizures Learning and memory ?Seizures
Glutamate and aspartate	Long neurons	Quisqualate – depolarizes membranes NMDA – depolarizes membranes Kainate – depolarizes membranes	Seizures ?Schizophrenia

Substances with a neuromodulatory effect on brain neurotransmitters by direct actions of specific receptors that modify the actions of the transmitters listed include: prostaglandins, adenosine, enkephalins, substance P, cholecystokinin, endorphins, endogenous benzodiazepine receptor ligands, and possibly histamine. CNS, central nervous system. NMDA, N-methyl-D-aspartate. Strych, strychnine.

Table 2.2. Criteria which must be fulfilled for a substance to be considered as a transmitter

---

- It should be present in a nerve terminal and in the vicinity of the area of the brain where it is thought to act.
- It should be released from the nerve terminal, generally by a calcium-dependent process, following stimulation of the nerve.
- The enzymes concerned in its synthesis and metabolism should be present in the nerve ending, or in the proximity of the nerve ending.
- It should produce a physiological response following its release by activating a postsynaptic receptor site. Such changes should be identical to those seen following the local application of the transmitter (e.g. by micro-ionophoresis).
- Its effects should be selectively blocked by a specific antagonist and mimicked by a specific agonist.

These criteria should be regarded as general guidelines, not specific rules.

---

four different transmitters can occur in the same neuron. In the vertebrate there is also increasing evidence from the seminal studies of Höckfelt and colleagues in Stockholm that some neurons in the central nervous system can also contain more than one transmitter. Such neurons appear to contain a peptide within monoamine-containing terminals. Peptide transmitters (usually referred to as neuropeptides) are contained in specific types of storage vesicles. Thus Dale's Law has to be modified to allow for the presence of neuropeptides in amine-containing nerve terminals, whose function is to act as a neuromodulator of the amine when it acts on the postsynaptic receptor.

There are several criteria which must be fulfilled for a substance to be considered as a transmitter. These are given in Table 2.2.

Neurotransmitter receptor mechanisms

Role of ion channels in nerve conduction

Ion channels are large proteins which form pores through the neuronal membrane. The precise structure and function of the ion channels depend on their physiological function and distribution along the dendrites and cell body. These include specialized neurotransmitter-sensitive receptor channels. In addition, some ion channels are activated by specific metal ions such as sodium or calcium. The structure of the voltage-dependent sodium channel has been shown to consist of a complex protein with both a hydrophilic and a hydrophobic domain, the former domain occurring within the neuronal membrane while the latter domain occurs both inside and outside the neuronal membrane.

Four regions containing the hydrophilic units are arranged in the membrane in the form of a pore, with two units forming the remaining sides of the pore. This allows the sodium ions to pass in a regulated manner as the diameter of the pore, and the electrical charges on the amino acids which comprise the proteins lining the pore, determine the selectivity of the ion channel for sodium.

Advances in molecular biology have shown that the DNA sequences which code for the proteins that make up the ion channels can enable the protein structure to be modified by point mutations. By changing the structure of the protein by even a single amino acid it is now apparent that the properties of the ion channel also change resulting, for example, in the opening and closing of the channel for longer or shorter periods of time or in carrying larger or smaller currents. As a consequence of molecular biological studies, it is now recognized that most ion channels of importance in neurotransmission are composed of three to five protein subunits. Their identification and characterization have now made it possible to map their location on specific neurons and to correlate their location with their specific function (Figure 2.2).

Synaptic transmission

The sequence of events that result in neurotransmission of information from one nerve cell to another across the synapses begins with a wave of depolarization which passes down the axon and results in the opening of the voltage-sensitive calcium channels in the axonal terminal. These channels are frequently concentrated in areas which correspond to the active sites of neurotransmitter release. A large (up to $100\,\mu M$) but brief rise in the calcium concentration within the nerve terminal triggers the movement of the synaptic vesicles, which contain the neurotransmitter, towards the synaptic membrane. By means of specific membrane-bound proteins (such as synaptobrevin from the neuronal membrane and synaptotagrin from the vesicular membrane) the vesicles fuse with the neuronal membrane and release their contents into the synaptic gap by a process of exocytosis. Once released of their contents, the vesicle membrane is reformed and recycled within the neuronal terminal. This process is completed once the vesicles have accumulated more neuro-transmitter by means of an energy-dependent transporter on the vesicle membrane (Table 2.3).

The neurotransmitters diffuse across the synaptic cleft in a fraction of a millisecond where, on reaching the postsynaptic membrane on an adjacent neuron, they bind to specific receptor sites and trigger appropriate physiological responses.

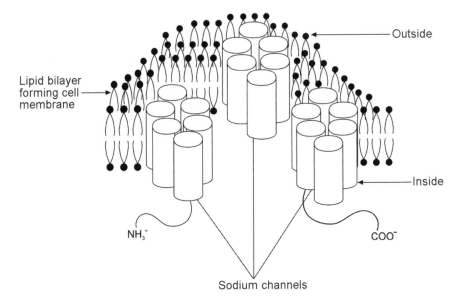

Figure 2.2 Diagram of a voltage-activated sodium channel protein. The channel is composed of a long chain of amino acids interconnected by peptide bonds. The amino acids perform specific functions within the ion channel. The cylinders represent amino acid assemblies located within the membrane of the nerve cell and responsible for the foundation of the ion pore.

Table 2.3. Stages of neurotransmission in the brain

1. Action potential depolarizes the axonal terminal.
2. Depolarization produces opening of voltage-dependent calcium channels.
3. Calcium ions diffuse into the nerve terminal and bind with specific proteins on the vesicular and neuronal membranes.
4. Vesicles move towards the presynaptic membrane and fuse with it.
5. Neurotransmitter is released into the synaptic cleft by a process of exocytosis and activates receptors on adjacent neurons.
6. The postsynaptic receptors respond either rapidly (ionotropic type) or slowly (metabotropic type) depending on the nature of the neurotransmitter.

There are two major types of receptor which are activated by neurotransmitters. These are the ionotropic and metabotropic receptors. The former receptor type is illustrated by the amino acid neurotransmitter receptors for glutamate, gamma-aminobutyric acid (GABA) and glycine, and the acetylcholine receptors of the nicotinic type. These are examples of fast transmitters in that they rapidly open and close the ionic channels in the neuronal membrane. Peptides are often co-localized with these fast transmitters but act more slowly and modulate the excitatory or inhibitory actions of the fast transmitters. By contrast to the amino acid neurotransmitters, the biogenic amine transmitters such as noradrenaline, dopamine and serotonin, and the non-amine transmitter acetylcholine acting on the muscarinic type of receptor, activate metabotropic receptors. These receptors are linked to intracellular second messenger systems by means of G (guanosine triphosphate-dependent) proteins. These comprise the slow transmitters because of the relatively long time period required for their physiological response to occur. It must be emphasized however that a number of metabotropic receptors have recently been identified that are activated by fast transmitters so that the rigid separation of these receptor types is somewhat blurred.

Over 50 different types of neurotransmitter have so far been identified in the mammalian brain and these may be categorized according to their chemical structure.

Presynaptic mechanisms

Another important mechanism whereby the release of a neurotransmitter may be altered is by *presynaptic inhibition*. Initially this mechanism was thought to be restricted to noradrenergic synapses, but it is now known to occur at GABA-ergic, dopaminergic and serotonergic terminals also.

In brief, it has been shown that at noradrenergic synapses the release of noradrenaline may be reduced by high concentrations of the transmitter in the synaptic cleft. Conversely, some adrenoceptor antagonists, such as phenoxybenzamine, have been found to enhance the release of the amine. It is now known that the subclass of adrenoceptors responsible for this process of autoinhibition are distinct from the α_1 adrenoceptors which are located on blood vessels, on secretory cells, and in the brain. These autoinhibitory receptors, or α_2 adrenoceptors, can be identified by the use of specific agonists and antagonists, for example clonidine and yohimbine respectively. Drugs acting as specific agonists or antagonists on α_1 receptors, for example the agonist methoxamine and the antagonist prazosin, do not affect noradrenaline release by this mechanism.

The inhibitory effect of α_2 agonists on noradrenaline release involves a hyperpolarization of the presynaptic membranes by opening potassium ion channels. The reduction in the release of noradrenaline following the administration of an α_2 agonist is ultimately due to a reduction in the concentration of free cytosolic calcium, which is an essential component of the mechanism whereby the synaptic vesicles containing noradrenaline fuse to the synaptic membrane before their release.

There is evidence that a number of closely related phosphoproteins associated with the synaptic vesicles, called synapsins, are involved in the short-term regulation of neurotransmitter release. These proteins also appear to be involved in the regulation of synapse formation, which allows the nerve network to adapt to long-term passage of nerve impulses.

Experimental studies have shown that the release of a transmitter from a nerve terminal can be decreased or increased by a variety of other neurotransmitters. For example, stimulation of 5-HT receptors on noradrenergic terminals can lead to an enhanced release of noradrenaline. While the physiological importance of such a mechanism is unclear, this could be a means whereby drugs could produce some of their effects. Such receptors have been termed *heteroceptors* (Figure 2.3).

In addition to the physiological process of autoinhibition, another mechanism of presynaptic inhibition has been identified in the peripheral nervous system, although its precise relevance to the brain is unclear. In the dorsal horn of the spinal cord, for example, the axon terminal of a local neuron makes axo-axonal contact with a primary afferent excitatory input, which leads to a reduction in the neurotransmitter released. This is due to the local neuron partly depolarizing the nerve terminal, so that when the axon potential arrives, the change induced is diminished, thereby leading to a smaller quantity of transmitter being released. In the brain, it is possible that GABA can cause presynaptic inhibition in this way.

Summary

It seems that the release of a transmitter from its nerve terminal is not only dependent upon the passage of an action potential but also on the intersynaptic concentration of the transmitter and the modulatory effects of other neurotransmitters that act presynaptically on the nerve terminal. The interrelationship between these different processes is illustrated in Figure 2.3.

Postsynaptic mechanisms

Neurotransmitters can either excite or inhibit the activity of a cell with which they are in contact. When an excitatory transmitter such as acetylcholine, or an inhibitory transmitter such as GABA, is released from a nerve terminal it diffuses across the synaptic cleft to the postsynaptic membrane, where it activates the receptor site. Some receptors, such as the nicotinic receptor, are directly linked to sodium ion channels, so that when acetylcholine stimulates the nicotinic receptor, the ion channel opens to allow an exchange of sodium and potassium ions across the nerve membrane. Such receptors are called *ionotropic* receptors.

The generation of action potentials by nerve axons and muscle fibres was first described by the German physiologist Emil DuBois-Reymond in 1849.

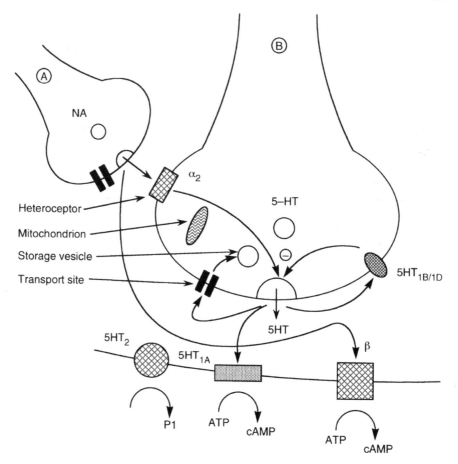

Figure 2.3. Modulation of 5-HT release by alpha-adrenergic heteroceptors.

However, it was not until over a century later that the underlying mechanism was explained in terms of the properties of the specific membrane proteins forming the voltage-gated ion channels of sodium and potassium ions.

Second messenger system

When receptors are directly linked to ion channels, fast excitatory postsynaptic potentials (EPSPs) or inhibitory postsynaptic potentials (IPSPs) occur. However, it is well established that slow potential changes also occur and that such changes are due to the receptor being linked to the ion channel indirectly via a *second messenger system*.

For example, the stimulation of β-adrenoceptors by noradrenaline results in the activation of adenylate cyclase on the inner side of the nerve membrane. This enzyme catalyses the breakdown of ATP to the very labile, high-energy compound cyclic 3,5-adenosine monophosphate (cyclic AMP). Cyclic AMP then activates a protein kinase which, by phosphorylating specific membrane proteins, opens an ion channel to cause an efflux of potassium and an influx of sodium ions. Such receptors are termed *metabotropic* receptors.

Many monoamine neurotransmitters are now thought to work by this receptor-linked second messenger system. In some cases, however, stimulation of the postsynaptic receptors can cause the inhibition of adenylate cyclase activity. For example, D_2 dopamine receptors inhibit, while D_1 receptors stimulate, the activity of the cyclase.

Such differences have been ascribed to the fact that the cyclase is linked to two distinct guanosine triphosphate (GTP) binding proteins in the cell membrane, termed G_I and G_S. The former protein inhibits the cyclase, possibly by reducing the effects of the G_S protein which stimulates the cyclase. The relationship between the postsynaptic receptor and the second messenger system is illustrated in Figure 2.4.

Recently there has been much interest in the possible role of the family of protein kinases which translate information from the second messenger to the membrane proteins. Many of these kinases are controlled by free calcium ions within the cell. It is now established that some serotonin (5-HT) receptors, for example, are linked via G proteins to the phosphatidyl inositol pathway which, by mobilizing membrane-bound diacylglycerol and free calcium ions, can activate a specific protein kinase C. This enzyme affects the concentration of calmodulin, a calcium sequestering protein that plays a key role in many intracellular processes.

Structurally G-proteins are composed of three sub-units termed alpha, beta and gamma. Of these, the alpha sub-units are structurally diverse so that each member of the G-protein super-family has a unique alpha sub-unit. Thus the multiplicity of the alpha, and to a lesser extent the beta and gamma, sub-units provides for the coupling of a variety of receptors to different second messenger systems. In this way, different receptor types are able to interact and regulate each other, thereby allowing for greater signal divergence, convergence or filtering than could be achieved solely on the basis of the receptor diversity (Table 2.4).

The functional response of a nerve cell to a transmitter can change as a result of the receptor becoming sensitized or desensitized following a decrease or increase, respectively, in the concentration of the transmitter at the receptor site. Among those receptors that are directly coupled to ion channels, receptor desensitization is often rapid and pronounced.

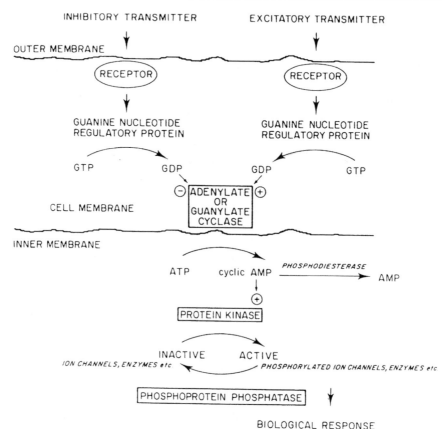

Figure 2.4. Relationship between the postsynaptic receptor and the secondary messenger system. GTP=guanosine triphosphate; GDP=guanosine diphosphate; ATP=adenosine triphosphate; AMP=adenosine monophosphate.

Most of the experimental evidence came initially from studies of the frog motor end-plate, where it was shown that the desensitization of the nicotinic receptor caused by continuous short pulses of acetylcholine was associated with a slow-conformational change in that the ion channel remained closed despite the fact that the transmitter was bound to the receptor surface.

A similar mechanism has also been shown to occur in brain cells. For example, continuous exposure of β-adrenoceptors on rat glioma cells *in vitro* results in a rapid reduction in the responsiveness of the receptors. This is followed by a secondary stage of desensitization, whereby the number of β-receptors decreases. It seems likely that the receptors are not lost but move into the cell and are therefore no longer accessible to the transmitter.

Table 2.4. The role of G-proteins in neurotransmission

1. An excitatory neurotransmitter such as noradrenaline or serotonin acts on its receptor and activates the intermembrane G-protein by converting GDP to GTP thereby linking the receptor to the second messenger system, usually adenylate cyclase.
2. The second messenger, for example cyclic adenosine monophosphate (cAMP), then activates cAMP-dependent protein kinase which modulates the function of a broad range of membrane receptors, intracellular enzymes, ion channels and transcription factors.
3. An inhibitory neurotransmitter activates an inhibitory G-protein thereby leading to a reduction in cAMP synthesis.
4. The termination of signal transduction results from the hydrolysis of GTP to GDP by GTPase thereby returning the G-protein to its inactive form.

The importance of the changes in receptor sensitivity to our understanding of the chronic effects of psychotropic drugs is discussed on pp. 45–47.

It must be emphasized that there is considerable integration and modulation between the various second messenger systems and these interactions lead to cross-talk between neurotransmitter systems. Such cross-talk between the second messenger systems may account for changes in the sensitivity of neurotransmitter receptors following prolonged stimulation by an agonist whereby a reduction in the receptor density is associated with a reduced physiological response (also termed receptor down-regulation).

Summary

Neurotransmitters can control cellular events by two basic mechanisms. First, they may be linked directly to sodium (e.g. acetylcholine acting on nicotinic receptors, or excitatory amino acids such as glutamate acting on glutamate receptors) or chloride (as exemplified by GABA) ion channels, thereby leading to the generation of fast EPSPs or IPSPs respectively. Second, the receptor may be linked to a second messenger system that mediates slower postsynaptic changes. These different mechanisms whereby neurotransmitters may change the activity of a postsynaptic membrane by fast, voltage-dependent mechanisms, or slower, second messenger-mediated mechanisms provide functional plasticity within the nervous system.

Co-transmission

During the mid-1970s, studies on such invertebrates as the mollusc Aplysia showed that at least four different types of transmitters could be liberated from the same nerve terminal. This was the first evidence that Dale's Law does not always apply. Extensive histochemical studies of the mammalian peripheral and central nervous systems followed, and it was shown that transmitters such as acetylcholine, noradrenaline and dopamine can co-exist with such peptides as cholecystokinin, vasoactive intestinal peptide, and gastrin-like peptides.

It is now evident that nerve terminals in the brain may contain different types of storage vesicles that store the peptide co-transmitters. Following their release, these peptides activate specific pre- or postsynaptic receptors, and thereby modulate the responsiveness of the membrane to the action of the traditional neurotransmitters such as acetylcholine or noradrenaline. In the mammalian and human brain, acetylcholine has been found to localize with vasoactive intestinal peptide; dopamine with cholecystokinin-like peptide, and 5-HT with substance P. In addition, there is increasing evidence that some peptides may act as neurotransmitters in their own right in the mammalian brain. These include the enkephalins, thyrotrophin-releasing hormone, angiotensin II, vasopressin, substance P, neurotensin, somatostatin, and corticotropin, among many others. With the advent of specific and sensitive immunocytochemical techniques, several more peptides are being added to this list every year. The similarities and differences between the peptide transmitters/co-transmitters and the "classical" transmitters such as acetylcholine are summarized in Table 2.5.

The peptide transmitters form the largest group of neurotransmitters in the mammalian brain, at least 40 different types having been identified so far. The mechanism governing their release differs from those of the non-peptide transmitters. Thus peptides are stored in large dense core vesicles which appear to require more prolonged and widespread diffusion of calcium into the nerve terminal before they can be released. In general, the peptide transmitters form part of the slow transmitter group as they activate metabotropic receptors.

Table 2.5.   Similarities and differences between the peptide transmitters/co-transmitters

---

1. Both neurotransmitters and peptides show high specificity for their specific receptors.
2. Neurotransmitters produce physiological responses in nano- or micromolar (10^{-9} to 10^{-6}) concentrations, whereas peptides are active in picomolar (10^{-12}) concentrations.
3. Neurotransmitters bind to their receptors with high affinity but low potency, whereas peptides bind with very high affinity and high potency.
4. Neurotransmitters are synthesized at a moderate rate in the nerve terminal, whereas the rate of synthesis of peptides is probably very low.
5. Neurotransmitters are generally of low molecular weight (200 or below) whereas peptides are of intermediate molecular weight (1000 to 10 000 or occasionally more).

Measuring neurotransmitter receptors in the brain

Little was known about the identity of neurotransmitter receptors in the brain until the early 1970s when several laboratories independently reported that a potent snake venom, alpha-bungarotoxin, could bind with high affinity to nicotinic receptors that occurred in the electric organs of certain species of fish. This laid the basis for *ligand receptor binding studies*. Such studies rely on the use of radiolabelled (generally with tritium or carbon-14) drugs or chemicals which have a high affinity for a specific receptor. Such ligands may be either agonists or antagonists that bind to the receptor, thereby enabling the number of receptors on a tissue to be determined by measuring the quantity of radioactive ligand that has been specifically bound.

In practice, pieces of brain tissue (e.g. membrane preparations or crude tissue homogenates) are incubated with the radioligand in a physiological buffer solution. The tissue is then filtered or centrifuged to separate the tissue from the incubation medium. The quantity of ligand bound to the tissue can then be estimated by solubilizing the tissue and counting the radioactivity in a liquid scintillation counter. As most radioligands also bind non-specifically to brain tissue, to the walls of the incubation tube and even to the filters used to separate the tissue from the incubation medium, it is essential to determine the amount of radioligand bound specifically to the receptor. This is done by incubating the tissue preparation in tubes containing the specific radioligand alone and also with the ligand together with another drug or compound which is not radioactively labelled but which also binds with high affinity to the same receptor. For example, to study the number of beta adrenoceptors in a brain or lymphocyte preparation, tritiated dihydroalprenolol ([³H]DHA) is used as the radioligand and DL-propranolol as the non-radioactive displacing agent. Thus propranolol will tend to displace all of the [³H]DHA bound to the beta receptor but is less effective in displacing any radioligand that is bound non-specifically, and possibly irreversibly, to other types of receptor or to non-receptor sites. The amount of radioactivity present in the tissue preparation that has been incubated with the radioligand alone and that remaining after the specifically bound ligand has been displaced by propranolol is then counted. The difference between the total (i.e. the radioactivity in the tube containing the radioligand alone) and the non-specifically bound activity (i.e. the radioactivity in the tube containing the radioligand and the displacing agent) gives a measure of the amount of radioactivity specifically bound to the beta adrenoceptor. This is illustrated in Figure 2.5.

The number of receptors in a tissue preparation may be determined by plotting the ratio of the bound to free radioligand against the total bound ligand. For one population of receptors in a tissue, this plot yields a straight line, the number of binding sites (termed the B_{max}) being determined from the point of intersection of the y axis. This is illustrated in Figure 2.6.

This method of expressing the results of radioligand binding assays is known as a *Scatchard plot*, after the chemist who used it to study the binding of small molecules to proteins. A non-linear Scatchard plot often implies that there are two or more binding sites, one of these sites to which the ligand binds with high affinity and low capacity (shown as B_{max1} in Figure 2.7) and the other to which the ligand binds with low affinity and high capacity (shown as B_{max2} in Figure 2.7).

The affinity of a ligand for a receptor can be calculated from the slope of the plot, 1/slope being known as the K_d value or the binding affinity.

Thus by means of this relatively simple technique it is possible to determine the number of binding sites in a piece of brain tissue, their homogeneity and the affinity of the ligand for these sites. This enables changes in the density of specific receptors to be determined following drug treatment or as a result of disease. However, it must be emphasized that a binding site for a radioligand is not necessarily a receptor. To classify a

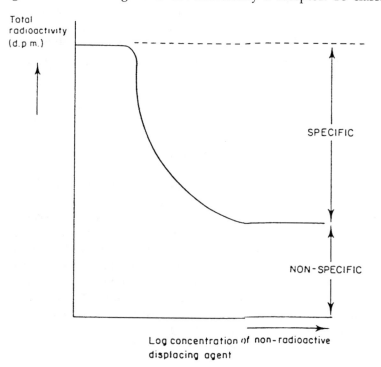

Figure 2.5. Diagrammatic representation of the binding of a radioactive ligand to a membrane preparation.

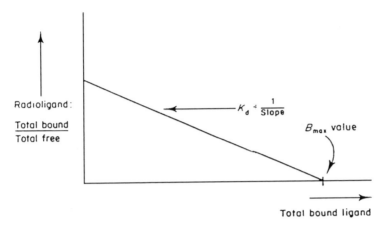

Figure 2.6. Scatchard plot of the binding of a radioligand to a membrane preparation containing two binding sites. In this diagram, B_{max1} represents a high affinity (K_{d1}) low capacity site, whereas B_{max2} represents a low affinity (K_{d2}) high capacity site.

binding site as a receptor it is essential to show that the binding site is linked to an ion channel or secondary messenger system or that an electro-physiological response occurs as a direct consequence of the activation of the binding site. It is possible, for example, that the ligand binds to a portion of the nerve membrane that is not involved in neurotransmission. Following the discovery that tritiated benzodiazepines bind with high specificity to nerve membranes it took several years of further research to show that occupation of the benzodiazepine-binding site could lead to the enhanced sensitivity of the GABA-A receptor to the effects of GABA. Only when the functional activity of the benzodiazepine receptor was established could the binding site be justifiably called a receptor site.

The application of ligand binding techniques to the quantification of receptor sites in the brain has had important implications for psychopharmacology. It has now been possible to correlate the therapeutic potencies of some drugs with their receptor occupancy. Neuroleptics are known to block dopamine receptors in the brain. By studying the binding of a series of neuroleptics to the different types of dopamine receptor in nerve membrane preparations, it has been found that there is a good correlation between the occupancy of the D_2 receptor subtype and the therapeutic potency. There does not appear to be a direct correlation between the binding of these drugs to adrenoceptors, histamine, 5-HT or acetylcholine receptors and their therapeutic potency. However, by considering the interaction of psychotropic drugs with these various receptors, it is possible to predict their side effects. For example, antagonism

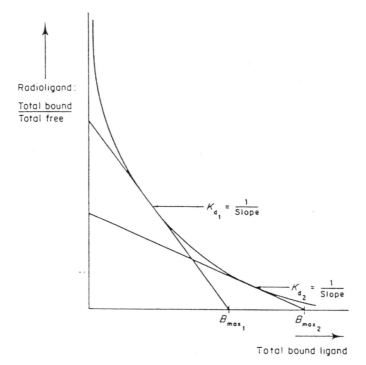

Figure 2.7. Method used to determine the receptor number and the ligand affinity for the receptor by the Scatchard plot.

of alpha$_1$ adrenoceptors, histamine$_1$ and muscarinic receptors is associated with postural hypotension, sedation and anticholinergic side effects respectively. Thus by using this relatively simple technique it is possible to gain an insight into the site(s) of action of most classes of psychotropic drug and to predict with reasonable accuracy what their side effects will be. Whether the receptor affinity of a drug *in vitro* necessarily provides information about its mode of action in the brain is quite another issue.

Quantitative autoradiography

In this method, thin tissue sections of the brain are incubated with a specific radioligand, the unbound ligand removed by washing and the resulting tissue section placed on a sensitive photographic film. The sites where the radioligand binds to the tissue fog the film, and following its development grain counts, densitometric analysis and photometric techniques can be used to quantify the extent of the binding of the radioligand to specific cell structures. More recently, the application of computerized image analysis has simplified the problem of visualization and quantification. The system most widely used consists of a television camera linked to an IBM personal computer. This system can colour code images to enhance contrast, modify images, subtract one image from another and average densities in specific regions of the visual field. The ability of this system to include and process autoradiographic standards enables the density of the radioligand binding to be quantified. Finally, the system can tabulate, store and calculate the B_{max} and K_d values of the radioligand.

One of the most important uses of autoradiography in psychopharmacology lies in enabling the sites in the brain where a drug acts to be identified. For example, the brain region or specific neuronal circuit that is affected by a drug may be visualized. Since most psychotropic drugs have multiple effects in the brain, autoradiographic methods have helped to explain the complexity of the effects by identifying the receptors and their distribution in the brain. Changes in receptor density may reflect neuronal function. Receptor mapping has therefore been applied to biopsy and autopsy samples from patients with Parkinsonism, Alzheimer's disease, schizophrenia and depression. The results of such studies have already begun to throw light on the possible biochemical changes that underlie such diseases. There are practical limitations to the autoradiographic technique however. The resolution using the light microscope is limited and it is seldom possible to readily identify specific cell structures that contain the receptors or to distinguish between functional and non-functional receptors to which the ligand is bound. It should be emphasized that this is also a problem with conventional radioligand techniques as applied to membrane preparations or to tissue homogenates. To overcome the problem of resolution, electron microscopic autoradiography may eventually prove to be of value, particularly when this is combined with immunohistochemical techniques to improve the resolution.

Imaging methods: their application to psychopharmacology

Introduction

Ten years ago, neuroimaging was largely restricted to determining the localization of pathological lesions in the human brain. Due to the rapid advances in magnetic resonance imaging (MRI) and related technologies, methods have now been developed to determine the precise functional importance of brain lesions, how cognitive operations are carried out within the brain and why they fail.

MRI is an example of the technological development that is no longer restricted to the crude location of a brain lesion. The recently introduced analytical approach enables the size of the image structures in the MRI to be determined, thereby enabling the investigator to track small changes in the structure over time. This permits the abnormal pattern of development in grey or white matter to be detected. For example, using such techniques it has been possible to track the distribution of grey and white matter during the onset of schizophrenia in children, and to show that the condition is characterized by an abnormal time course in the reduction in grey matter in several brain regions. Such changes suggest that there are abnormalities in synaptic pruning which normally takes place during the early stages of neurodevelopment. A further extension of the MRI technique, the diffusion-tensor technique (whereby the diffusibility of water molecules is rendered visible by the preferential orientation of their movement in neurons), has enabled the researcher to track major fibre bundles in white matter.

Another important change has been the shift from positron emission tomography (PET) to MRI-based techniques for the indirect measurement of neuronal activity. Nevertheless, PET and single photon emission computed tomography (SPECT) remain the only viable techniques for studying ligand binding in the human brain and the increasing resolution of PET is constantly improving as new detectors are developed. Recently, new radiotracers have enabled signal transduction mechanisms and gene expression to be evaluated in the human brain.

Specific molecules can now be determined in the human brain by means of magnetic resonance spectroscopy (MRS). Such methods have enabled the glutamate–GABA system to be assessed during neuronal activation and have shown how this pathway is defective in depression and altered by pharmacological treatments. Unlike most of the techniques described here, MRS is also applicable to analysing changes in energy metabolism and the glutamate/GABA pathway in the rat brain.

Undoubtedly, one of the most important advances has been in functional magnetic resonance imaging (fMRI), which enables the researcher to distinguish between the encoding and retrieval phases of memory. An additional application of the fMRI technique in the study of mood and emotion has revealed that the systems involved are widely distributed throughout the brain. However, despite these improvements it will never be possible using fMRI to approach the accuracy of event-related potential (ERP) methods which can quantify events occurring over milliseconds. ERP methods have now been combined with fMRI so that it is possible, for example, to measure signals that occur in visual tasks when they arrive at the cortex, how the signals are modulated by attention and how they are decoded into semantic information. Once these intricate processes have been elucidated in normal behaviour, it should be possible to apply them to specific psychiatric disorders such as schizophrenia where there appears to be a major deficit in the processing of visual stimuli.

Finally, it has now become possible to use imaging methods to study the functional interaction between different brain regions. This has been made possible by the development of effective connectivity mapping which is based on moment-to-moment relationships between fMRI signals in different brain regions to create equations which enable the contribution of the activity of one brain region with another to be quantified. Another approach has been to combine fMRI with transcranial magnetic stimulation (TMS). In this technique, areas of the brain are directly stimulated by magnetic currents and the resulting changes in brain regions quantified by fMRI.

To date, these techniques have been applied almost entirely to man. Over the next decade it will be equally important to further refine them so they may become applicable to the brains of experimental animals, particularly rodents. So far it has only been possible to determine gross structural changes in the rat, for example, using MRI.

Some examples of the application of new imaging methods to psychopharmacology

(a) Application of MRS

It is well known that GABA is the major inhibitory neurotransmitter in the mammalian cerebral cortex and that the functional activity of the GABAergic system is disrupted in several neurological and psychiatric disorders. Furthermore, several classes of psychotropic drugs are known to specifically affect the GABAergic system. Thus MRS should be an ideal method for assessing changes in the glutamate–GABA system in both man and animals.

The initial studies using MRS were performed in rats following the administration of the antiepileptic drug, and GABA transaminase inhibitor, vigabatrin and subsequently in epileptic patients being treated with the drug. In the MRS studies on epileptic patients, it was shown that vigabatrin failed to raise the GABA concentration at a dose that exceeded 3 g/day (an antiepileptic dose). This led to a detailed analysis of the mechanism regulating the GABA concentration in the brain. The enzyme synthesizing GABA from glutamate, glutamate decarboxylase (GAD), exists in two major isoforms (GAD 67 and 65) in the brain and these are products of separate genes, differentially distributed (GAD 67 in the cytoplasm and GAD 65 in synaptic terminals) and have different kinetic properties. Using MRS, it was found that GAD 67 activity was reduced in response to the elevated GABA concentration and that, in rats, vigabatrin selectively inhibited the GAD 67 isoform. Other studies using the MRS technique have shown that several antiepileptic drugs with no known action on the GABAergic system (for example, GABApentin, topiramate and lamotrigine) also increase the concentration of GABA *in vivo*. MRS studies also showed that the regulation of GABA metabolism was closely integrated with GABAergic function. In epileptic patients, these studies showed that the GABA concentration was decreased and that it was the cytosolic GABA concentration which was important in the suppression of seizures by antiepileptic drugs. Chronic vigabatrin administration was shown to reduce the seizure frequency in parallel with the rise in cytosolic GABA.

In addition to epilepsy, reduced GABA has been recorded in patients with unipolar depression, following alcohol withdrawal and in hepatic encephalopathy. The finding that the concentration of GABA is reduced in depression is unexpected as there is no evidence that the disorder is associated with an increased cortical excitability. One possibility is that the reduction in GABA is a reflection of a decreased availability in its excitatory amino acid precursor glutamate.

(b) Application of TMS

A fundamental problem with conventional functional imaging has been an inability to probe the causal relationship between regional brain activity and behaviour. For example, if a brain region utilizes more glucose or oxygen while the subject performs a behavioural task, it is only possible to conclude that the change in regional activity correlates with the behaviour; a causal relationship between the metabolic and behavioural changes can only be inferred. By combining TMS with fMRI it is now possible to directly test how information flows within the brain.

With TMS, a brief but powerful electric current is passed through a small coil held against the scalp of a conscious patient. This generates a powerful local magnetic field which passes unimpeded through the skull and induces a weaker, less focused electric current within the brain. Due to the non-invasive nature of this method, the important physiological effects of TMS are likely to be a consequence of the density of the electric current and the electric field which is induced in the cortex. It is believed that the induced electrical fields cause neuronal depolarization which changes the neurotransmitter release mechanisms.

TMS has now been combined with glucose utilization studies and fMRI.

Repetitive TMS, unlike electroconvulsive therapy (ECT), uses subconvulsive stimuli to treat depression. Compared to ECT, TMS has a potential to target specific brain regions and to stimulate brain areas thought to be primarily involved in depression while sparing areas like the hippocampus, thereby reducing the probability of cognitive side effects. However, the therapeutic efficacy of TMS as a treatment for depression is, unlike ECT, modest. Most TMS studies use high-frequency, fast stimulation (> 10 Hz) over the left dorsolateral prefrontal cortex, an area which has been shown to be hypofunctional in PET and electroencephalogram (EEG) studies of depressed patients. Most "open" and double-blind studies have confirmed that TMS has a modest antidepressant response in non-psychotically depressed patients. No seizures or cognitive side effects have so far been reported following fast TMS, pain at the treatment site being the only recorded problem.

Hopefully the combination of TMS with fMRI will enable the more precise location of the regional dysfunction in depression to be located and thereby enable the neuronal pathways concerned to be identified. To date, the early studies of TMS with fMRI have shown that the effects of TMS occur in brain regions distant from the site of stimulation, including the caudate, orbitofrontal cortex and the cerebellum.

Classification of neurotransmitter receptors

The British physiologist Langley, in 1905, was first to postulate that most drugs, hormones and transmitters produce their effects by interacting with specific sites on the cell membrane which we now call *receptors*. Langley's postulate was based on his observation that drugs can mimic both the specificity and potency of endogenous hormones and neurotransmitters, while others appear to be able to selectively antagonize the actions of such substances. Thus, substances which stimulate the receptor, or mimic the action of natural ligands for the receptor, are called *agonists*, while those substances blocking the receptor are called *antagonists* (this is expanded upon in Chapter 5). This revolutionary hypothesis was later extended by Hill, Gaddum and Clark, who quantified the ways in which agonists and antagonists interacted with receptors both *in vitro* and *in vivo*. More recently the precise structures of a large number of different types of transmitter receptors have been determined using cloning and other techniques, so that it is now possible to visualize precisely how an agonist or antagonist interacts with certain types of receptor.

To date, different types of cholinergic, β-adrenergic and serotonergic receptors have been cloned, and their essential molecular features identified. In addition, a number of peptide receptors such as the insulin, gonadotrophin, angiotensin, glucagon, prolactin and thyroid stimulating hormone receptors have also been identified and their key structures determined. The location and possible functional importance of the different types of neurotransmitter receptors which are of relevance to the psychopharmacologist are summarized below. It must be emphasized that this list is by no means complete and that many of these receptor types are likely to be further subdivided as a result of the development of highly selective ligands.

Cholinergic receptors

Sir Henry Dale noticed that the different esters of choline elicited responses in isolated organ preparations which were similar to those seen following the application of either of the natural substances muscarine (from poisonous toadstools) or nicotine. This led Dale to conclude that, in the appropriate organs, acetylcholine could act on either *muscarinic* or *nicotinic receptors*. Later it was found that the effects of muscarine and nicotine could be blocked by atropine and tubocurarine, respectively. Further studies showed that these receptors differed not only in their molecular structure but also in the ways in which they brought about their physiological responses once the receptor has been stimulated by an agonist. Thus nicotinic receptors were found to be linked directly to an ion channel and their activation always caused a rapid increase in cellular permeability to sodium and potassium ions. Conversely, the responses to muscarinic receptor stimulation were slower and involved the activation of a second messenger system which was linked to the receptor by G-proteins.

Muscarinic receptors

To date, five subtypes of these receptors have been cloned. However, initial studies relied on the pharmacological effects of the muscarinic antagonist pirenzepine which was shown to block the effect of several muscarinic agonists. These receptors were termed M_1 receptors to distinguish them from those receptors for which pirenzepine had only a low affinity and therefore failed to block the pharmacological response. These were termed M_2 receptors. More recently, M_3, M_4 and M_5 receptors have been identified which, like the M_1 and M_2 receptors occur in the brain. Recent studies have shown that M_1 and M_3 are located postsynaptically in the brain whereas the M_2 and M_4 receptors occur presynaptically where they act as inhibitory autoreceptors that inhibit the release of acetylcholine. The M_2 and M_4 receptors are coupled to the inhibitory Gi protein which reduces the formation of cyclic adenosine monophosphate (cyclic AMP) within the neuron. By contrast, the M_1, M_3 and M_5 receptors are coupled to the stimulatory Gs protein which stimulates the intracellular hydrolysis of the phosphoinositide messenger within the neuron (see Figure 2.8).

The cholinergic system has the capacity to adapt to changes in the physiological environment of the brain. Thus the density of the cholinergic receptors is increased by antagonists and decreased by agonists. The reduction in the density of the receptors is a result of their rapid internalization into the neuronal membrane (receptor sequestration) followed by their subsequent destruction. This phenomenon may have a bearing on the long-term efficacy of cholinomimetic drugs and anti-cholinesterases which are currently used in the symptomatic treatment of

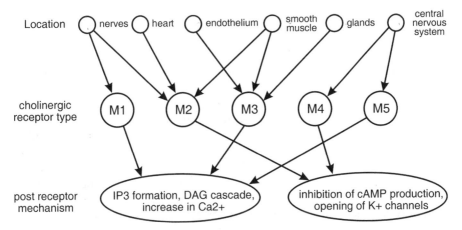

Figure 2.8. Location of muscarinic receptors and their link to second messenger systems.

Alzheimer's disease. While it is widely believed that the relapse in the response to treatment is due to the continuing neurodegenerative changes in the brain which are unaffected by cholinomimetic drugs, it is also possible that such treatments could impair cholinergic function by causing an increased sequestration and destruction of muscarinic receptors. The possible detrimental effect of cholinergic agonists on memory is supported by the observation that the chronic administration of physostigmine or oxotremorine to rats decreases the number of muscarinic receptors and leads to an impairment of memory when the drugs are withdrawn. Conversely chronic treatment with a cholinergic antagonist such as atropine increases the number of cholinergic receptors and leads to a memory improvement when the drug is withdrawn. Whether these effects in experimental animals are relevant to the clinical situation in which cholinomimetic agents are administered for several months is unknown.

Although other transmitters such as noradrenaline, serotonin and glutamate are involved, there is now substantial evidence to suggest that muscarinic receptors play a key role in learning and memory. It is well established that muscarinic antagonists such as atropine and scopolamine impair memory and learning in man and that their effects can be reversed by anticholinesterases. Conversely, muscarinic agonists such as arecoline improve some aspects of learning and memory. However, cholinomimetic drugs such as carbachol which stimulate the inhibitory autoreceptors impair memory by blocking the release of acetylcholine in the hippocampus and cortex; the selective autoreceptor antagonist secoverine has the opposite effect.

Comment on the use of cholinomimetic drugs in the treatment of Alzheimer's disease

In addition to the accumulation of senile plaques (abnormal beta amyloid containing proteins) and neurofibrillary tangles (modified microtubular associated proteins) which characterize the disease, the most consistent neuropathological finding in patients with Alzheimer's disease is a degeneration of the projections from the main cholinergic cell body which comprise the nucleus basalis of Meynert. The degenerative changes involve the loss of M_1 and M_2 receptors and a reduction in the activity of choline acetyltransferase (CAT), the rate-limiting enzyme for the synthesis of acetylcholine. The reduction in CAT and the associated neuronal loss in the basal forebrain are the most consistent correlates of cognitive impairment seen in Alzheimer's disease. The treatment strategies are primarily aimed at increasing cholinergic transmission. These include the centrally acting reversible inhibitors of acetylcholinesterase such as tacrine, donepezil, rivastigmine, galanthamine and metrofinate. Physostigmine has also been used but its efficacy and peripheral side effects have limited its widespread clinical use. Such drugs have beneficial effects in about 40% of patients; the patients show an improved score in several tests of cognitive function. However, even in those patients who do show some improvement following the administration of these drugs at an early stage in the development of the disease, the benefit is limited to approximately 18 months. Furthermore gastrointestinal side effects are often problematic.

Nicotinic receptors

Following studies of the actions of specific agonists and antagonists on the nicotinic receptors from skeletal muscle and sympathetic ganglia, it was soon apparent that not all nicotinic receptors are the same. The heterogeneity of the nicotinic receptors was further revealed by the application of molecular cloning techniques. This has led to the classification of nicotinic receptors into N-m receptors and N-n receptors, the former being located in the neuromuscular junction, where activation causes end-plate depolarization and muscle contraction, while the latter are found in the autonomic ganglia (involved in ganglionic transmission), adrenal medulla (where activation causes catecholamine release) and in the brain, where their precise physiological importance is currently unclear. Of the specific antagonists that block these receptor subtypes, and which have clinical applications, tubocurarine and related neuromuscular blockers inhibit the N-m type receptor while the antihypertensive agent trimethaphan blocks the N-n receptor.

In contrast to the more numerous muscarinic receptors, much less is known about the function of nicotinic receptors in the brain. In addition to

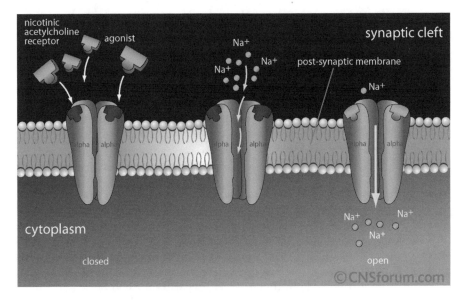

Figure 2.9. Diagrammatic representation of an ionotropic nicotinic receptor.

their distribution in the neuromuscular junction, ganglia and adrenal medulla, nicotinic receptors occur in a high density in the neocortex.

Nicotinic receptors are of the ionotropic type which, on stimulation by acetylcholine, nicotine or related agonists, open to allow the passage of sodium ions into the neuron. There are structural differences between the peripheral and neuronal receptors, the former being pentamers composed of two alpha and one beta, gamma and delta sub-units while the latter consist of single alpha and beta sub-units. It is now known that there are at least four variants of the alpha and two of the beta sub-units in the brain. In Alzheimer's disease it would appear that there is a selective reduction in the nicotinic receptors which contain the alpha 3 and 4 sub-units (Figure 2.9). Unlike the muscarinic receptors, repeated exposure of the neuronal receptors to nicotine, both *in vivo* and *in vitro*, results in an increase in the number of receptors; similar changes are reported to occur after physostigmine is administered directly into the cerebral ventricles of rats. These changes in the density of the nicotinic receptors are accompanied by an increased release of acetylcholine. Following the chronic administration of physostigmine, however, a desensitization of the receptors occurs. Functionally nicotinic receptors appear to be involved in memory formation; in clinical studies it has been shown that nicotine can reverse the effects of scopolamine on short-term working memory and both nicotine and arecholine have been shown to have positive, though modest, effects on cognition in patients with Alzheimer's disease.

Adrenergic receptors

Ahlquist, in 1948, first proposed that noradrenaline could produce its diverse physiological effects by acting on different populations of adrenoceptors, which he termed α and β receptors. This classification was based upon the relative selectivity of adrenaline for the α receptors and isoprenaline for the β receptors; drugs such as phentolamine were found to be specific antagonists of the α, and propranolol for the β receptors.

Alpha receptors

It later became possible to separate these main groups of receptors further, into α_1 and α_2 based on the selectivity of the antagonists prazosin, the antihypertensive agent that blocks α_1 receptors, and yohimbine, which is an antagonist of α_2 receptors.

At one time it was thought that α_1 receptors were postsynaptic and the α_2 type were presynaptic and concerned with the inhibitory control of noradrenaline release. Indeed, novel antidepressants like mianserin, and more recently the highly selective α_2 receptor antagonist idazoxan, or yohimbine, were thought to act by stimulating the relase of noradrenaline from central noradrenergic synapses. It is now established, however, that the α_2 receptors also occur postsynaptically, and that their stimulation by such specific agonists as clonidine leads to a reduction in the activity of the vasomotor centre, thereby leading to a decrease in blood pressure. Conversely, the α_2 antagonist yohimbine enhances noradrenaline release (see Figure 2.10).

The α_1 receptors are excitatory in their action, while the α_2 receptors are inhibitory, these activities being related to the different types of second messengers or ion channels to which they are linked. Thus, α_2 receptors hyperpolarize presynaptic membranes by opening potassium ion channels, and thereby reduce noradrenaline release. Conversely, stimulation of α_1 receptors increases intracellular calcium via the phosphatidyl inositol cycle which causes the release of calcium from its intracellular stores; protein kinase C activity is increased as a result of the free calcium, which then brings about further changes in the membrane activity.

Both types of receptor occur in the brain as well as in vascular and intestinal smooth muscle: α_1 receptors are found in the heart whereas α_2 receptors occur on the platelet membrane (stimulation induces aggregation) and nerve terminals (stimulation inhibits release of the transmitter). It is now recognized that there are several subtypes of α_1 and α_2 receptors, but their precise function is unclear.

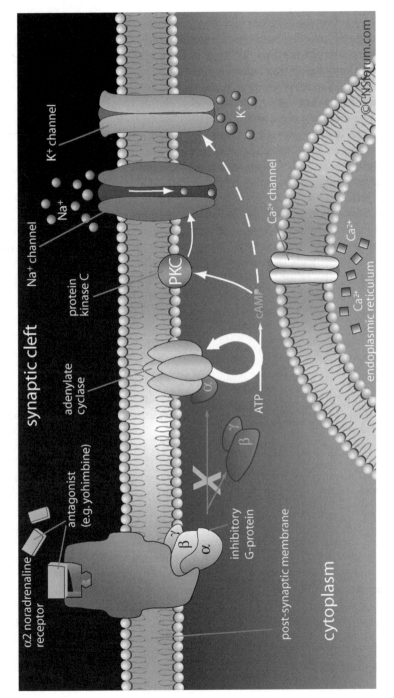
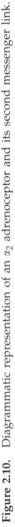

Figure 2.10. Diagrammatic representation of an α_2 adrenoceptor and its second messenger link.

Beta receptors

So far three subtypes of β receptors have been identified and cloned. They differ in their distribution, the β_1 type being found in the heart, the β_2 in lung, smooth muscle, skeletal muscle and liver, while the β_3 type occurs in adipose tissue. There is evidence that β_2 adrenoceptors occur on the lymphocyte membrane also but the precise function there is unknown.

The antihypertensive drug metoprolol is a clinically effective example of a β_1 antagonist. All the β receptor subtypes are linked to adenylate cyclase as the second messenger system. It seems that both β_1 and β_2 receptor types occur in the brain and that their activation leads to excitatory effects. Of particular interest to the psychopharmacologist is the finding that chronic antidepressant treatment leads to a decrease in the functional responsiveness of the β receptors in the brain, and in the density of these receptors on lymphocytes, which coincides with the time necessary for the therapeutic effects of the drugs to be manifest. Such changes have been ascribed to the drugs affecting the activity of the G-proteins that couple the receptor to the cyclase sub-unit.

The adrenergic receptors have been purified and their genes cloned. They have seven membrane-spanning units, which are involved in binding the selective agonists and antagonists.

Dopamine receptors

Two types of dopamine receptors have been characterized in the mammalian brain, termed D_1 and D_2. This subtyping largely arose in response to the finding that while all types of clinically useful neuroleptics inhibit dopaminergic transmission in the brain, there is a poor correlation between reduction in adenylate cyclase activity, believed to be the second messenger linked to dopamine receptors, and the clinical potency of the drugs. This was particularly true for the butyrophenone series (e.g. haloperidol) which are known to be potent neuroleptics and yet are relatively poor at inhibiting adenylate cyclase.

Detailed studies of the binding of ^{3}H-labelled haloperidol to neuronal membranes showed that there was a much better correlation between the therapeutic potency of a neuroleptic and its ability to displace this ligand from the nerve membrane. This led to the discovery of two types of dopamine receptor that are both linked to adenylate cyclase but whereas the D_1 receptor is positively linked to the cyclase, the D_2 receptor is negatively linked. It was also shown that the D_1 receptor is approximately 15 times more sensitive to the action of dopamine than the D_2 receptor; conversely, the D_1 receptor has a low affinity for the butyrophenone and atypical neuroleptics such as clozapine, whereas the D_2 receptor appears to have a high affinity for most therapeutically active neuroleptics.

There is still some controversy over the precise anatomical location of the dopamine receptor subtypes, but there is now evidence that the D_2 receptors are located presynaptically on the corticostriatal neurons and postsynaptically in the striatum and substantia nigra. Conversely, the D_1 receptors are found presynaptically on nigrostriatal neurons, and postsynaptically in the cortex. It is possible to differentiate these receptor types on the basis of their agonist and antagonist affinities.

In addition to these two subtypes, there is also evidence that the release of dopamine is partially regulated by feedback inhibition operating via the dopamine autoreceptor.

With the development of D_1 and D_2 agonists, however, emphasis has become centred on the pharmacological characteristics of the specific drug in order to determine whether an observed effect is mediated by D_1 or D_2 receptors. It is now apparent that dopamine receptors with the same pharmacological characteristics do not necessarily produce the same functional responses at the same receptor. For example, D_2 receptors are present in both the striatum and the nucleus accumbens, but cause an inhibition of adenylate cyclase only in the striatum. Furthermore, recent studies indicate that dopamine receptors can influence cellular activities through mechanisms other than adenylate cyclase. These may include direct effects on potassium and calcium channels, as well as modulation of the phosphatidyl inositol cycle. To complicate the picture further, D_1 and D_2 receptors have opposite effects on some behaviours (e.g. chewing in rats) but are synergistic in causing other behaviours (e.g. locomotor activity and some types of stereotypy). The precise clinical importance of these interactions is unclear.

The densities and functional activities of dopamine receptors have been shown to change in response to chronic drug treatment and in disease. Thus an increase in the dopamine receptor density in the nigrostriatal pathway appears to be related to the behavioural supersensitivity observed following unilateral destruction of the dopaminergic system in the striatum. Dopamine receptor antagonists, such as the "classical" neuroleptics like chlorpromazine, are also known to increase the density of dopamine receptors in the striatal region. This contributes to the extrapyramidal side effects of such drugs, which frequently follows their prolonged use and reflects the drug-induced functional deficit of dopamine in the brain. Abrupt withdrawal of a neuroleptic following its prolonged administration is frequently associated with tardive dyskinesia, a disorder which may be partly due to the sudden activation of supersensitive dopamine receptors. Despite the appeal of this hypothesis, it should be emphasized that many other factors, such as brain damage and prior exposure to tricyclic antidepressants, may also predispose patients to this condition.

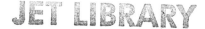

With regard to the change in dopamine receptor activity in disease, there is some evidence from post-mortem studies that the density of D_2 receptors is increased in the mesocortical areas of the schizophrenic brain, and in the putamen and caudate nucleus in neuroleptic-free patients. Positron emission tomography of schizophrenic patients has, however, failed to confirm these findings. There is also evidence that the link between the D_1 and D_2 receptors is defective in some patients with diseases in which the dopaminergic system might be involved. Thus the well-known loss of dopaminergic function in patients with Parkinson's disease is associated with a compensatory rise in the density of postsynaptic D_1 and D_2 receptors. The long-term treatment of Parkinson's disease with L-dopa reduces the receptor density to normal (so-called receptor "down-regulation"). Similarly, the densities of D_1 and D_2 receptors are reduced in the striata of patients with Huntington's chorea, as is the linkage between these receptors.

Dopamine has been implicated in a number of psychiatric conditions of which schizophrenia and the affective disorders are the most widely established. Five major subtypes of dopamine receptors have now been cloned. These are divided into two main groups, D_1 and D_2 respectively. The D_1 receptors consist of D_1 and D_5 types and are positively linked to the adenylate cyclase second messenger system, while the D_2 group consists of the D_2, D_3 and D_4 receptors which are negatively linked to the adenylate cyclase system.

The D_1 receptors have been subdivided into the D_{1A} and D_{1B} types and are coded by genes located on chromosomes 5 and 4 respectively. Several selective antagonists of the D_1 receptors have been developed (for example, SCH 31966, SCH 23390 and SKF 83959), none of which have so far been developed for therapeutic use.

Apomorphine is an agonist at both the D_1 and D_2 receptors. From the pathological viewpoint, a malfunction of the D_1 receptors has been implicated in the negative symptoms of schizophrenia but as there is a close interaction between these receptor types it is difficult to conclude whether the changes seen in schizophrenia are attributable to a primary decrease in D_1 receptor function or an increase in D_2 receptor function. The function of the D_5 receptors is unclear; these receptors, though widely distributed in the brain, are only present in a relatively low density in comparison to the other dopamine receptor types.

The D_2 receptor types, besides being subdivided into D_3 and D_4 types, are further divided into the D_2 long and D_2 short forms. D_2 antagonists, in addition to virtually all therapeutically active neuroleptics, also include such novel drugs as raclopride, eticlopride and sniperone while quinpirole is an example of a specific D_2 receptor agonist. The latter drugs are not available for therapeutic use. A malfunction of the D_2 receptors has been associated with psychosis, extrapyramidal side effects and hyperprolactinaemia.

The human D_3 gene has produced two variants, D_3 and D_3s. So far there do not appear to be any selective agonists or antagonists of the D_3 receptor which enable the function of this receptor to be clearly distinguished from that of the D_2 receptor. The D_3 receptors are located in the ventral and limbic regions of the brain but absent from the dorsal striatum. This suggests that specific antagonists of the D_3 receptors may be effective antipsychotics but without causing extrapyramidal side effects.

The D_4 receptor has eight polymorphic variants in the human. However, even though several specific antagonists of this receptor type have been developed and shown to have antipsychotic activity in animal models of schizophrenia, the clinical findings have been disappointing. Because of the high density of the D_4 receptors in the limbic cortex and hippocampus, but their absence from the motor regions of the brain, it was anticipated that such drugs have antipsychotic efficacy without the motor side effects. In support of this view, it has been shown that the atypical antipsychotic clozapine has a high affinity for the D_4 receptors; other studies have also indicated that many of the atypical, and some of the typical, antipsychotics have similar affinities for these receptors.

In addition to the postsynaptic receptors, dopamine autoreceptors also exist on the nerve terminals, dendrites and cell bodies. Experimental studies have shown that stimulation of the autoreceptors in the somatodendritic region of the neuron slows the firing rate of the dopaminergic neuron while stimulation of the autoreceptors on the nerve terminal inhibits both the release and the synthesis of the neurotransmitter. Structurally, the autoreceptor appears to be of the D_2 type. While several experimental compounds have been developed that show a high affinity for the autoreceptors, to date there is no convincing evidence for their therapeutic efficacy.

5-Hydroxytryptamine receptors

Gaddum and Picarelli, in 1957, were the first investigators to provide evidence for the existence of two different types of 5-HT receptor in peripheral smooth muscle. These receptors were termed D (for dibenzyline, an α_1 adrenoceptor antagonist which also blocked 5-HT receptors) and M (for morphine, which blocked the contractile response mediated through the myenteric plexus in the intestinal wall). Studies undertaken in the 1980s revealed the existence of multiple binding sites for 5-HT receptors. The 5-HT_D receptor was shown to have the characteristics of the 5-HT_2 receptor, while the M receptor has been shown to be identical to the 5-HT_3 receptor in the brain and gastrointestinal tract.

This biogenic amine transmitter contributes to the regulation of a variety of psychological functions which include mood, arousal, attention, impulsivity, aggression, appetite, pain perception and cognition, In addition, serotonin plays a crucial role in regulating the sleep–wake cycle and in the control of brain maturation. It is therefore understandable that a dysfunction of the serotonergic system has been implicated in a variety of psychiatric disorders such as schizophrenia, depression, alcoholism and in phobic states. Undoubtedly interest in the role of the serotonergic system in psychiatry has been stimulated by the therapeutic success of the selective serotonin reuptake inhibitors (SSRIs) which have proven to be effective in alleviating the symptoms of many of these disorders. The complexity of the serotonergic system lies in the number of different serotonin receptors within the brain. These are classified into seven distinct types that are heterogeneously distributed in the brain, each with its specific physiological function. The function of the serotonin receptors is a reflection of their structure. Thus the 5-HT$_3$ receptors are ionotropic in nature whereas the remainder are metabotropic, coupled to specific G-proteins and share a common seven-membrane domain structure. These receptors have been cloned and their physiological activity shown to be associated with the activation of either phospholipase C (5-HT$_2$ receptors) or adenylate cyclase (5-HT$_4$–5-HT$_7$). The 5-HT$_{1A, 1B}$ and $_{1D}$ receptors are also coupled to adenylate cyclase but they inhibit the function of this second messenger system. Although the precise physiological activity of the different serotonin receptors is still the subject of ongoing studies, links between specific receptor subtypes and their possible involvement in specific neurological and psychiatric disorders have been identified. For example, the antimigraine drug sumatriptan decreases headache by activating the inhibitory 5-HT$_{1B}$ receptors located presynaptically on perivascular nerve fibres. This blocks the release of pain-causing neuropeptides and the conduction in the trigeminal vascular neurons. With regard to the 5-HT$_{1A}$ receptors, agonists such as buspirone and ipsapirone act as anxiolytics while the antidepressant effects of the SSRIs have been associated with an indirect reduction in the activity of the 5-HT$_{1A}$ receptors. Conversely the sexual side effects of the SSRIs are attributed to their indirect action on 5-HT$_{2C}$ receptors which follows the enhanced serotonergic function; these receptors may also be involved in the regulation of food intake which could help to explain the antibulimic action of the SSRIs.

Several different types of serotonin receptor (for example, 5-HT$_{1A}$, 5-HT$_{2A}$, 5-HT$_{2C}$, 5-HT$_{1B/1D}$) have been associated with the motor side effects of the SSRIs which may arise should these drugs be administered in conjunction with a monoamine oxidase inhibitor. The 5-HT$_3$ receptor is an example of a non-selective cation channel receptor which is permeable to both sodium and potassium ions and, because both calcium and magnesium ions can modulate its activity, the 5-HT$_3$ receptor resembles the glutamate–NMDA receptor. Antagonists of the 5-HT$_3$ receptor, such as ondansetron, are effective antiemetics and are particularly useful when nausea is associated with the administration of cytotoxic drugs or some anaesthetic agents. However, they are ineffective against the nausea of motion sickness or that induced by apomorphine, suggesting that the $5-HT_3$ receptors function at the level of the vomiting centre in the brain. In addition, there is evidence from experimental studies that these receptors are involved in anxiety and in cognition. $5-HT_3$ antagonists have both anxiolytic and cognitive enhancing properties but it still remains to be proven that such properties are therapeutically relevant.

The precise function of the $5-HT_{4,5,6}$ and $_7$ receptors is less certain. All these receptors have been cloned and their distribution in the brain determined. There is some evidence that $5-HT_4$ receptors act as heteroceptors on cholinergic terminals and thereby modulate the release of acetylcholine. While the physiological role of the $5-HT_{5,6}$ and $_7$ receptors is unclear, it is of interest to note that several atypical neuroleptics, such as clozapine, and several antidepressants have a good affinity for these receptors. There is also evidence that selective agonists and antagonists, such as zacopride, ergotamine, methysergide and LSD, have a high affinity for the $5-HT_4$ and $5-HT_5$ receptors but how these effects relate to their pharmacological actions is presently unknown. Figure 2.11 summarizes the possible sites of action of different classes of psychotropic drugs on the serotonin receptors in the brain.

Clearly, much remains to be learned about the distribution and functional activity of these receptor subtypes before their possible roles in mental illness can be elucidated. A summary of the distribution of the different types of 5-HT receptors and their agonists is shown in Table 2.6.

Amino acid receptors

There are two amino acid neurotransmitters, namely GABA and glutamate, which have been of major interest to the psychopharmacologist because of the potential therapeutic importance of their agonists and antagonists. The receptors upon which GABA and glutamate act to produce their effects differ from the "classic" transmitter receptors in that they seem to exist as receptor complexes that contain sites for agonists, in addition to the amino acid transmitters; these sites, when occupied, modulate the responsiveness of the receptor to the amino acid. For example, the benzodiazepines have long been known to facilitate inhibitory transmission, and their therapeutic properties as anxiolytics and anticonvulsants are attributable to such an action. It is now apparent that benzodiazepines occupy a receptor site on the GABA receptor complex which enhances the responsiveness of the GABA receptor to the inhibitory action of GABA. Similarly, it has recently been shown that the inhibitory transmitter glycine can act on a strychnine-insensitive site on the N-methyl-D-aspartate (NMDA) receptor, and thereby modify its responsiveness to glutamate.

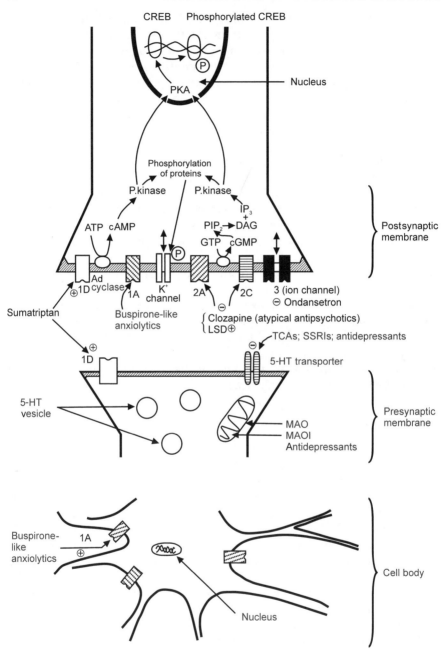

Figure 2.11. The presumed sites of action of some psychotropic drugs which modulate central serotonergic function.

Knowledge of the mechanisms whereby the amino acid transmitters produce their effects has been valuable in the development of psychotropic drugs that may improve memory, reduce anxiety, or even counteract the effects of post-stroke hypoxia on brain cell survival. Some of these aspects are considered later.

GABA receptors

The major amino acid neurotransmitters in the brain are GABA, an inhibitory transmitter, and glutamic acid, an excitatory transmitter. GABA is widely distributed in the mammalian brain and has been calculated to contribute to over 40% of the synapses in the cortex alone. While it is evident that a reduction in GABAergic activity is associated with seizures, and most anticonvulsant drugs either directly or indirectly facilitate GABAergic transmission, GABA also has a fundamental role in the brain by shaping, integrating and refining information transfer generated by the excitatory transmitters. Indeed, because of its wide anatomical distribution, GABA may be involved in such diverse functions as vigilance, consciousness, arousal, thermoregulation, learning, food consumption, hormonal control, motor control and the control of pain.

At the cellular level, GABA is located in the interneurons. GABAergic neurons project both locally and, by long axons, to more distant regions of the brain. For example, GABAergic neurons project from the neostriatum to the substantia nigra. As with the biogenic amine neurotransmitters, the synthesis of GABA is highly regulated. GABA is synthesized by glutamate decarboxylase from glutamate. This enzyme acts as the rate-limiting step as its activity is dependent on the pyridoxal phosphate cofactor; it has been estimated that at least 50% of glutamate decarboxylase present in the brain is not bound to cofactor and is therefore inactive. Newly synthesized GABA is stored in vesicles in the nerve terminal and, following its release, its action is terminated by a reuptake mechanism into the glial cells which surround the neuron, and also into the nerve terminal. GABA is then metabolized by GABA transaminase to succinic semialdehyde, a component of the GABA-shunt pathway, and thence to the tricarboxylic acid cycle to generate metabolic energy. Thus GABA differs substantially from the conventional biogenic amine transmitters in that it is largely metabolized once it has been released during neurotransmission.

Of the many drugs that have been developed which modulate GABA function, the inhibitors of GABA transaminase have been shown to be effective anticonvulsants. These are derivatives of valproic acid that not only inhibit the metabolism of GABA but may also act as antagonists of the GABA autoreceptor and thereby enhance the release of the neurotransmitter. GABA-uptake inhibitors have also been developed (for example, derivatives

Table 2.6. Summary of the properties of 5-HT receptor subtypes in the mammalian brain

	5-HT_{1A}	5-HT_{1B}[a]	5-HT_{1C}[b]	5-HT_{1D}[a]	5-HT_{2}[c]
Second messenger system	↓ Cyclic AMP	↓ Cyclic AMP	↑ PI	↓ Cyclic AMP	↑ PI
Location	Hippocampus, raphé, cortex		Choroid plexus		Cortex, olfactory system, claustrum
Ligands	8-OH-DPAT, *Ipsapirone, gepirone*, *Buspirone*[d], *Pindolol*[d]	?	*Methiopin*[d], *Mesulergine*[d], *Ritanserin*[d]	*Metergoline*[d]	DOI, DOM, LSD, *Ketanserin*, Sergolexole
Physiological/ Pathological Effects	Anxiety, depression, Appetite, aggression, Pain, sexual behaviour		Appetite, anxiety, Mood	Vasoconstriction, Appetite	

[a] 5-HT_{1B} and 5-HT_{1D} receptors are structurally and functionally similar and act as inhibitory presynaptic receptors. 5-HT_{1B} receptors occur in most mammalian brains whereas 5-HT_{1D} receptors are located in primates and the guinea pig brain.
[b] Now classified as 5-HT_{2C}.
[c] Now classified as 5-HT_{2A}.
[d] Indicates ligand is non-selective and also acts on other 5-HT, and possibly non-5-HT, receptors. Italic indicates compounds are in therapeutic use. PI, phosphatidyl inositol. DOI, (2,5-dimethoxy-1-iodophenyl)-2-aminopropane. DOM, dimethoxy-methamphetamine.

Table 2.6. (continued)

	5-HT$_3$	5-HT$_4$	5-HT$_5$	5-HT$_{5B}$	5-HT$_6$	5-HT$_7$
Second messenger system	Ion channel	↓ Cyclic AMP	?	?	cAMP	cAMP
Location	Area postrema Cortex (low density) vagal efferents	Superior colliculi Hippocampus	Cortex, Hippocampus Olfactory bulb Cerebellum	Habenula Hippocampus	Striatum Amygdala Cortex	Hypothalamus Hippocampus Cortex Olfactory bulb
Ligands	M-chlorophenyl-biguanide Ondansetron Granisetron Raclopride	ICS 205-930 Renzapride Cisapride Metoclopramide[d] 5-Methoxy tryptamine	2-Bromo-LSD Ergotamine Methysergide	LSD Dihydroergotamine Methysergide Methiothepin	Clozapine Amoxapine Clomipramine Amitriptyline	LSD Clozapine Loxapine Amitriptyline
Physiological/ pathological effects	Emesis Anxiety Pain, cognition?	Arrhythmia Atrial fibrillation Cognition?	Similar to 5-HT$_{1D}$	?	?	?

of nipecotic acid, guvacine) which also have anticonvulsant activity at least in experimental animals. However, the major development in the pharmacology of the GABAergic system has been in drugs which facilitate the functioning of the GABA-A receptors. These will be discussed later.

There are three types of GABA receptor, A, B and C. Unlike the ionotropic GABA-A receptors, the GABA-B receptors are metabotropic and coupled via inhibitory G-proteins to adenylate cyclase. Not only do the GABA-B receptors inhibit the second messenger but they also modulate potassium and calcium channels in the neuronal membrane. Baclofen, the antispastic drug, owes its therapeutic efficacy to its agonistic action on these receptors while phaclofen, an experimental drug, acts as an antagonist. Unlike drugs that act on GABA-A receptors, GABA-B receptor agonists have antinociceptive properties which may account for the efficacy of drugs like baclofen in the treatment of trigeminal neuralgia. Experimental studies suggest that GABA-B antagonists may have antiepileptic activity. GABA-B receptors are widely distributed throughout the brain and in several peripheral organs. Their distribution differs from the GABA-A receptors. In the cortex and several other brain regions, GABA-B receptors occur on the terminals of both GABA and non-GABA neurons where they modulate neurotransmitter release.

GABA-C receptors have only recently been identified and their function is still uncertain. There is evidence that, besides GABA, the GABA receptor agonists muscimol and isogucacine have a high affinity for these receptors. A high density of GABA-C receptors has been detected in the retina where they appear to be involved in the development of retinal rod cells. In the brain, there is evidence that GABA-C receptors are concentrated in the superior colliculus where they have a disinhibitory role. There is also evidence that they play an important role in some aspects of neuro-endocrine regulation both in the gastrointestinal tract and in the secretion of thyroid stimulating hormone.

The GABA-A receptors have been cloned and the structures of some of the 10 subtypes of this receptor have been described. As these subtypes appear to be heterogeneously distributed throughout the brain, it may ultimately be possible to develop drugs that will affect only one specific species of GABA-A receptor, thereby optimizing the therapeutic effect and reducing the possibility of non-specific side effects. It seems likely that this will be an important area for psychotropic drug development in the near future.

The GABA-A receptor is directly linked to chloride ion channels, activation of which results in an increase in the membrane permeability to chloride ions, and thereby the hyperpolarization of cell bodies. GABA-A receptors are also found extrasynaptically where, following activation, they can depolarize neurons. The convulsant drug bicuculline acts as a specific antagonist of GABA on its receptor site, while the convulsant drug picrotoxin binds to an adjacent site on the GABA-A receptor complex and

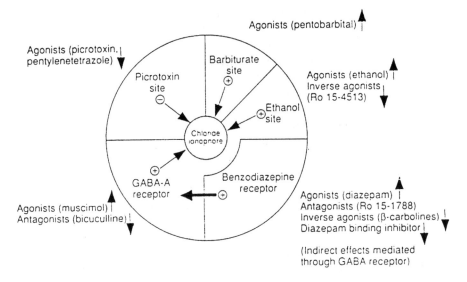

Figure 2.12. Diagrammatic representation of the GABA-benzodiazepine supramolecular complex. Compounds that increase inhibitory transmission may do so either by directly activating the GABA receptor site (e.g. muscimol) or by acting directly on the chloride ionophore (e.g. barbiturates). Benzodiazepines (e.g. diazepam) enhance the sensitivity of the GABA-A receptor to GABA. Compounds that decrease inhibitory transmission may do so by activating the picrotoxin site, which closes the chloride ionophore, or by blocking the GABA-A receptor.

directly decreases chloride ion flux; barbiturates have the opposite effect on the chloride channel and lock the channel open.

The inhibitory effect of GABA is mediated by the chloride ion channel (Figure 2.12). When the GABA-A receptor is activated by GABA or a specific agonist such as muscimol, the frequency of opening of the channel is increased and the cell is hyperpolarized. Barbiturates, such as phenobarbitone, and possibly alcohol, also facilitate the chloride ion influx, but these drugs increase the duration, rather than the frequency, of the channel opening. Recently, novel benzodiazepine receptor ligands have been produced which, like the typical benzodiazepines, increase the frequency of chloride channel opening. The cyclopyrrolone sedative/hypnotic zopiclone is an example of such a ligand. Some glucocorticoids are also known to have sedative effects which may be ascribed to their ability to activate specific steroid receptor facilitatory sites on the GABA-A receptor.

In addition to the benzodiazepine receptor agonists which, depending on the dose administered, have anxiolytic, anticonvulsant, sedative and amnestic properties, benzodiazepines have also been developed which block the action of agonists on this receptor. Such antagonists may be exemplified by flumazenil. Other compounds have a mixture of agonist and antagonist properties and are termed partial agonists or antagonists. However, the complexity of the benzodiazepine receptor only became fully apparent recently when a series of compounds were discovered that had the opposite effects of the "classic" benzodiazepines when they activated the receptor. These inverse agonists were found to have anxiogenic, proconvulsant, stimulant, spasmogenic and promnestic properties in man and animals. Such compounds were found to decrease GABA transmission.

Naturally occurring inverse agonists called the β-carbolines have been isolated from human urine, but it now seems probable that these compounds are byproducts of the extraction procedure. Thus the benzodiazepine receptor is unique in that it has a bidirectional function. This may be of considerable importance in the design of benzodiazepine ligands which act as partial agonists (see Chapter 5). Such drugs may combine the efficacy of the conventional agents with a lack of unwanted side effects, such as sedation, amnesia and dependence. Partial inverse agonists have also been described. Such drugs appear to maintain the promnestic properties of the full inverse agonists without causing excessive stimulation and convulsions which can occur with full inverse agonists. The presence of a specific benzodiazepine site in the mammalian brain also raises the possibility that endogenous substances are present that modulate the activity of the site. While the precise identity of such natural ligands remains an enigma, there is evidence that substances like tribulin, nephentin and the diazepam-binding inhibitor could have a physiological and pathological function. There is also evidence that trace amounts of benzodiazepines (such as nordiazepine and lorazepam) occur in human brain, human breast milk and also in many plants, including the potato. Such benzodiazepines have been found in post-mortem brains from the 1940s and 1950s before the discovery of the benzodiazepine anxiolytics (see Chapter 19 for further details).

Modulation of GABA-A receptors

During brain development, the RNA expression of the sub-units which comprise the GABA-A receptor change so that each sub-unit exhibits a unique regional and temporal profile. Such changes may reflect the increase in the sensitivity of the foetal brain to GABA, and its decreased sensitivity to the benzodiazepines which indirectly enhance GABA-A receptor function. Thus during the later stages of development of the foetal brain, at a stage when the synapses are present, GABA acts as a neurotrophic factor that promotes neuronal growth and differentiation, synaptogenesis and the synthesis of GABA-A receptors. This may account for the increased sensitivity of these receptors to the actions of GABA as the concentration of the transmitter in the developing brain is relatively low. Thus as GABA has to diffuse to receptors which are relatively distant from the neurons from which it is released, the increased sensitivity of the GABA-A receptors ensures that they are activated even by a low concentration of the transmitter.

Changes have also been reported to occur in the sub-unit composition of the GABA-A receptor following chronic exposure to barbiturates, neurosteroids, ethanol and benzodiazepine agonists. These changes may underlie the development of tolerance, physical dependence and the problems which are associated with the abrupt withdrawal of such drugs.

Excitatory amino acid receptors: glutamate receptor

It has long been recognized that glutamic and aspartic acids occur in uniquely high concentrations in the mammalian brain and that they can cause excitation of nerve cells. However, these amino acids have only recently been identified as excitatory neurotransmitters because of the difficulty that arose in dissociating their transmitter from their metabolic role in the brain. For example, glutamate is an important component of brain proteins, peptides and a precursor of GABA. As a result of microdialysis and micro-iontophoretic techniques, in which the release and effect of local application could be demonstrated, and the synthesis and isolation of specific agonists for the different types of excitatory amino acid receptor (e.g. quisqualic, ibotenic and kainic acids), it is now generally accepted that glutamic and aspartic acids are excitatory transmitters in the mammalian brain.

Glutamate is uniformly distributed throughout the mammalian brain. Unlike the biogenic amine transmitters, glutamate has an important metabolic role as well as a neurotransmitter role in the brain being linked to the synthesis of GABA, where it acts as a precursor, and to the tricarboxylic acid cycle where it is metabolized to alpha-ketoglutaric acid. In nerve terminals, glutamate is stored in vesicles and released by calcium-dependent exocytosis. Specific glutamate transporters remove the amino acid from the synaptic cleft into both the nerve terminals and the surrounding glial cells.

Four main types of glutamate receptor have been identified and cloned. These are the ionotropic receptors (NMDA and alpha-amino-3-hydroxy-5-methylisoxazole, AMPA, and kainate types) and a group of metabotropic receptors of which eight types have been discovered. The AMPA and kainate receptors are involved in fast excitatory transmission whereas the NMDA receptors mediate slower excitatory responses and play a more complex role in mediating synaptic plasticity.

The ionotropic receptors have a pentameric structure. The most important of these, the NMDA receptors, are assembled from two sub-units, NR_1 and NR_2, each of which can exist in different isoforms thereby giving rise to structurally different glutamate receptors in the brain. The functional significance of these different receptor types is presently unclear. The sub-units comprising the AMPA and kainate receptors, termed $GluR_{1-7}$ and $KA_{1,2}$ are closely related.

The NMDA receptors are unique among the ligand-gated cation channel receptors in that they are permeable to calcium but blocked by magnesium, the latter acting at a specific receptor site within the ion channel. The purpose of the voltage-dependent magnesium blockade of the ion channel is to permit the summation of excitatory postsynaptic potentials. Once these have reached a critical point, the magnesium blockade of the ion channel is terminated and calcium flows into the neuron to activate the calcium-dependent second messengers. Such a mechanism would appear to be particularly important for the induction of long-term potentiation, a process which underlies short-term memory formation in the hippocampus (Figure 2.13).

With regard to the action of psychotropic drugs on the NMDA receptors, there is evidence that one of the actions of the anticonvulsant lamotrigine is

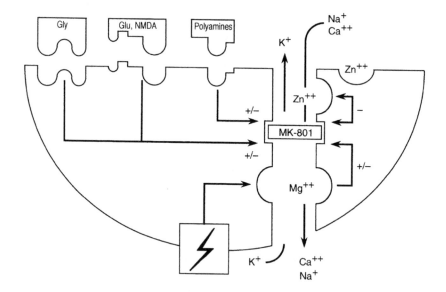

Figure 2.13. Schematic model of the NMDA receptor. The flow of ions through the channel of the NMDA receptor can be regulated by a variety of factors. Glycine (Gly) and glutamate (Glu) must both bind to the NMDA receptor to cause opening of the ion channel. Polyamines bind to a distinct recognition site on the receptor to regulate the opening of the ion channel. Compounds such as MK-801 appear to bind in the open channel. At physiological concentrations of Mg^{++}, the channel is blocked unless the membrane is depolarized. Zn^{++} also regulates the opening of the ion channel.

to modulate glutamatergic function; the antidementia drug memantine also has similar action. Thus the therapeutic efficacy of some of the newer drugs used to treat epilepsy and Alzheimer's disease owe their efficacy to their ability to modulate a dysfunctional glutamatergic system.

Some of the hallucinogens related to the dissociation anaesthetic ketamine, such as phencyclidine, block the ion channel of the NMDA receptor. Whether the hallucinogenic actions of phencyclidine are primarily due to this action is uncertain as the putative anticonvulsant dizocilpine (MK 801) is also an NMDA ion channel inhibitor but is not a notable hallucinogen. Presumably the ability of phencyclidine to enhance dopamine release, possibly by activating NMDA heteroceptors on dopaminergic terminals, and also its action on sigma receptors which it shares with benzomorphan – like hallucinogens – contribute to its hallucinogenic activity.

In contrast to the ionotropic receptors, the metabotropic receptors are monomeric in structure and unique in that they show no structural similarity to the other G-protein-coupled neurotransmitter receptors. They are located both pre- and postsynaptically and there is experimental evidence that they are involved in synpatic modulation and excitotoxicity, functions which are also shared with the NMDA receptors. To date, no drugs have been developed for therapeutic use which are based on the modulation of these receptors.

The NMDA receptor complex has been extensively characterized and its anatomical distribution in the brain determined. The NMDA receptor is analogous to the GABA-A receptor in that it contains several binding sites, in addition to the glutamate site, whereby the movement of sodium and calcium ions into the nerve cell can be modulated.

These sites include a regulatory site that binds glycine, a site which is insensitive to the antagonistic effects of strychnine. This contrasts with the action of glycine on glycine receptors in the spinal cord where strychnine, on blocking the receptor, causes the characteristic tonic seizures.

In addition to the glutamate and glycine sites on the NMDA receptor, there also exist polyamine sites which are activated by the naturally occurring polyamines spermine and spermidine. Specific divalent cation sites are also associated with the NMDA receptor, namely the voltage-dependent magnesium site and the inhibitory zinc site. In addition to the excitatory amino acids, the natural metabolite of brain tryptophan, quinolinic acid, can also act as an agonist of the NMDA receptor and may contribute to nerve cell death at high concentrations.

Interest in the therapeutic potential of drugs acting on the NMDA receptor has risen with the discovery that epilepsy and related convulsive states may occur as a consequence of a sudden release of glutamate. Sustained seizures of the limbic system in animals result in brain damage that resembles the changes seen in glutamate toxicity. Similar changes are seen at autopsy in patients with intractable epilepsy. It has been shown that the non-competitive NMDA antagonists such as phencyclidine or ketamine can block glutamate-induced damage. The novel antiepileptic drug lamotrigine would also appear to act by this mechanism, in addition to its ability to block sodium channels, in common with many other types of antiepileptic drugs.

In addition to epilepsy, neuronal death due to the toxic effects of glutamate has also been implicated in cerebral ischaemia associated with multi-infarct dementia and possibly Alzheimer's disease. With the plethora of selective excitatory amino acid receptor antagonists currently undergoing development, some of which are already in clinical trials, one may expect definite advances in the drug treatment of neurodegenerative disorders in the near future.

Nitric oxide – an important gaseous neurotransmitter

The discovery that mammalian cells generate nitric oxide (NO), a gas until recently considered to be an atmospheric pollutant, is providing new insights into a number of regulatory processes in the nervous system. There is evidence that NO is synthesized in the vascular epithelium where it is responsible for regulating the vascular tone of the blood vessels. When released from neurons in the brain, NO acts as a novel transmitter one of whose functions is in memory formation. In the periphery, the non-adrenergic non-cholinergic nerves synthesize and release NO which is responsible for neurogenic vasodilatation and the regulation of various gastrointestinal, respiratory and genitourinary tract functions. In addition, NO is also involved in platelet aggregation. These numerous actions of NO are attributed to its direct stimulatory action on soluble guanylate cyclase, thereby enabling it to act as a modulator of conventional neurotransmitters. In all tissues, NO is synthesized by the action of nitric oxide synthase on the amino acid arginine.

In the brain, nitric oxide synthase activity has been detected in all brain regions, the highest activity being located in the cerebellum. One of the main physiological roles of NO is in memory formation. There is evidence that in the hippocampus NO is released from postsynaptic sites to act on presynaptic neurons as a retrograde transmitter to release glutamate. This leads to a stable increase in synaptic transmission and forms the basis of long-term potentiation and the initiation of memory formation. Inhibition of nitric oxide synthase activity has been shown experimentally to impair memory formation. Other roles for NO include the development of the cortex and in vision where it assists in the transduction of light signals in the retinal photoreceptor cells. Other roles include feeding behaviour, nociception and olfaction. Recent evidence

Table 2.7.   Nitric oxide and carbon monoxide as mediators

	Nitric oxide (NO)	Carbon monoxide (CO)
Formation		
Precursor	Arginine	Haem
Enzyme	NO Synthase (NOS)	Haem oxygenase
Inhibited by	L-NMMA	Zn protoporphyrin
	L-NAME	
Activated by	Intracellular Ca^{2+}	Not known
Effect	Activates soluble guanylate cyclase	Activates soluble guanylate cyclase
	Increases cGMP	Increases cGMP
Inactivated by	Haemoglobin	Haemoglobin
Implicated in	Vasodilatation	?LTP
	Smooth muscle relaxation	
	LTP/LTD	
	Neuroprotection/ neurotoxicity	

L-NMMA=N^G-monomethyl-L-arginine; L-NAME=N^G-monomethyl-L-arginine; LTP=long-term potentiation; LTD=long-term depression.

suggests that the microglia cells in the brain, which form part of the monocyte/macrophage system, express an inducible form of nitric oxide synthase. Overactivity of these cells has been implicated in the pathogenesis of a number of neurological diseases such as multiple sclerosis, Alzheimer's disease and Parkinson's disease. Presumably drugs will be developed in the near future to counteract the degenerative effects caused by NO. It is also of interest to note that carbon monoxide also acts as a gaseous transmitter in the brain but its function is uncertain (see Table 2.7).

Biochemical pathways leading to the synthesis and metabolism of the major neurotransmitters in the mammalian brain

No attempt will be made to give an overview of the main pathways of the several dozen neurotransmitters, neuromodulators and co-transmitters which are possibly involved in the aetiology of mental illness. Instead a summary is given of the relevant pathways involved in the synthesis and metabolism of those transmitters which have conventionally been considered to be involved in the major psychiatric and neurological diseases and through which the psychotropic drugs used in the treatment of such diseases are believed to operate.

Acetylcholine

Acetylcholine has been implicated in learning and memory in all mammals, and the gross deficits in memory found in patients suffering from Alzheimer's disease have been ascribed to a defect in central cholinergic transmission. This transmitter has also been implicated in the altered mood states found in mania and depression, while many different classes of psychotropic drugs are known to have potent anticholinergic properties which undoubtedly have adverse consequences for brain function.

Acetylcholine is synthesized within the nerve terminal from choline (from both dietary and endogenous origins) and acetyl coenzyme A (acetyl CoA) by the enzyme choline acetyltransferase. Acetyl CoA is derived from glucose and other intermediates via the glycolytic pathway and ultimately the pyruvate oxidase system, while choline is selectively transported into the cholinergic nerve terminal by an active transport system. There are believed to be two main transport sites for choline, the high affinity site being dependent on sodium ions and ATP and which is inhibited by membrane depolarization, while the low affinity site operates by a process of passive diffusion and is therefore dependent on the intersynaptic concentration of choline. The uptake of choline by the high affinity site controls the rate of acetylcholine synthesis, while the low affinity site, which occurs predominantly in cell bodies, appears to be important for phospholipid synthesis. As the transport of choline by the active transport site is probably optimal, there seems little value in increasing the dietary intake of the precursor in an attempt to increase acetylcholine synthesis. This could be one of the reasons why feeding choline-rich diets (e.g. lecithin) to patients with Alzheimer's disease has been shown to be ineffective.

As with all the major transmitters, acetylcholine is stored in vesicles within the nerve terminal from which it is released by a calcium-dependent mechanism following the passage of a nerve impulse. The inter-relationship between the intermediary metabolism of glucose, phospholipids and the uptake of choline is summarized in Figure 2.14.

It is well established that acetylcholine can be catabolized by both *acetylcholinesterase* (AChE) and *butyrylcholinesterase* (BChE); these are also known as "true" and "pseudo" cholinesterase, respectively. Such enzymes may be differentiated by their specificity for different choline esters and by their susceptibility to different antagonists. They also differ in their anatomical distribution, with AChE being associated with nervous tissue while BChE is largely found in non-nervous tissue. In the brain there does not seem to be a good correlation between the distribution of cholinergic terminals and the presence of AChE, choline acetyltransferase having been found to be a better marker of such terminals. An assessment of cholinesterase activity can be made by examining red blood cells, which contain only AChE, and plasma,

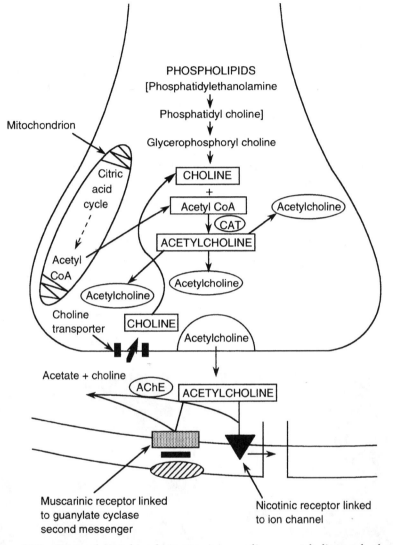

Figure 2.14. Inter-relationship between intermediary metabolism of glucose, phospholipids and acetylcholine synthesis. Acetyl CoA=acetyl coenzyme A; CAT=catechol-*O*-methyltransferase; AChE=acetylcholinesterase.

which contains only BChE. Of the *anticholinesterases*, the organophosphorus derivatives such as diisopropylfluorophosphonate are specific for BChE, while drugs such as ambenonium inhibit AChE.

Most cholinesterase inhibitors inhibit the enzyme by acylating the esteratic site on the enzyme surface. Physostigmine and neostigmine are examples of *reversible anticholinesterases* which are in clinical use. Both act in similar ways but they differ in terms of their lipophilicity, the former being able to penetrate the blood–brain barrier while the latter cannot. The main clinical use of these drugs is in the treatment of glaucoma and myasthenia gravis.

Irreversible anticholinesterases include the organophosphorus inhibitors and ambenonium, which irreversibly phosphorylate the esteratic site. Such drugs have few clinical uses but have been developed as insecticides and nerve gases. Besides blocking the muscarinic receptors with atropine sulphate in an attempt to reduce the toxic effects that result from an accumulation of acetylcholine, the only specific treatment for organophosphate poisoning would appear to be the administration of 2-pyridine aldoxime methiodide, which increases the rate of dissociation of the organophosphate from the esteratic site on the enzyme surface.

Anatomical distribution of the central cholinergic system

The cholinergic pathways in the mammalian brain are extremely diffuse and arise from cell bodies located in the hindbrain and the midbrain. Of these areas, there has been considerable interest of late in the nucleus basalis magnocellularis of Meynert because this region appears to be particularly affected in some patients with familial Alzheimer's disease. As the projections from this area innervate the cortex, it has been speculated

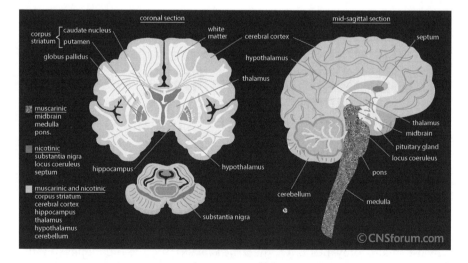

Figure 2.15. Distribution of muscarinic and nicotinic receptors in the human brain. Note the very restricted distribution of the nicotinic receptors. Cholinergic tracts arising from the magnocellular cholinergic nuclei innervate large areas of the cortex and subcortical regions.

that a disruption of the cortical cholinergic system may be responsible for many of the clinical features of the illness. The use of cholinomimetic drugs of various types to treat such diseases is discussed in a later chapter.

Figure 2.15 illustrates the distribution of the main cholinergic receptors in the human brain.

The catecholamines

Much attention has been paid to the catecholamines noradrenaline and dopamine following the discovery that their depletion in the brain leads to profound mood changes and locomotor deficits. Thus noradrenaline has been implicated in the mood changes associated with mania and depression, while an excess of dopamine has been implicated in schizophrenia and a deficit in Parkinson's disease.

Noradrenaline is the main catecholamine in postganglionic sympathetic nerves and in the central nervous system; it is also released from the adrenal gland together with adrenaline. Recently *adrenaline* has also been shown to be a transmitter in the hypothalamic region of the mammalian brain so, while the terms "noradrenergic" and "adrenergic" are presently used interchangeably, it is anticipated that they will be used with much more precision once the unique functions of adrenaline in the brain have been established.

The catecholamines are formed from the dietary amino acid precursors phenylalanine and tyrosine, as illustrated in Figure 2.16.

The rate-limiting step in the synthesis of the catecholamines from tyrosine is tyrosine hydroxylase, so that any drug or substance which can reduce the activity of this enzyme, for example by reducing the concentration of the tetrahydropteridine cofactor, will reduce the rate of synthesis of the catecholamines. Under normal conditions tyrosine hydroxylase is maximally active, which implies that the rate of synthesis of the catecholamines is not in any way dependent on the dietary precursor tyrosine. Catecholamine synthesis may be reduced by *end product inhibition*. This is a process whereby catecholamine present in the synaptic cleft, for example as a result of excessive nerve stimulation, will reduce the affinity of the pteridine cofactor for tyrosine hydroxylase and thereby reduce synthesis of the transmitter. The experimental drug alpha-methyl-*para*-tyrosine inhibits the rate-limiting step by acting as a false substrate for the enzyme, the net result being a reduction in the catecholamine concentrations in both the central and peripheral nervous systems.

Drugs have been developed which specifically inhibit the L-aromatic amino acid decarboxylase step in catecholamine synthesis and thereby lead to a reduction in catecholamine concentration. Carbidopa and benserazide are examples of decarboxylase inhibitors which are used clinically to

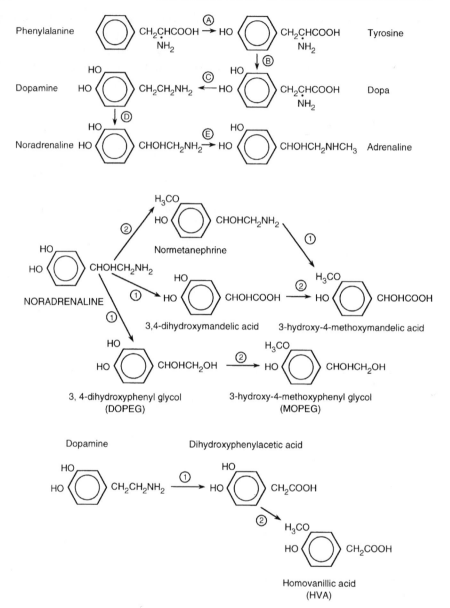

Figure 2.16. Pathways for the synthesis and metabolism of the catecholamines. A=phenylalanine hydroxylase+pteridine cofactor+O_2; B=tyrosine hydroxylase+ tetrahydropteridine+$Fe^{++}+O_2$; C=dopa decarboxylase+pyridoxal phosphate; D= dopamine beta-oxidase+ascorbate phosphate+$Cu^{++}+O_2$; E=phenylethanolamine N-methyltransferase+S-adenosylmethionine; 1=monoamine oxidase and aldehyde dehydrogenase; 2=catechol-O-methyltransferase+S-adenosylmethionine.

prevent the peripheral catabolism of L-dopa (levodopa) in patients being treated for parkinsonism. As these drugs do not penetrate the blood–brain barrier they will prevent the peripheral decarboxylation of dopa so that it can enter the brain and be converted to dopamine by dopamine beta-oxidase (also called dopamine beta-hydroxylase).

Dopamine beta-oxidase inhibitors are only of limited clinical use at the present time, probably due to their relative lack of specificity. Diethyldithiocarbamate and disulfiram are examples of drugs that inhibit dopamine beta-oxidase by acting as copper-chelating agents and thereby reducing the availability of the cofactor for this enzyme. Whether their clinical use in the treatment of alcoholism is in any way related to the reduction in brain catecholamine concentrations is uncertain. The main action of these drugs is to inhibit liver aldehyde dehydrogenase activity, thereby leading to an accumulation of acetaldehyde, and the onset of nausea and vomiting, should the patient drink alcohol.

Two enzymes are concerned in the metabolism of catecholamines, namely *monoamine oxidase*, which occurs mainly intraneuronally, and *catechol-O-methyltransferase*, which is restricted to the synaptic cleft. The importance of the two major forms of monoamine oxidase, A and B, will be considered elsewhere.

The process of oxidative deamination is the most important mechanism whereby all monoamines are inactivated (i.e. the catecholamines, 5-HT and the numerous trace amines such as phenylethylamine and tryptamine). Monoamine oxidase occurs in virtually all tissues, where it appears to be bound to the outer mitochondrial membrane. Whereas there are several specific and therapeutically useful monoamine oxidase inhibitors, inhibitors of catechol-O-methyltransferase have found little application. This is mainly due to the fact that at most only 10% of the monoamines released from the nerve terminal are catabolized by this enzyme. The main pathways involved in the catabolism of the catecholamines are shown in Figure 2.16.

Anatomical distribution

One of the first demonstrations of the central monoamine pathways in the mammalian brain was by a fluorescence technique in which thin sections of the animal brain were exposed to formaldehyde vapour which converted the amines to their corresponding fluorescent isoquinolines. The distribution of these compounds could then be visualized under the fluorescent microscope. Using this technique it has been possible to map the distribution of the noradrenergic, dopaminergic and serotonergic pathways in the animal and human brain.

The central noradrenergic system. This is not so diffusely distributed as the cholinergic system. In the lower brainstem, the neurons innervate the medulla oblongata and the dorsal vagal nucleus, which are thought to be important in the central control of blood pressure. Other projections arising from cell bodies in the medulla descend to the spinal cord where they are believed to be involved in the control of flexor muscles. However, the most important noradrenergic projections with regard to psychological functions arise from a dense collection of cells in the locus coeruleus and ascend from the brainstem to innervate the thalamus, dorsal hypothalamus, hippocampus and cortex. The ventral noradrenergic bundle occurs caudally and ventrally to the locus coeruleus and terminates in the hypothalamus and the subcortical limbic regions. The dorsal bundle arises from the locus coeruleus and innervates the cortex. Both the dorsal and ventral noradrenergic systems appear to be involved psychologically in drive and motivation, in mechanisms of reward and in rapid eye movement (REM) sleep. As such processes are severely deranged in the major affective disorders it is not unreasonable to speculate that the central noradrenergic system is defective in such disorders. The distribution of the noradrenergic tracts in the human brain is shown in Figure 2.17.

The central dopaminergic systems. These are considerably more complex than the noradrenergic system. This may reflect the greater density of dopamine-containing cells, which have been estimated to be 30–40 000 in number compared with 10 000 noradrenaline-containing cells. There are several dopamine-containing nuclei as well as specialized dopaminergic neurons localized within the retina and the olfactory bulb. The dopaminergic system within the mammalian brain can be divided according to the length of the efferent fibres into the intermediate and long length systems.

The intermediate length systems include the tuberoinfundibular system, which projects from the arcuate and periventricular nuclei into the intermediate lobe of the pituitary and the median eminence. This system is responsible for the regulation of such hormones as prolactin. The interhypothalamic neurons send projections to the dorsal and posterior hypothalamus, the lateral septal nuclei and the medullary periventricular group, which are linked to the dorsal motor nucleus of the vagus; such projections may play a role in the effects of dopamine on the autonomic nervous system.

The *long length fibres* link the ventral tegmental and substantia nigra dopamine-containing cells with the neostriatum (mainly the caudate and the putamen), the limbic cortex (the medial prefrontal, cingulate and entorhinal areas) and with limbic structures such as the septum, nucleus accumbens, amygdaloid complex and piriform cortex. These projections are usually called the *mesocortical* and *mesolimbic dopaminergic systems*, respectively, and are functionally important in psychotic disorders and in the therapeutic effects of neuroleptic drugs. Conversely, changes in the functional activity of the dopaminergic cells in the neostriatum are primarily responsible for movement disorders such as Parkinsonism and Huntington's chorea.

The central adrenergic system.   It is only recently that immunohistochemical methods have been developed to show that adrenaline-containing cells occur in the brain. Some of these cells are located in the lateral tegmental area, while others are found in the dorsal medulla. Axons from these cells innervate the hypothalamus, the locus coeruleus and the dorsal motor nucleus of the vagus nerve. While the precise function of adrenergic system within the brain is uncertain, it may be surmised that adrenaline could play a role in endocrine regulation and in the central control of blood pressure. There is evidence that the concentration of this amine in cerebrospinal fluid

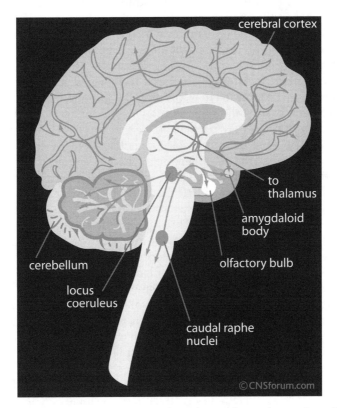

Figure 2.17. Diagrammatic representation of central noradrenergic pathways.

is reduced in depression, which might imply that it is also concerned in the control of mood.

5-HT

5-HT, together with noradrenaline, has long been implicated in the aetiology of depression. Indirect evidence has been obtained from the actions of drugs which can either precipitate or alleviate the symptoms of depression and from the analysis of body fluids from depressed patients. Recently, the development of novel anxiolytic drugs which appear to act as specific agonists for a subpopulation of 5-HT receptors (the 5-HT$_{1A}$ type) suggests that this amine may also play a role in anxiety. To add to the complexity of the role of 5-HT, there is evidence that impulsive behaviour as exhibited by patients with obsessive–compulsive disorders and bulimia may also involve an abnormality of the serotonergic system. Whether 5-HT is primarily involved in this disparate group of disorders or whether it functions to "fine tune" other neurotransmitters which are causally involved is presently unclear.

5-HT is an indoleamine transmitter which is synthesized within the nerve ending from the amino acid L-tryptophan. Tryptophan, which is obtained from dietary and endogenous sources, is unique among the amino acids concerned in neurotransmitter synthesis in that it is about 85% bound to plasma proteins. This means that it is only the unbound portion that can be taken up by the brain and is therefore available for 5-HT synthesis. In the periphery, tryptophan may be metabolized in the liver via the *kynurenine* pathway, and it must be emphasized that the pathway that leads to the synthesis of 5-HT in the periphery (e.g. in platelets and the enterochromaffin cells of the gastrointestinal tract) or as a neurotransmitter in the brain is relatively minor. It is known that the activity of the kynurenine pathway, also known as the tryptophan pyrrolase pathway, in the liver can be increased by steroid hormones. Thus natural or synthetic glucocorticoids can induce an increase in the activity of this pathway and thereby increase the catabolism of plasma free tryptophan. Other steroids, such as the oestrogens used in the contraceptive pill, can also induce pyrrolase activity. This has been proposed as a mechanism whereby the contraceptive pill, particularly the high oestrogen type of pill which has now largely been withdrawn, may predispose some women to depression by reducing the availability of free tryptophan for brain 5-HT synthesis. Despite the plausible belief that the availability of plasma free tryptophan determines the rate of brain 5-HT synthesis, it now seems unlikely that such an important central transmitter would be in any way dependent on the vagaries of diet to sustain its synthesis! Nevertheless, changes in liver tryptophan pyrrolase activity, which may be brought about by endogenous steroids, insulin, changes in diet and by the circadian rhythm, may play a secondary role in regulating brain 5-HT synthesis. Furthermore, there is evidence that a tryptophan-deficient diet can precipitate depression in depressed patients who are in remission. Thus when such patients are given a drink containing high concentrations of amino acids but which lacks tryptophan, a depressive episode rapidly occurs.

Free tryptophan is transported into the brain and nerve terminal by an active transport system which it shares with tyrosine and a number of other essential amino acids. On entering the nerve terminal, tryptophan is hydroxylated by tryptophan hydroxylase, which is the rate-limiting step in the synthesis of 5-HT. Tryptophan hydroxylase is not bound in the nerve terminal and optimal activity of the enzyme is only achieved in the presence of molecular oxygen and a pteridine cofactor. Unlike tyrosine hydroxylase, tryptophan hydroxylase is not usually saturated by its substrate. This implies that if the brain concentration rises then the rate of 5-HT synthesis will also increase. Conversely, the rate of 5-HT synthesis will decrease following the administration of experimental drugs such as *para*-chlorophenylalanine, a synthetic amino acid which irreversibly inhibits the enzyme. *Para*-chloramphetamine also inhibits the activity of this enzyme, but this experimental drug also increases 5-HT release and delays its reuptake thereby leading to the appearance of the so-called "serotonin syndrome", which in animals is associated with abnormal movements, body posture and temperature.

Following the synthesis of 5-hydroxytryptophan (5-HTP) by tryptophan hydroxylase, the enzyme aromatic amino acid decarboxylase (also known as 5-HTP or dopa decarboxylase) then decarboxylates the amino acid to 5-HT. L-Aromatic amino acid decarboxylase is approximately 60% bound in the nerve terminal and requires pyridoxal phosphate as an essential enzyme.

There is evidence that the compartmentalization of 5-HT in the nerve terminal is important in regulating its synthesis. It appears that 5-HT is synthesized in excess of normal physiological requirements and that some of the amine which is not immediately transported into the storage vesicle is metabolized by intraneuronal monoamine oxidase. Another autoregulatory mechanism governing 5-HT synthesis relies on the rise in the intersynaptic concentration of the amine stimulating the autoreceptor of the nerve terminal.

5-HT is metabolized by the action of monoamine oxidase by a process of oxidative deamination to yield 5-hydroxyindoleacetic acid (5-HIAA). In the *pineal gland*, 5-HT is *o*-methylated to form melatonin. While the physiological importance of this transmitter in the regulation of the oestrus cycle in ferrets would appear to be established, its precise role in man is unknown. Nevertheless, it has been speculated that melatonin plays some role in regulating the circadian rhythm, which may account for the occurrence of low plasma melatonin levels in depressed patients.

A summary of the major steps that lead to the synthesis of 5-HT, and of the minor pathway whereby the trace amine tryptamine is synthesized from tryptophan by the action of tryptophan hydroxylase, is shown in Figure 2.18.

Anatomical distribution of the central serotonergic system

Neurons containing 5-HT are restricted to clusters of cells around the midline of the pons and upper brainstem; this is known as the raphé area of the midbrain. In addition, according to studies of rat brain, cells containing 5-HT are located in the area postrema and in the caudal locus coeruleus, which forms an anatomical basis for a direct connection between the serotonergic and noradrenergic systems. The more caudal groups of cells in the raphé project largely to the medulla and the spinal cord, the latter projections being physiologically important in the regulation of pain perception at the level of the dorsal horn. Conversely, the more rostral cells of the dorsal and median raphé project to limbic structures such as the hippocampus and, in particular, to innervate extensively the cortex. Unlike the noradrenergic cortical projections, there does not appear to be an organized pattern of serotonergic terminals in the cortex. In general, it would appear that the noradrenergic and serotonergic systems are co-localized in most limbic areas of the brain, which may provide the anatomical basis for the major involvement of these transmitters in the affective disorders.

The distribution of the serotonergic system in the human brain is shown in Figure 2.19.

Amino acid neurotransmitters

Unlike for the "classical" neurotransmitters such as acetylcholine and noradrenaline, it has not been possible to map the distribution of the amino acid transmitters in the mammalian brain. The reason for this is that these transmitters are present in numerous metabolic pools in the brain and are not restricted to one particular type of neuron as occurs with the "classical" transmitters. As an example, glutamate is involved in peptide and protein synthesis, in the detoxification of ammonia in the brain (by forming glutamine), in intermediary metabolism, as a precursor of the inhibitory transmitter GABA and as an important excitatory transmitter in its own right. While the evidence in favour of the amino acids glutamate, aspartate, glycine and GABA as transmitters is good, it is not yet possible to describe their anatomical distribution in detail.

With regard to the possible role of these neurotransmitters in psychiatric and neurological diseases, there is growing evidence that

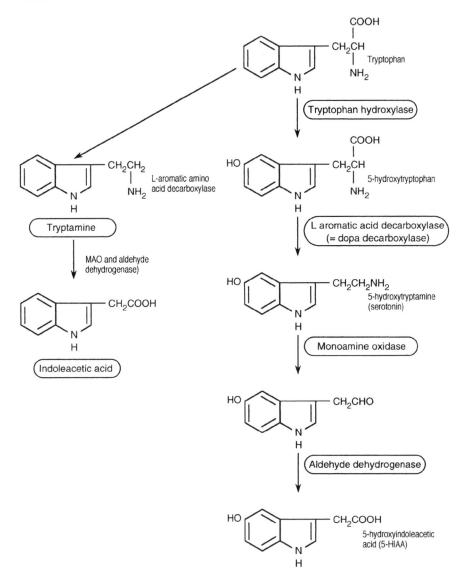

Figure 2.18. The major pathway leading to the synthesis and metabolism of 5-hydroxytryptamine (5-HT). Metabolism of tryptophan to tryptamine is a minor pathway which may be of functional importance following administration of a monoamine oxidase (MAO) inhibitor. Tryptamine is a trace amine. L-Aromatic amino acid decarboxylase is also known to decarboxylate dopa and therefore the term "L-aromatic amino acid decarboxylase" refers to both "dopa decarboxylase" and "5-HTP decarboxylase".

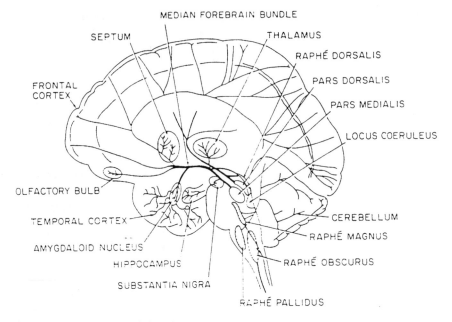

Figure 2.19.   Anatomical distribution of the serotonergic pathways in human brain.

glutamate is causally involved in the brain damage that results from cerebral anoxia, for example following stroke, and possibly in epilepsy. Conversely, GABA deficiency has been implicated in anxiety states, epilepsy, Huntington's chorea and possibly parkinsonism. The roles of the excitatory amino acid aspartate and the inhibitory transmitter glycine in disease are unknown.

The principal amino acid transmitters and their metabolic inter-relationships are shown in Figure 2.20.

Glycine

Glycine is structurally the simplest amino acid. There is evidence that it acts as an inhibitory transmitter in the hindbrain and spinal cord. The seizures that occur in response to strychnine poisoning are attributable to the convulsant-blocking glycine receptors in the spinal cord. Recent evidence also suggests that glycine can modulate the action of the excitatory transmitter glutamate on the major excitatory amino acid receptor complex in the brain, the so-called N-methyl-D-aspartate (NMDA) receptor. As the density of NMDA receptor sites is high in the cortex, amygdala and basal ganglia, this might explain the relatively high concentration of glycine which also occurs in these brain regions.

Aspartate and glutamate

Aspartate and glutamate are the most abundant amino acids in the mammalian brain. While the precise role of aspartate in brain function is obscure, the importance of glutamate as an excitatory transmitter and as a precursor of GABA is well recognized. Despite the many roles which glutamate has been shown to play in intermediary metabolism and transmitter function, studies on the dentate gyrus of the hippocampal formation, where glutamate has been established as a transmitter, have shown that the synthesis of glutamate is regulated by feedback inhibition and by the concentration of its precursor glutamine. Thus the neuronal regulation of glutamate synthesis would appear to be similar to that of the "classical" transmitters. In the brain, there appears to be an inverse relationship between the concentration of glutamate and of GABA, apart from the context where both amino acids are present in low concentrations.

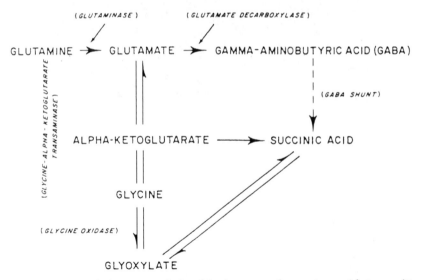

Figure 2.20. Metabolic inter-relationship between the amino acid transmitters glutamate, GABA and glycine. The diagram shows how glutamate and glycine synthesis are linked via the succinic acid component of the citric acid cycle. GABA, formed by the decarboxylation of glutamate, may also be metabolized to succinate via the "GABA shunt". Alpha-ketoglutarate acts as an intermediate between glutamate and glycine synthesis; the transfer of the $-NH_2$ group from glycine to alpha-ketoglutarate leads to the synthesis of glutamate and glyoxylate.

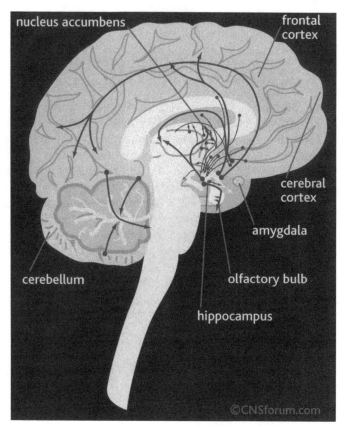

Figure 2.21. Diagrammatic representation of the distribution of GABA in the human brain.

GABA

GABA is also present in very high concentrations in the mammalian brain, approximately 500 µg/g wet weight of brain being recorded for some regions! Thus GABA is present in a concentration some 200–1000 times greater than neurotransmitters such as acetylcholine, noradrenaline and 5-HT.

GABA is one of the most widely distributed transmitters in the brain and it has been calculated that it occurs in over 40% of all synapses. Nevertheless, its distribution is quite heterogeneous, with the highest concentrations being present in the basal ganglia, followed by the hypothalamus, the periaqueductal grey matter and the hippocampus; approximately equal concentrations are present in the cortex, amygdala and

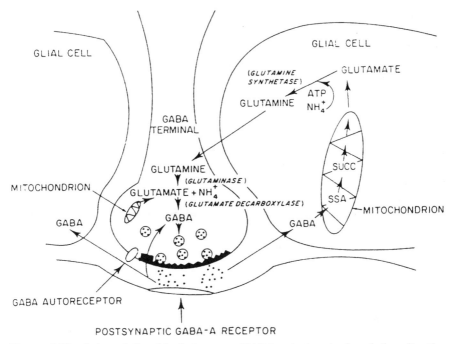

Figure 2.22. Inter-relationship between a GABAergic terminal and the glia: the GABA shunt. The diagram shows the synthesis of GABA in the nerve terminal from glutamine and glutamate. Glutamine synthesis is essential for the transport of the GABA precursor from the glial cell to the nerve terminal. Glutamate is synthesized in mitochondria by the action of GABA transaminase. Following its release from the nerve terminal, GABA can be transported into the nerve terminal by a specific active transport system or taken up into glial cells where, under the influence of GABA transaminase, it is converted to glutamate. Glutamate is also synthesized from citric acid cycle intermediates in the mitochondria. SSA=succinic semi-aldehyde; SUCC=succinic acid; ATP=adenosine triphosphate.

thalamus. The distribution of GABAergic tracts in the human brain is shown in Figure 2.21.

GABA is present in storage vesicles in nerve terminals and also in the glia that are densely packed around nerve terminals, where they probably act as physical and metabolic "buffers" for the nerve terminals. Following its release from the nerve terminal, the action of GABA may therefore be terminated either by being transported back into the nerve terminal by an active transport system or by being transported into the glia. This is shown diagrammatically in Figure 2.22.

The rate of synthesis of this transmitter is determined by glutamate decarboxylase, which synthesizes it from glutamate. A feedback inhibitory mechanism also seems to operate whereby an excess of GABA in the synaptic cleft triggers the GABA autoreceptor on the presynaptic terminal, leading to a reduction in transmitter release. Specific GABA-containing neurons have been identified as distinct pathways in the basal ganglia, namely in interneurons in the striatum, in the nigrostriatal pathway and in the pallidonigral pathway.

Conclusions

In this chapter, no attempt has been made to give a complete overview of neurotransmission. Those wishing to obtain a fuller account of this rapidly growing area are recommended to consult the key review articles and monographs. This brief discourse on the nature of the adrenergic, cholinergic, serotonergic, dopaminergic and amino acid receptors should provide the reader with the basis upon which the actions of the various drugs mentioned in subsequent chapters may be better understood.

3 Pharmacokinetic Aspects of Psychopharmacology

Introduction

Pharmacokinetics is concerned with the bioavailability, distribution and excretion of drugs. For many classes of drugs there is a direct relationship between the pharmacological and toxicological effects of a drug and its concentration in the body. For most lipophilic drugs, which would include psychotropic agents, there is a positive relationship between the concentration of the drugs in the blood and its concentration at the site of action. Pharmacokinetics also enables the relationship between the efficacy of the drug and the dose administered to the patient to be determined.

The *bioavailability* of a drug is defined as the fraction of the unchanged drug that reaches the systemic circulation following administration by any route. For an intravenously administered drug this equals unity, whereas for an orally administered drug this will be less than unity. This is due to factors such as incomplete absorption, metabolism by the liver and incomplete reabsorption of the drug following enterohepatic cycling.

When assessing the bioavailability of a drug it is also possible to determine the rate at which a given dose reaches the general circulation. Thus by plotting a graph of the blood concentration against the time following administration, the rate at which the peak drug concentration is reached may be calculated from the graph and the bioavailability can be calculated from the area under the curve. The duration of the pharmacological effect is a function of the length of time that the blood concentration is above the minimum effective concentration, while the intensity of the pharmacological effect is directly related to the degree to which the drug concentration exceeds the minimum effective concentration.

There are two further terms which are important in pharmacokinetics – the *clearance* and the *volume of distribution*. The volume of distribution (V_d) relates the quantity of drug in the body to that in the blood or plasma. This

Fundamentals of Psychopharmacology. Third Edition. By Brian E. Leonard
© 2003 John Wiley & Sons, Ltd. ISBN 0 471 52178 7

factor reflects the space available in the general circulation or within the tissues. Depending on the dissociation constant (pK_a) of the drug in the various body fluids, the lipophilicity, the degree of protein binding to serum and tissue proteins, the V_d of drugs may vary widely. For example, the antimalarial drug quinacrine (mepacrine) has an apparent V_d of 50 000 litres, while drugs that are extensively plasma protein bound have V_d values of as little as 7 litres. The tricyclic antidepressants have a high V_d value despite their strong protein binding; this may be related to their lipophilicity and to the fact that their binding to brain proteins is greater than to plasma proteins.

The clearance of a drug is usually defined as the rate of elimination of a compound in the urine relative to its concentration in the blood. In practice, the clearance value of a drug is usually determined for the kidney, liver, blood or any other tissue, and the total systemic clearance calculated from the sum of the clearance values for the individual tissues. For most drugs clearance is constant over the therapeutic range, so that the rate of drug elimination is directly proportional to the blood concentration. Some drugs, for example phenytoin, exhibit saturable or dose-dependent elimination so that the clearance will not be directly related to the plasma concentration in all cases.

The rate of elimination of a drug from a specific organ can be calculated from the blood flow to and from the organ and the blood concentration. If a drug is largely metabolized in the liver, the clearance of the drug will be largely dependent on the hepatic blood flow; many classes of psychotropic drug are almost completely metabolized by the liver. Small changes in the hepatic circulation or in the rate of liver metabolism will therefore have a dramatic effect on the drug clearance.

Once the clearance rate for a drug is known, the frequency of dosing may be calculated. It is usually desirable to maintain drug concentrations at a steady-state level within a known therapeutic range. This will be achieved when the rate of drug administration equals the total rate of clearance.

Another term which is important in pharmacokinetics is the *half-life* ($t_{1/2}$) of a drug. This value is related to the V_d and the total clearance. If it is assumed that the body is a single compartment in which the size of the compartment equals the V_d, the $t_{1/2}$ may be calculated from the equation:

$$t_{1/2} = 0.693 \, \frac{V_d}{Cl}$$

where Cl is the total clearance. The $t_{1/2}$ is defined as the time required for the drug to obtain 50% of the steady-state level, or to decay 50% from the steady-state concentration after the drug administration has ceased. It must be emphasized that disease states can profoundly affect both the V_d

and the clearance, so the $t_{1/2}$ value of a drug is not a reliable indicator of drug disposition unless the functional state of the liver, kidneys, etc. is normal.

This short introduction to the terms used in pharmacokinetics is intended to provide a general overview of the subject. Those wishing to obtain a proper grounding in this important subject are recommended to consult a standard textbook of pharmacology.

Relationship between plasma neuroleptic concentrations and the therapeutic response

Controversy still rages regarding the value of measuring the plasma drug concentrations of psychotropic drugs as a means of assessing the therapeutic response of the patient to treatment. A number of factors determine the value of such information. These include:

1. The reliability of the assay method used to determine the concentration of the drug and its possible metabolites.
2. The homogeneous nature of the patient population and the number of patients in the sample.
3. The use of fixed doses of the drugs so that the plasma levels remain independent of clinical impression or improvement.
4. The use of double-blind conditions and ensuring that the drug is administered for an adequate period of time.
5. Ensuring that other drugs or treatments are not administered which may interact with the psychotropic drug under investigation (e.g. lithium, electroconvulsive therapy).
6. Use of appropriate statistical methods for the analysis of the data.

Unfortunately, few of the studies that have attempted to relate the blood concentrations of neuroleptics to therapeutic response have fulfilled all these criteria. There is a suggestion that a *"therapeutic window"* exists for some phenothiazine neuroleptics. A therapeutic window is a range of concentrations of a drug measured in the blood that are associated with a good therapeutic response. Plasma concentrations outside this range are either too low to ensure a therapeutic response or so high that they induce toxic side effects. Despite the numerous studies of the relationship between the plasma concentration and the therapeutic response for a number of "standard" neuroleptics, it would appear that such correlations rarely account for more than 25% of the variance in clinical response to treatment. The existence of a therapeutic window for neuroleptics would therefore appear to be unproven. However, there could be ranges of plasma concentrations associated with optimal antipsychotic action, but these must be defined separately for each drug. There is also evidence that some non-responders to treatment may improve when the plasma drug concentration is reduced rather than raised.

Besides the poor specificity of many of the assays used to determine plasma drug concentrations, another problem which has arisen from these studies has been the length of the "wash-out" period necessary before the patient is given the neuroleptic under investigation. As a result of the prolonged duration of blockade of dopamine receptors in the brain by conventional neuroleptics and their metabolites, it is necessary to allow a wash-out period of several weeks before the patients are subject to a pharmacokinetic study. This raises serious ethical questions. Perhaps with the advent of new imaging techniques it may be possible in the near future actually to determine the rate of disappearance of neuroleptics from the brain of the patient. This may enable the relationship between plasma concentration and clinical response to be accurately determined.

Relationship between plasma antidepressant concentrations and the therapeutic response

Over the past 20 years there has been widespread interest in monitoring plasma antidepressant, particularly tricyclic, levels to optimize the response to treatment. One aspect of this research that is universally agreed upon concerns the extensive interindividual variability among patients, but it is still uncertain whether a knowledge of the plasma drug concentration is of clinical value.

For the tricyclic antidepressants (TCAs) the two major oxidative pathways that occur in the liver are desmethylation and hydroxylation, the latter pathway being the main rate-limiting step that governs the renal excretion of these drugs. *First-pass metabolism*, whereby the drug passes via the portal system directly to the liver, is much greater following oral rather than intravenous administration of such drugs. For the major TCAs, first-pass metabolism accounts for approximately 50% or more of the drug concentration which enters the portal circulation. Such extensive first-pass metabolism probably occurs with the newer antidepressants that also undergo oxidation and desmethylation in the liver. It seems possible that the presence of high concentrations of the therapeutically inactive hydroxylated metabolites of the TCAs in the brain could result in a reduction in the therapeutic activity of the parent compound. The presence of desmethylated metabolites of the tertiary antidepressants such as nor-chlorimipramine and desipramine undoubtedly contribute to the anti-depressant effects of the parent compound. Whereas the tertiary precursors show some selectivity for inhibiting the uptake of 5-hydroxytryptamine

(5-HT) into the nerve terminal, the desmethylated metabolites show selectivity as noradrenaline uptake inhibitors. Thus no TCA can be considered to be selective in inhibiting the uptake of either of these biogenic amines. In the case of TCA overdose, the normal oxidative pathways in the liver are probably saturated, which leads to a disproportionately high concentration of the desmethylated metabolite. The practical consequence of this finding is that toxic plasma concentrations of a TCA are very likely to occur if the dose of the drug is increased in those patients who fail to respond to normal therapeutic doses of the drug. Such a transition to toxic doses could occur suddenly.

There is good evidence that *genetic differences* in hepatic metabolism are responsible for the large interindividual variation in the metabolism of TCAs, including maprotiline and the monoamine oxidase inhibitors. Such genetic factors have been investigated using pharmacogenetic probes. Drugs such as antipyrine (phenazone) and debrisoquine have been investigated in patients treated with TCAs to see if the clearance of such drugs correlates with the metabolism of the antidepressants. It has been found that the clearance of antipyrine correlated well with the metabolism of the benzodiazepines but not with all of the TCAs. Those individuals who showed a deficient hydroxylation of debrisoquine also differed from the normal population in their metabolism of TCAs. However, at the present level of knowledge, it would appear that despite overall similarities in the metabolic pathways for most antidepressants, specific drugs are subject to specific metabolic processes that limit the application of pharmacokinetic phenotyping compounds such as debrisoquine. If the pharmacokinetic properties of an antidepressant in an individual patient need to be known, a test dose of the drug should be given. However, to date there is no convincing evidence that such information improves the frequency of the therapeutic response!

It may be concluded that, so far, a pharmacokinetic analysis of antidepressants is of limited clinical value because of:

1. Large interindividual variability in plasma concentrations which reflect genetically determined metabolic differences.
2. The effects of variables such as age, sex, race and drug interactions on the pharmacokinetics of the antidepressant.
3. The presence of therapeutically active metabolites that may contribute to the pharmacodynamic and toxic effects.

In contrast to the limited value of pharmacokinetics to the use of antidepressants, knowledge of the kinetics of *lithium* has been important in defining the therapeutic and toxic range in unipolar or bipolar manic patients. Prediction of the dose required by the individual patient by giving a single dose of the drug and measuring the erythrocyte/plasma lithium ratio has been shown to be useful, and non-compliance of a patient can be readily detected. The pharmacokinetic profiles of the various types of normal- and slow-release preparations now enable adjustment of the dosage to the needs of the individual patient. Such knowledge has also led to the clinical practice of maintaining the patient on the lowest plasma concentration of lithium for long periods of time, thereby prolonging the remission of both manic and depressive symptoms.

Pharmacokinetic aspects of TCAs

All TCAs are fairly well absorbed following oral administration. Although it is recommended that TCAs are administered in divided doses initially, their relatively long half-lives (12–20 hours) and relatively wide dose range (50–300 mg) mean that a once daily dose at night is often preferred. However, it must be remembered that, due to the structure of the drugs, the higher therapeutic doses have potent anticholinergic effects which lead to a reduction in gastrointestinal tract activity and gastric emptying. As a consequence, the absorption of the antidepressant is impeded, as is that of any drug given concurrently. The plasma concentration of most TCAs reaches a peak 2–8 hours after oral administration and once absorbed the drugs are widely distributed. As these drugs are highly protein bound, and also bind to tissue proteins, they have a high apparent volume of distribution. This implies that plasma drug monitoring to ensure optimal therapeutic response is of questionable value, even though it is often recommended that the most satisfactory antidepressant response occurs in the plasma concentration range of 50–300 ng/ml, toxic effects becoming apparent when the drug concentration reaches 0.5–1.0 μg/ml.

The metabolism and elimination of TCAs takes several days to occur, the elimination half-life ranging from 20 hours for amitriptyline to 80 hours for protriptyline. The half-life values for the desmethylated metabolites such as desmethylimipramine and nortriptyline are approximately twice those of the parent compounds imipramine and amitriptyline. It is also well established that the half-life values of the TCAs are considerably greater in the elderly, which predisposes such patients to a greater possibility of severe side effects.

Pharmacokinetic aspects of MAOIs

All the commonly used MAOIs (monoamine oxidase inhibitors), exemplified by phenelzine, isocarboxazid and pargyline, are irreversible inhibitors of both forms of the enzyme, forming covalent bonds with the active sites on the enzyme surface. This is the reason why the effects of these drugs last for many days even though their blood concentrations are undetectable. This can result in an accumulation of the drugs following their long-term use as they can also inhibit their own metabolism. These drugs are metabolized in the liver largely by a process of acetylation. Because of the relevance of the genetic status of the patient to the rate of metabolism of many drugs that are acetylated (the half-life of a drug that is acetylated rapidly being shorter and therefore less likely to accumulate than one that is slowly acetylated), it was hypothesized that the acetylator status of patients being treated with the older type of MAOIs may be an important determinant of their therapeutic effects. Recent clinical studies, however, have failed to show that the acetylator status is an important determinant of the therapeutic action of the phenelzine type of drug.

Because the long duration of action of the older irreversible inhibitors of MAO could be responsible for drug and dietary interactions, different types of MAOIs have been synthesized which are reversible inhibitors of the enzyme. Such compounds have the advantage that their action on the enzyme can be terminated by the presence of the high concentration of a natural substrate. Thus, should a patient on such a reversible inhibitor inadvertently take a tyramine-rich food, the tyramine would overcome the inhibitory effect of the drug on the MAO in the gastrointestinal wall and be metabolized. The tyramine would not then be absorbed and lead to the chance of a hypertensive episode. However, the MAO activity in other tissues, including the brain, would remain inhibited by the drug so that the therapeutic benefits would be maintained. In addition to the advantage of being less likely to interact with dietary amines, reversible MAOIs have a shorter duration of action than the irreversible inhibitors. Brofaromine, for example, has a half-life of 12 hours in the brain, in contrast to several days in the case of the phenelzine type of MAOI. A further advantage of the reversible and selective inhibitors lies in their effects on brain amines. Initially an irreversible inhibitor such as clorgyline may show selectivity, but will lose this following chronic treatment due to its long duration of action and possible accumulation. Such an effect is less likely to occur with the reversible MAOIs, which will be metabolized more readily, will not accumulate and will therefore be less likely to inhibit the non-preferred isoenzyme. Several selective MAO-A type inhibitors have now been synthesized (e.g. brofaromine, cimoxatone, moclobemide and toloxatone) which have proven to be clinically effective antidepressants. There is evidence that some of these inhibitors, for example moclobemide, act as pro-drugs in that they form active metabolites *in vivo* which have a greater affinity for MAO-A than the parent compound. Of the selective and reversible MAO-B inhibitors, caroxazone and Ro 16-6491 are currently undergoing development.

Relationship between plasma anxiolytic concentrations and the therapeutic response

While the individual drugs in the benzodiazepine group differ in potency, all benzodiazepines in common use have anxiolytic, sedative-hypnotic, anticonvulsant and muscle-relaxant activity in ascending order of dose. The main clinical difference between the individual drugs lies in the time of onset of their therapeutic effect, and the intensity and duration of their clinical activity.

All benzodiazepines are derived from weak organic acids and some, such as midazolam, form water-soluble salts at a low pH. However, at normal physiological pHs, all benzodiazepines are lipophilic, the lipid solubility varying from highly lipophilic in the case of drugs like midazolam, flurazepam, diazepam and triazolam to slightly lipophilic for drugs such as clonazepam, bromazepam and lormetazepam. The benzodiazepines are also highly protein bound, so that at the plasma pH the proportion of the drug in the free form will vary from only 2% in the case of diazepam to about 30% with alprazolam. However, for most benzodiazepines the percentage of the drug in the pharmacologically active free form is independent of the total plasma concentration over a wide therapeutic range.

Transport of the benzodiazepines into the brain is rapid, the rate of uptake being determined by the physicochemical properties of the drug. Absorption from the gastrointestinal tract, or from an injection site, is the rate-limiting step governing the speed of onset of the therapeutic response. Oral absorption is more rapid when the drug is taken on an empty stomach.

The activity of benzodiazepines may be terminated when the drug is removed from the benzodiazepine receptor site and diffuses into peripheral adipose tissue sites and then metabolized in the liver, or when there is a decrease in the sensitivity of the benzodiazepine receptors following chronic exposure to the drug (termed *acute tolerance*). The rate of development of acute tolerance appears to vary with the different benzodiazepines, making it difficult to relate the changes in therapeutic response to the changes in plasma concentration.

Pharmacokinetic factors do play a role in terminating the pharmacological effects of these drugs however. It would appear that the distribution of the drug rather than its clearance is the most important factor governing the termination of action. The extent of peripheral distribution of a benzodiazepine increases according to the lipophilicity of the drug. This phase is usually rapid and leads to the termination of the therapeutic effects of the drug; the apparent elimination $t_{1/2}$ of the drug is usually much slower and is not necessarily related to the time course of the pharmacological effects. This means that drugs with apparently long half-lives may have very short durations of action due to their extensive distribution throughout the body, whereas those drugs that are less lipophilic have a smaller V_d and therefore a longer duration of action, particularly after a single dose. Midazolam is an unusual benzodiazepine in that it is very lipophilic, has a large V_d and is rapidly metabolized and excreted. Both clearance and distribution therefore contribute to the cessation of its therapeutic effect.

The extent of accumulation of an anxiolytic will depend on the elimination half-life in relation to the dosing interval. Thus drugs with long half-lives will have cumulative sedative effects, and may impair cognition, following repeated administration. However, despite increasing blood and presumably brain concentrations of the drug, central depression does not increase in parallel because of the development of tolerance to the non-specific depressant actions of the drug. Long half-life anxiolytics are slowly eliminated whereas short half-life drugs tend to be eliminated rapidly. This means that the dose of the latter type of drug must be tapered slowly to avoid withdrawal effects at the end of a period of treatment.

Oxidation and *conjugation* are the principal mechanisms whereby the benzodiazepines are metabolized. Nitroreduction is an additional pathway that is involved in the metabolism of nitrazepam, flunitrazepam and clonazepam. Aliphatic hydroxylation and *N*-dealkylation are the main oxidative routes and often lead to active metabolites (e.g. diazepam gives rise to desmethyldiazepam, oxazepam and temazepam as active metabolites). The second main mechanism is hepatic conjugation to glucuronic acid. Drugs such as oxazepam, lorazepam, temazepam and lormetazepam are inactivated in this way. The main oxidative pathways are influenced by physiological factors such as age, by pathological factors such as hepatitis and by drugs such as the oestrogens and cimetidine which affect hepatic oxidative metabolism.

The relative contribution of the active metabolites of the benzodiazepines to the overall therapeutic effect of the parent compound will depend on the concentration of the metabolite formed, its agonist potency at central benzodiazepine receptors and its lipophilicity. For example, after the chronic administration of diazepam, desmethyldiazepam accumulates in the brain. As this metabolite has potency at the benzodiazepine receptors equal to diazepam, the metabolite probably plays an important part in the overall action of diazepam. In the case of clobazam, however, even though the active metabolite desmethylclobazam is present in higher concentrations than the parent compound after chronic administration, it has a lower potency than clobazam and therefore is of less importance than the parent compound with regard to the anxiolytic effect.

Of the *non-benzodiazepines* that have been introduced recently for the treatment of anxiety and insomnia, buspirone and zopiclone have been the most extensively investigated so far. The pharmacokinetic characteristics of zopiclone have been studied in healthy subjects, in the elderly and in patients with renal and hepatic malfunction. It would appear that the kinetics of this drug only alter appreciably in patients in the terminal stages of renal or hepatic disease; in the elderly only a slight increase in the half-life of the drug was observed. Zopiclone is a short (approximately 5 hours) half-life hypnotic which is converted to another short half-life active metabolite, zopiclone N-oxide. The kinetics of the drug are not apparently altered by repeated daily dosing. Buspirone and its close analogue gepirone form the active metabolite 1-piperazine (1-PP). There is also extensive metabolism of the parent compound by hydroxylation and oxidation. The 1-PP metabolite is lipophilic and rapidly enters the brain, where it has an apparent $t_{1/2}$ of about 2.5 hours. This metabolite also accumulates in the brain after chronic dosing, thereby suggesting that it contributes to the anxiolytic action of the parent compound.

The importance of drug pharmacokinetics to drug interactions

Genetic polymorphism

In pharmacokinetics, genetic polymorphism refers to differences between individuals' ability to metabolize drugs. More than 25 years ago it was shown that the steady-state plasma concentration of the TCA nortriptyline was related to the genetic characteristics of the patient. Thus homozygous, but not heterozygous, twins had similar blood nortriptyline concentrations. Since that time it has become clear that many of the liver enzymes concerned with drug metabolism exhibit genetic polymorphism. This may be particularly important when depressed patients receiving antidepressant therapy are also given other drugs which compete for the same hepatic enzyme.

The most important group of liver enzymes that are responsible for the oxidative metabolism of most drugs are the microsomal cytochrome P_{450} oxidases. There are many subtypes (termed isozymes).

Each cytochrome P450 isoenzyme is the product of a separate gene, and so far more than 200 such genes have been identified. Furthermore, a number of cytochrome P450 genes have been shown to have different alleles which have resulted from mutation. Where such a mutation exists in more than 1% of the population, the term "genetic polymorphism" is applied. Many of the polymorphic forms of the cytochrome P450 enzyme appear to be of minor significance in drug metabolism. Substrates and inhibitors of these isoenzymes are presented in Table 3.1.

In some individuals an isoenzyme may be absent. This is an inherited trait which can vary in incidence according to racial background.

Table 3.1. Characteristics, substrates and inhibitors of some cytochrome P450 isoenzymes

Isoenzyme	Polymorphism	Substrate	Inhibitor
1A2	Probably not, but very wide inter-patient variability	Warfarin, propranolol, phenacetin, clozapine, theophylline, TCAs (desmethylation)	Fluvoxamine
2C19	2–3% of Caucasians 15–25% of Orientals 4% of Blacks	Diazepam, tolbutamide, phenytoin, TCAs (desmethylation)	Fluvoxamine, fluoxetine, sertraline
2D6	5–8% of Caucasians Lower in other races	Codeine, dextromethorphan, haloperidol, thioridazine, perphenazine, nortriptyline, desipramine, fluoxetine, norfluoxetine, TCAs (hydroxylation), beta-blockers such as timolol and metoprolol, type 1C antiarrhythmics encainide, flecainide	Fluoxetine, paroxetine, sertraline, fluphenazine
3A4	Unknown	TCAs (desmethylation), triazolam, alprazolam, midazolam, carbamazepine, terfenadine, quinidine, lidocaine, erythromycin, cyclosporin	Very likely all SSRIs (norfluoxetine particularly), nefazodone, ketoconazole

Depending on whether the isoenzyme is absent or present, individuals are classified as extensive or poor metabolizers of the reference compound.

The clinical importance of genetic polymorphism depends on factors such as the health status of the patient and the concomitant administration of any drugs which might act as a substrate or inhibitor of a particular isoenzyme. For example, a depressed patient who metabolizes an SSRI (selective serotonin reuptake inhibitor) slowly will have higher plasma concentrations of that drug than another patient who metabolizes the drug at the normal rate. However, this is unlikely to be clinically significant given the high therapeutic index of the SSRIs. In contrast, TCAs have a low therapeutic index and the active metabolites of amitriptyline (nortriptyline) and imipramine (desipramine) are usually hydroxylated via the cyto-chrome P450 2D6 pathway. Slow metabolizers of desmethylated TCAs will experience TCA accumulation, which may result in potentially toxic cardiovascular effects. Conversely, patients who are fast metabolizers may experience subtherapeutic plasma drug concentrations.

Another factor which should be considered is the relative importance of the defective metabolic pathway in the overall metabolism of a drug. For example, paroxetine is metabolized by at least two pathways and the suboptimal activity of one enzyme has a relatively minor effect on the elimination of the drug. For the other SSRIs, the hepatic enzymes responsible for oxidization have not been clearly identified. However, these agents have a high affinity for the cytochrome P450 system and drug–drug interactions may be important under certain circumstances.

The biochemical basis of important drug interactions

Introduction

The biotransformation of a drug may either lead to the termination of its pharmacological activity or, occasionally, to its activation to a pharmacologically effective entity. It is also possible that a drug may be metabolized to form pharmacologically or toxicologically active metabolites. Whatever the outcome, the biotransformation of a drug ultimately involves its conversion to a more hydrophilic form thereby facilitating its excretion into the urine. However, some lipophilic drugs and their metabolites are excreted via the bile into the intestine while others, that are volatile, pass into the lungs and are thereby excreted in the expired air.

The biotransformation of drugs occurs in two main phases which are summarized in Table 3.2. Phase 1 involves the oxidative catabolism of the drug. The end products of the phase 1 reactions are generally conjugated by uridine diphosphorylglucuronyl transferase, sulphatase or N-acetyltransferase to form polar, water-soluble products which are then excreted into the urine. These are the products of the phase 2 reactions. While it is well known that products of the phase 1 reactions are often pharmacologically active (for example, norfluoxetine which is a metabolic product of fluoxetine), it is also possible that the end product of phase 2 reactions can also be pharmacologically active. For example, morphine-6-glucuronide is as pharmacologically active as the parent compound.

These stages can be illustrated schematically as shown in Figure 3.1. The primary site of biotransformation is the liver although the gastrointestinal tract, kidneys and the skin also contribute to a minor extent.

Drugs that are orally administered often undergo first-pass metabolism. This involves their (generally partial) metabolism in the liver following their entry from the gastrointestinal tract via the portal circulation. This

Table 3.2.   Biotransformation of drugs by phase 1 and phase 2 reactions

Phase 1 reactions	Oxidative reactions involving N- and O-dealkylation, aliphatic and aromatic hydroxylation, N- and S-oxidation, deamination.
Phase 2 reactions	Biotransformation reactions involving glucuronization, sulphation, acetylation.

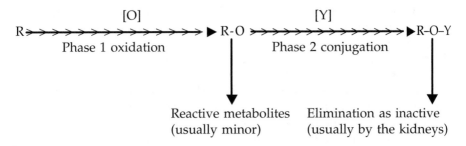

[Y]=glucuronide, sulphate or acetyl group.

Figure 3.1. Relationship between the phase 1 and 2 biotransformation reactions.

inevitably leads to a reduction in the effective blood concentration and must therefore be taken into account when the dose of the drug to be administered is calculated.

In the liver, the microsomal enzymes that are responsible for catalysing the oxidative reactions are the cytochrome P450 family of enzymes. These enzymes are haem-containing membrane proteins that are bound to the smooth endoplasmic reticulum of the hepatocytes. Of the 12 gene families of the cytochrome P450 system that have been identified in man, those classified as cytochrome P450 types 1, 2 and 3 account for most of the drug biotransformations. In addition to the oxidative reactions undertaken by the P450 enzymes (also known as isozymes), hydrolytic reactions are carried out by epoxide hydrolase and several amidases, esterases, proteases and peptidases.

There are several important factors which may influence biotransformation reactions. Thus some drugs or toxins may induce the synthesis of microsomal oxidases by the liver (for example, a barbiturate) and thereby enhance the metabolism of the drug, or any other drug given concurrently which is metabolized by the same enzyme system (for example, warfarin). Nicotine in tobacco smoke is known to increase the activity of the cytochrome P450 1A2 isozyme which may predispose some individuals to a greater risk of cancer. Some drugs produce hepatotoxic metabolites which thereby impair the biotransformation of other drugs or toxins which may be present. For example, chronic alcohol intake can lead to the formation of hepatotoxic metabolites. Drugs may also selectively inhibit individual isozymes of the P450 system, thereby causing an unexpected rise in the blood and tissue concentrations of any drug given concurrently which is also metabolized by that isozyme. The SSRI antidepressants for example have been shown to act as inhibitors of some P450 isozymes, thereby not only reducing their own metabolism but also those of other drugs given concurrently (see p. 89). Some foods may also inhibit the P450 isozymes and thereby enhance the toxicity, or the duration and magnitude of the therapeutic response of a drug given concurrently. Grapefruit juice, for example, is a significant inhibitor of the P450 isozyme 3A4, an enzyme which is widely involved in the metabolism of psychotropic drugs (see p. 89).

It is self-evident that biotransformation will be reduced in patients with liver or kidney disease, in the elderly and also in neonates. In addition, pharmacogenetic differences play a considerable role in the way an individual patient metabolizes a drug. Such differences often result from polymorphisms in the cytochrome P450 family of microsomal enzymes.

Classification of the cytochrome P450 enzymes

These enzymes have been classified according to the degree of structural similarity in their amino acid structures (the so-called sequence homology). Thus the closer the enzymes are from both the phylogenic and functional point of view, the more likely they are to be a member of the same enzyme family with a sequence homology of at least 40%. The enzymes are further grouped into subfamilies (isozymes) which are designated by the letters A, B, C, D, E, F. All enzymes in the same subfamily have a sequence homology of at least 55%. The final number designates the gene that codes for a specific enzyme (1, 2, 3, 4, 5, 6, 7, etc.). With regard to the metabolism of the psychotropic drugs, cytokines 1A2, 2C19, 2D6, 3A3/4 are of primary importance.

The cytochrome P450 enzymes are divided into two major groups, namely the "steroidogenic" enzymes (which are the phylogenically older type and are responsible for the synthesis of steroids and related compounds comprising the cell wall) and the "xenobiotic" type (located in the smooth endoplasmic reticulum and involved in the metabolism of foreign, or xenobiotic, compounds which include all drugs). The following list summarizes the types of compounds metabolized by the main groups of P450 enzymes:

- Steroidogenic type – steroids, bile acids, cholesterol, prostaglandin biosynthesis.
- Xenobiotic type – drugs, toxins, carcinogens, mutagens.

It should be noted that the genetic information for the P450 enzymes is present throughout in all tissues, but knowledge of the role of the enzymes in tissues other than the liver and gastrointestinal tract is unclear. For example, cytochrome P450 2D6 is found in the brain where it is linked to the dopamine transporter. Whether a deficit in the activity of this enzyme is responsible for predisposing some individuals to Parkinson's disease is a matter of conjecture.

Table 3.3.   Main types of drug metabolized by cytochrome P450 isozymes

CypP450 1A2	Antidepressants – tricyclics, mirtazepine, fluoxetine* Antipsychotics – clozapine, haloperidol, olanzapine, phenothiazines Sedative/hypnotics – zopiclone Beta-blockers – propranolol, warfarin, theophylline
CypP450 2C19	Antidepressants – amitriptyline, clomipramine, imipramine, moclobemide, citalopram Antipsychotics – olanzapine Mood stabilizers – phenytoin, valproate, topiramate Sedative/anxiolytics – diazepam, barbiturates Beta-blockers – propranolol
CypP450 2D6	Antidepressants – tricyclics, fluoxetine*, paroxetine*, sertraline*, mirtazepine, venlafaxine, mianserin Antipsychotics – phenothiazines, haloperidol, clozapine, olanzapine, quetiapine Antiarrhythmics – encainide, flecainide, mexiletine Beta-blockers – alprenolol, metoprolol, propranolol, timolol Opiates – codeine, dextromethorphan, ethylmorphine
CypP450 3A3/4	Antidepressants – tricyclics, nefazodone*, fluoxetine*, fluvoxamine*, citalopram, mirtazepine, venlafaxine Antipsychotics – chlorpromazine, clozapine, pimozide, quetiapine, risperidone Anxiolytics – clonazepam, diazepam, temazepam, triazolam, alprazolam, midazolam, buspirone Anticonvulsants – ethosuximide, carbamazepine Calcium channel blockers – diltiazem, felodipine, nifedipine, verapamil Antibiotics – clarithromycin, erythromycin Others – omeprazole, cisapride, dapsone, lavastatin

*Also inhibits this enzyme.

A summary of the main classes of psychotropic drugs metabolized by the P450 enzymes, together with some of the drugs of other classes with which they may interact, is given in Table 3.3.

Drug–drug interactions

There are two main types of drug interactions, pharmacodynamic and pharmacokinetic. Pharmacodynamic interactions arise when one drug increases or decreases the pharmacological effect caused by a second drug that may be given concurrently. Pharmacokinetic interactions occur when one drug alters a pharmacokinetic component of another drug thereby causing a change in its effective concentration at its site of action. The relationship between the pharmacodynamic and pharmacokinetic characteristics and the subsequent therapeutic response can be summarized by the following equations:

$$\text{Magnitude of therapeutic response} = \text{drug pharmacodynamics} + \text{drug pharmacokinetics} + \text{individual biological variation}$$

$$\text{Magnitude of clinical response} = \text{potency at site of action} + \text{drug concentration at site of action} + \text{biological status of the patient}$$

With regard to the differences between the pharmacodynamic and pharmacokinetic drug interactions, it would appear that pharmacokinetic interaction produces the same result as a change in the dose of the drug. For example, combining the SSRI antidepressant fluoxetine with a sub-therapeutic dose of a tricyclic antidepressant could result in a two- to threefold elevation in the blood concentration of the tricyclic as fluoxetine inhibits its metabolism via the 2D6/3A4 isozymes. However this change in the pharmacodynamic response to the tricyclic antidepressant could (a) result in unexpected cardiotoxicity due to the abrupt increase in the concentration of the drug in the cardiac tissue resulting in the block of the fast sodium channels and (b) prolong the elimination half-life of the tricyclic antidepressant thereby resulting in a cumulative toxicity of the drug. Thus the SSRI, by inhibiting the metabolism of the tricyclic, has changed the clearance of the drug as illustrated by the equation:

$$\text{Rate of dosing/Clearance} \rightarrow \text{Steady-state concentration} \rightarrow \text{Therapeutic response}$$

By decreasing the clearance due to cytochrome P450 inhibition, but maintaining the same dose and rate of dosing, the steady-state concentration of the tricyclic antidepressant increases thereby enhancing the therapeutic or toxicological response. In clinical practice, pharmacokinetic drug interactions may be dismissed as an idiosyncrasy of the patient rather than a potential drug hazard.

Another practical example of a pharmacokinetic drug interaction concerns the incidence of seizures in patients given a standard (300 mg/day) dose of clozapine. Should the patient be given an SSRI antidepressant (such as fluoxetine, fluvoxamine, sertraline or paroxetine) concurrently then the clearance of clozapine could be reduced by up to 50%, an effect which would be comparable with a doubling of the dose. This could lead to a threefold increase in the risk of the patient suffering a seizure.

In addition to the above examples, toxicity problems can also arise when one drug induces the metabolism of the second drug. Toxic metabolites, which are not normally present in a sufficiently high concentration to be noticeable, may increase due to the increase in their concentration as a consequence of enzyme induction. For example, carbamazepine induces P450 3A3/4 which enhances the metabolism of valproate. This leads to the increased production of the 4-ene metabolite of valproate which is hepatotoxic.

Hopefully these few examples will serve to emphasize the importance of a knowledge of the pharmacokinetic features of psychotropic drugs in order to avoid the potentially serious side effects that can result from drug interactions.

Enantiomers: their importance in psychopharmacology

Introduction

The majority of naturally occurring drugs and biologically active compounds are asymmetrical in their chemical structure. This means that the molecule is structured around one or more carbon atoms in such a way that the molecule is distributed mostly on the right (R=rectus) or left (S=sinister) of the symmetrical carbon atom, the so-called chiral centre of the molecule. Thus a large proportion of psychotropic drugs in current use possess one or more chiral centres and therefore exist in pairs of enantiomers which differ in terms of their three-dimensional structures. However, it must be remembered that chirality can apply not only to molecules but also to anatomical structures. For example, the left and right hands are chiral structures as is evident when one attempts to put a left-handed glove on the right hand and vice versa!

At the cellular level, the various types of receptor, transporter, enzyme and ion channel are all chiral in form. Thus although the enantiomers of a drug may have identical physicochemical properties, the way in which they may interact with chiral targets at the level of the cell will give rise to different pharmacodynamic and pharmacokinetic properties. A few simple examples will illustrate how taste and olfactory receptors can differentiate between enantiomers. Thus R-carvone tastes like spearmint whereas the S-isomer tastes like caraway. Similarly, R-limolene smells like lemon whereas the S-enantiomer tastes of orange.

In psychopharmacology, interest in the properties of enantiomers has been aided by the need to improve the therapeutic efficacy and decrease the side effects and toxicity of drugs. For example, if the therapeutic activity resides entirely in one enantiomer (called a eutomer) then giving a racemic mixture which contains the active and the inactive enantiomer is clearly wasteful. Thus using the single enantiomer (isomer or eutomer) should enable the dose of the drug to be lowered, reduce the interpatient variability in the response and, hopefully, reduce the side effects and toxicity of the drug (see Table 3.4).

Table 3.4.   Possible advantages of the single stereoisomer over the racemic mixture

1.   Reduction in the therapeutic dose.
2.   Reduction in the interpatient variability in metabolism and in response to treatment.
3.   Simplification of the relationship between the dose and the response to treatment.
4.   Reduction in the toxicity and side effects due to the greater specificity of action of the isomer with the relevant biological processes.

In addition to the possible advantages of the single enantiomer, the pharmacologically inactive enantiomer may reduce the efficacy of the active isomer by reducing its activity at its site of action or by interfering with its metabolism. Thus separating a racemic mixture into its enantiomers, and assessing the individual properties of the isomers would seem to be a reasonable approach to improving the clinical profile of many well-established psychotropic drugs. The process whereby a racemic mixture is reintroduced as a single enantiomer is termed "chiral switching".

While there appears to be a compelling argument for using single enantiomers whenever possible in order to improve the efficacy and safety of a racemic drug, there is no certainty that chiral switching will always be beneficial. For example, in 1979 seven cases of inadvertent injection of the local anaesthetic racemic bupivacaine resulted in cardiovascular collapse in a few patients. The toxicity appeared to reside entirely in the R-isomer so that, by chiral switching, a safer and less toxic local anaesthetic was produced. Other examples have not been so successful however. For example, the chiral switching of racemic fenfluramine to its R-enantiomer, dexfenfluramine (the nomenclature has changed recently so that D-enantiomers, Dex enantiomers, are now termed R-enantiomers while the L-enantiomers, levoenantiomers, become S-enantiomers) was at first heralded as a successful new appetite suppressant. However, it was soon shown that, despite its improved efficacy, the R-enantiomer was more likely to cause pulmonary hypertension. This has resulted in the withdrawal of the drug.

Some examples of the properties of single enantiomers in psychopharmacology

(1) Analgesics – methadone

This synthetic opiate was introduced in 1965 to manage opioid dependence and has been successfully used as an aid to abstinence since that time. Methadone is a racemate, the R-enantiomer being the pharmacologically active form of the drug. This isomer shows a 10-fold higher affinity for the mu and delta opioid receptors, and nearly 50 times the antinociceptive activity of the S-enantiomer. In addition, the R-isomer is less plasma protein bound than the S-form; the latter isomer being more tightly bound to alpha-1 acid glycoprotein. The plasma clearance of the R-form is slower than the S-isomer. Patients treated with the isomers of methadone showed considerable individual variability, with some parameters reaching 70%: this would not have been detected if the racemate had been administered. These pharmacokinetic differences could be crucially important when patients are being treated with methadone as part of an opiate withdrawal programme as relatively small decreases in the plasma concentration could produce marked changes in mood, thereby undermining the positive benefit of the methadone withdrawal programme.

(2) Sedative/hypnotics – zopiclone

Zopiclone is widely used as a sedative–hypnotic. It is metabolized to an inactive N-desmethylated derivative and an active N-oxide compound, both of which contain chiral centres. S-Zopiclone has a 50-fold higher affinity for the benzodiazepine receptor site than the R-enantiomer. This could be therapeutically important, particularly if the formation and the urinary excretion of the active metabolite benefits the S-isomer, which appears to be the case. As the half-life of the R-enantiomer is longer than that of the S-form, it would seem advantageous to use the R-isomer in order to avoid the possibility of daytime sedation and hangover effects which commonly occur with long-acting benzodiazepine receptor agonists.

(3) Neuroleptics – thioridazine

Thioridazine is a complex first-generation antipsychotic agent that is metabolized to two other pharmacologically active drugs (mesoridazine and sulphoridazine) which have been introduced as neuroleptics in their own right. All three neuroleptics have chiral centres. Interest in thioridazine has arisen in recent years because of the higher incidence in sudden death, due to cardiotoxicity, found in patients who had been prescribed the drug. Thioridazine-5-sulphoxide would appear to be the metabolite responsible for the cardiotoxicity. This metabolite alone has four chiral centres and knowledge is lacking concerning the toxicity of these enantiomers which serves to illustrate the complexity of the problem.

Regarding the pharmacological activity of thioridazine, the R-enantiomer has been shown to be at least three times more potent than the R-isomer in binding to the D_2 dopamine receptors and nearly five times more potent than an alpha-1 receptor antagonist. Conversely, the S-isomer has a 10-fold greater affinity for the D_1 receptor than the R-form. Thus the pharmacological consequences of using a single enantiomer of thioridazine are, unlike the other three examples given, very complex. Thus if the S-enantiomer was selected, while the potency would undoubtedly increase (due to its D_2 antagonism), the chances of postural hypotension (due to the alpha-1 receptor antagonism) would also be greater. Furthermore, the relative activity and toxicity of the individual enantiomers and their metabolites is unknown. With regard to the extrapyramidal side effects for example, experimental studies have shown that the R-isomer is more likely to cause catalepsy and is, in addition, far more toxic than the S-form. Dose–response relationships have also been undertaken on the individual enantiomers versus the racemate form of thioridazine and show that the racemate is 12 times more potent than the S-isomer and three times more potent than the R-isomer.

(4) Antidepressants

It is widely agreed that there is little difference in the therapeutic efficacy between any of the first- and second-generation antidepressants. However, in terms of their tolerability and safety, the second-generation drugs are superior. Of these, the SSRI antidepressants are the most widely used but, despite their clear advantages over the tricyclic antidepressants which they have largely replaced in industrialized countries, they have such side effects as nausea and sexual dysfunction which can affect compliance. While there are clearly differences in the frequency of side effects between the SSRIs, no clear overall advantage emerges for any one of the drugs.

Many currently used antidepressants are chiral drugs (for example, tricyclic antidepressants, mianserin, mirtazepine, venlafaxine, reboxetine, fluoxetine, paroxetine, sertraline, citalopram), some of which are administered as racemates (such as the tricyclics, mianserin, mirtazepine, fluoxetine, reboxetine, venlafaxine, citalopram) while others are given as single isomers (paroxetine and sertraline).

The relative benefits of the enantiomers of antidepressants vary greatly. For example, when the therapeutic properties of the enantiomers are complementary (for example, mianserin) then use of the racemate is an advantage. However, if there are qualitative, but not quantitative, similarities then it would be beneficial to develop the active isomer. This has recently occurred with the development of citalopram.

The S-enantiomer of citalopram (escitalopram) is over 100 times more potent in inhibiting the reuptake of 5-HT into brain slices than the R-form and is devoid of any activity at the neurotransmitter of other receptor types (racemic citalopram has an affinity for histamine receptors and causes sedation). In *in vivo* studies, escitalopram is more potent than the R-form or the racemate in releasing 5-HT in the cortex of conscious rats; it has been shown to have antidepressant and anti-anxiety properties in both animal models and in patients. With regard to its side effects, the frequency of nausea and ejaculatory dysfunction after escitalopram is approximately the same as that of the racemate. From the results of the published clinical studies, it would appear that the tolerability of escitalopram is slightly better than the racemate and the time of onset of the clinical response may be slightly faster but this needs confirmation. In general, the adverse effects were mild and transient with a low patient withdrawal rate. Early clinical trials suggest that escitalopram is as effective as citalopram in the treatment of depression and anxiety disorders.

In CONCLUSION, current evidence suggests that for many psychotropic drugs there are functional differences between the enantiomers and the racemate which could have important clinical implications. However, it is apparent that the possible advantages of developing a single enantiomer must be considered on a drug-by-drug basis. For example, fluoxetine, like most SSRIs, exists in a chiral form but the most active enantiomer found in experimental studies caused cardiotoxicity in some patients. In general, however, it would appear that knowledge of the stereochemistry of psychotropic drugs will help in the development of new, and hopefully more effective, molecules in the near future.

Drug–protein interactions

In addition to metabolic interactions, consideration should be given to drug–protein binding interactions, although there is little clinical evidence to suggest that such interactions are of any consequence with the SSRIs. It must be stressed that many liver enzymes are non-specific for their substrates and that most drugs are metabolized by multiple pathways. Good therapeutic practice demands that drug interactions should be considered carefully, particularly in subpopulations of depressed patients such as the elderly or those with hepatic dysfunction or a history of alcoholism.

In SUMMARY, it would appear that a detailed knowledge of the pharmacokinetics of the main groups of psychotropic drugs is only of very limited clinical use. This is due to limitations in the methods for the detection of some drugs (e.g. the neuroleptics), the presence of active metabolites which make an important contribution to the therapeutic effect, particularly after chronic administration (e.g. many antidepressants, neuroleptics and anxiolytics), and the lack of a direct correlation between the plasma concentration of the drug and its therapeutic effect. Perhaps the only real advances will be made in this area with the development of brain imaging techniques whereby the concentrations of the active drug in the brain of the patient may be directly measured. Until such time as the kinetics of psychotropic drugs in the brain can be properly assessed, it can be concluded that the routine determination of plasma levels of psychotropic drugs is of very limited value.

Despite the limited value of measuring plasma psychotropic drug concentrations to assess clinical response, a knowledge of the pharmaco-kinetics of such a drug can be of value in predicting drug interactions.

4 Clinical Trials and their Importance in Assessing the Efficacy and Safety of Psychotropic Drugs

Prior to 1962, trials of new medications were largely based on a series of uncontrolled testimonials by clinicians associated with the studies. The change in the conduct of clinical trials arose largely in response to the public concern, and that of the medical profession, expressed as a result of the thalidomide disaster in which thousands of women in Europe produced offspring with serious limb deformations which occurred after taking the drug for the treatment of morning sickness during the first trimester of pregnancy. This tragedy resulted in the establishment of regulatory authorities in most European countries who established legal guidelines, mainly based on those of the Food and Drug Administration in the USA, which ensured that all new drugs would be subjected to adequate pre-clinical and clinical assessment before they could be marketed. This is not the place to describe in detail the pre-clinical and clinical studies which are now required by the Medicine Boards which were established by the European Commission to ensure that optimal standards are reached before any drug is made available for clinical use. However, the following summary will hopefully serve to illustrate the procedures involved in ensuring the efficacy and safety of drugs.

Pre-clinical testing

Drug discovery, almost without exception, is dependent on the pharmaceutical industry. This is understandable due to the enormous costs involved. Although there have been major developments in drug design (particularly with the application of combinatorial chemistry which enables the random synthesis of low molecular weight compounds by automated technology) that have helped to rationalize the methods used to identify novel compounds, the discovery of genuinely original drugs is still largely

Fundamentals of Psychopharmacology. Third Edition. By Brian E. Leonard
© 2003 John Wiley & Sons, Ltd. ISBN 0 471 52178 7

dependent on serendipity. Nowhere is this more apparent than in the area of psychopharmacology where, with few exceptions, the application of structure–activity relationships for the synthesis of new drugs has been disappointing. Thus it is still necessary for a lead compound to undergo extensive *in vitro* and *in vivo* testing to determine whether it will justify clinical development. Once it has been established that the compound is pharmacologically active at doses that do not cause major adverse side effects in rodents, and that it may offer benefits over the drugs that are already available, the compound is then submitted to extensive toxico-logical testing. This requires an assessment of the dose-related toxicity in at least two different species of mammal so that a risk–benefit assessment may be made regarding its suitability for further clinical development. In addition, information is obtained regarding the pharmacokinetic character-istics of the compound with regard to its bioavailability, metabolism, excretion and the occurrence of potentially toxic metabolites. Details of the manufacturing processes involved, together with details of the final dosage form which will be used in the initial clinical studies, must also be provided by the pharmaceutical company to the Medicines Board before the compound can undergo further testing. The processes involved in pre-clinical testing can take at least 5–7 years to complete in the case of a novel chemical entity but the period can be shorter if the compound is structurally related to a drug which is already in therapeutic use.

One of the major problems facing the researcher who is attempting to discover novel drugs to treat psychiatric disorders lies in the difficulty of obtaining relevant animal models of the human disorder. It is self-evident that only man appears to suffer from any of the major psychiatric disorders, which therefore restricts the researcher to studying changes in behavioural parameters that show some similarity to those observed in the model following drug treatment (accurately predict its activity in the patient?), face validity (are the behavioural or physiological changes observed in the model similar to those seen in the patient?) and construct validity (are the causes of the changes observed in the model similar to those causing the disorder in man?). As the biological basis of all major psychiatric disorders, and most neurological disorders, is far from certain and the behavioural repertoire of most animals is quite different from that of humans, it is understandable why no animal model meets the optimum criterion. Despite these limitations it is still possible to obtain information by studying the effects of novel compounds on animals (usually rodents) that offer some predictive validity. The introduction of "knock-out" mice, or mice in which specific receptors, neurotransmitters or toxic proteins (such as the human beta-amyloid protein) are over-expressed (see p. 128), has helped in understanding the relationship between the changes in central neurotransmitter function and abnormalities in behaviour which are amenable to drug treatment. Those interested in a more detailed overview of the use of animal models for the discovery of novel psychotropic drugs are referred to the list of publications at the end of the book.

Use of human brain tissue in drug discovery

Despite the success in using animal models to develop drugs which have similar pharmacological properties to those drugs in clinical use, they are much less successful in detecting novel compounds that have pharmacological properties, and possible therapeutic indications, that differ from the drugs that are currently available. In an attempt to improve the chance of discovering novel drugs and, at the same time, reduce the cost and increase the number of compounds which may be screened for their potential therapeutic activity, *in vitro* models have recently been introduced in pharmaceutical and biotechnological companies based on sequences from the human genome. Such an approach has been encouraged by the need to introduce models based on human brain tissue at a much earlier stage in drug development. In support of this view, it has been estimated that man and chimpanzees share more than 98.9% of their genes in common. However, the expression of genes in the brain was more than fivefold greater in man than in the chimpanzee, whereas the differences in gene expression in the liver and blood were small. Differences between the gene expression of man and rodents were much greater than between man and primates. This suggests that whereas it is possible to model drug metabolism and distribution in such primates, it is less likely that disorders of higher mental function (such as depression and schizophrenia) could be modelled with the same degree of certainty.

Drug discovery in recent years has moved away from the development of specific drugs (such as the SSRIs, 5-HT$_{1A}$ partial agonists, D$_4$ receptor antagonists) which were presumed to act at single targets, to the realization that complex psychiatric disorders require multiple targets for their effective treatment. This change in emphasis in drug discovery is due to an increased knowledge of the interactions that take place between physiological processes in order to maintain homeostasis and the fact that diseases arise as a consequence of a loss of homeostasis. In addition, it is now recognized that many physiological systems have an inbuilt redundancy, whereby the effects of a drug on one system can be compensated by an adaptive change in a closely related system.

In an attempt to model such interactions, cDNA microassays have been developed. Microassay technologies are particularly suited for use with human tissues, including brain tissue, because the widest availability of genes on microchip assemblies has been obtained thanks to the human genome project. Rat and mouse microassays are now also becoming commercially available.

Drug targets are usually proteins. To date, the high-throughput proteomic technologies are not as advanced as the microassay technologies in terms of their sensitivity and number of items which can be determined simultaneously. However, while neither proteomics nor gene expression analysis by microassays are ideal, they are powerful methods particularly when used in combination with *in situ* hybridization, antibody localization and PCR methods (see Chapter 5 for a discussion of these methods). With regard to the use of human tissues for drug development, stem cells offer a unique advantage over blood cells which have been used as targets for drug discovery in the recent past. Stem cells have a unique property of being able to develop into any cell type, including brain cells. Stem cells have already been used for cell therapy and transplantation therapy (for example, in Parkinson's disease) and more recently they have been used for target identification in drug discovery programmes. As a complementary approach, an analysis of the changes in gene expression using microassay assemblies that occur following the action of known drugs that have been administered acutely or chronically could lead to the development of new classes of drugs with improved therapeutic profiles. A further discussion of the application of these *in vitro* methods for the discovery of novel psychotropic drugs is given in the reference section at the end of the book.

Clinical trials

Once a decision has been made to develop a compound further following the extensive pre-clinical pharmacological and toxicological studies, approval for the first clinical studies must be sought from the regulatory authority (Medicines Board in Europe or the Food and Drug Administration in the USA). A clinical trial of a new drug is, in the words of Bradford Hill (in his *Principles of Medical Statistics*):

a carefully, and ethically, designed experiment with the aim of answering some precisely framed questions. In its most vigorous form it demands equivalent groups of patients concurrently treated in different ways. These groups are formed by the random allocation of patients to one or other treatment. In principle, the method is applicable to any disease or type of treatment. It may also be applied on any scale.

Thus the purpose of a clinical trial is to describe (a) whether the new treatment is of therapeutic value, (b) how it compares with a "standard" drug, (c) what type of patient would benefit from the new drug, (d) what is the best route of administration, how frequently and in what dose range should it be used, (e) what are the side effects and disadvantages of the new drug. For the classical randomized control trial, the following points should be stressed:

(a) The use of equivalent groups of patients by random (chance) allocation to a placebo, standard drug or novel drug group. It is self-evident that if the treatment groups differ with respect to age, gender, race, duration and severity of the disease it will not be possible to attribute differences in outcome to the novel treatment. The randomization of patients is therefore used to eliminate systematic bias and to permit the use of appropriate statistical methods to correct for any bias.
(b) Time and place of treatment. Treatment must be undertaken concurrently and concomitantly. Using control data from past clinical studies (historical controls) is almost always unacceptable.
(c) Precisely formulated questions. These must be formulated before the start of the trial. For example, "is drug A capable of treating depression more rapidly and effectively, and with fewer side effects, than drug B?".

Some important concepts in evaluating clinical trials

The null hypothesis postulates that there is no difference in outcome between a new and a standard drug. Thus when two groups of patients have been treated separately with the drugs (between-patient comparisons) or when each patient has received both drugs (within-patient comparisons) and the result of the outcome of treatment is apparently better with one drug than the other, it is essential to determine if this difference is statistically significant.

The test of statistical significance will enable the researcher to determine whether the differences observed between the two treatments are due to chance. In practice, it is generally agreed that if the difference between the two groups occurs five times, or less, in 100 trials then the null hypothesis is unlikely to hold true and there is a real difference between the treatment groups. The level of statistical significance which is usually considered to be acceptable is at the 5% level, or less. This is represented by a probability value $P < 0.05$ (the percentage divided by 100). If the probability of a result occurs only once in 100 trials then it is highly significant at $P < 0.001$.

The confidence interval is a measure of the degree of assurance, or confidence, one may have in the process or power of the result. The confidence interval is expressed as a range of values about the mean and within which it is 95% certain that the true value of the result lies. The range may be wide, indicating uncertainty, or narrow, indicating relative certainty. If a result lacks statistical significance at the 5% level or less, it can only be interpreted as meaning that there is no clinically or experimentally useful difference between the treatments. Small numbers in experimental groups inevitably mean low precision or statistical power. Often small clinical trials are published without any statement of statistical power or the inclusion of confidence intervals which reveal their inadequacy.

Types of error

Type 1 errors arise when a difference is found between treatments when, in reality, the groups do not differ, whereas Type 2 errors commonly arise when treatments do differ but no statistical differences are found. It must be emphasized that statistical tests do not prove that there is a difference between two groups, but merely that there is a probability of this being the case. However, a difference may be statistically significant and have narrow confidence limits but yet be biologically insignificant. For example, there is experimental evidence to show that beta adrenoceptors on lymphocytes change by over 50% between midday and midnight in healthy adults yet such changes would appear to have no clinical significance. Similarly, the activity of the serotonin transporter on the platelet membrane is one-third greater at noon than at 6 a.m. without having any apparent effect on physiological functions. Thus the statistical significance of a result in any area of neuroscience must always be considered in conjunction with the biological relevance of the change. This is often overlooked, particularly when considering the variables that are linked to psychiatric and neurological disorders.

Types of clinical trial: single and double-blind trials

Because both the clinician and the patient are subject to bias as a result of their expectations of the outcome of the trial of a new drug, the double-blind technique is usually applied to evaluate the efficacy of a new drug. In such a trial the randomized groups of patients are given identical capsules or tablets (containing either a placebo, unknown drug or standard comparator); the clinician undertaking the clinical assessment is also "blind" to the distribution of the different treatments. Occasionally a double-blind technique cannot be applied as, for example, when the side effects of one of the drugs is greater than that of the placebo or the second drug.

A non-blinded clinical trial (i.e. lacking a placebo or standard comparator) is called an "open" trial and is usually used for the first clinical exposure of a novel compound once it has been approved for clinical trial by the regulatory authority. "Open" trials are useful for obtaining the dose range for a new drug and the frequency of side effects;

healthy volunteers are usually involved in the first exposure to a new drug. Once the relative safety of the drug has been assessed, an "open" trial on a small group of well-defined patients is undertaken so that an idea of the therapeutic efficacy of the drug can be obtained. These are termed Phase 1 studies and they are followed by Phase 2 studies, which are double-blind and involve a comparator as a standard, and Phase 3 studies (usually multi-centred studies involving a large number of patients under double-blind conditions). The Phase 1–Phase 3 studies would normally take at least 6 years to complete. It has also been estimated that it takes at least 12 years from the initial chemical synthesis of a novel compound to its clearance for clinical use by the regulatory authorities at a cost in excess of $230 million. In addition, for every 10 000 chemical entities that are synthesized, approximately 10 million will enter Phase 1 trials but only one would be expected to obtain regulatory approval.

Use of placebos in clinical trials

While serious ethical objections have been raised regarding the use of placebos in trials of drugs used in the treatment of psychiatric disorders (largely based on the possibility that the patients may commit suicide if they are inadequately treated, although such patients are usually excluded from placebo controlled trials), all regulatory authorities insist on properly conducted, placebo controlled trials as a basis for registering a new drug.

The placebo is useful in (a) distinguishing the pharmacodynamic effects of a drug from the psychological impact of the medication and the environment in which it is given (the "halo" effect of the enthusiastic, or pessimistic, research clinician). It is well known, for example, that the placebo effect in major depression is as high as 30% while that of an effective antidepressant is approximately 60% of the optimal response. This statistic illustrates the importance of placebo-based studies in evaluating the efficacy of a new psychotropic drug.

The placebo also distinguishes drug effects from fluctuations in the disease, which is particularly relevant in the case of psychiatric disorders. Lastly, the placebo allows false negatives to be excluded. For example, if a placebo is compared to a novel drug and a standard drug and the outcome of all three treatments is the same, the conclusion reached would be that the trial design (for example, number of patients in each group) is incapable of distinguishing between an active and inactive drug and therefore should be modified. If a standard drug is not included, however, it can only be concluded that the new medication is inactive at the dose used or that the end point used for the clinical assessment is inadequate.

Informed consent must always be obtained from a patient participating in any clinical trial. In the trial of a psychotropic drug, the mental status examination is critical for determining the capacity of the patient to consent and the ability to communicate is an absolute prerequisite. Both the memory and the orientation of the patient must be substantially intact if the patient is to give informed consent.

Such studies may be undertaken in chronic, stable diseases that cannot be cured but whose symptoms may improve following drug treatment, for example, Parkinson's disease and the dementias. In such cases, each patient is subject to the new drug and placebo in a random order, the patients acting as their own control. In such studies, it is important to ensure that any "carry-over" effects of the active drug are taken into account when the placebo, or a lower dose of the active drug, follows the highest dose of the drug.

The number of patients to be included in any trial is usually decided by a statistician. In the fixed-number type of trial, the total number of patients to be recruited is agreed before the start of the study and must be adhered to even if the result of the study does not quite reach an acceptable level of statistical significance. In such circumstances it is not permissible to add additional patients to the study in the hope that the 5% level of significance will be reached as this will not allow chance and the effect of treatment to be the sole factors involved in deciding the outcome of the study. To avoid this situation, trials are now designed so that the number of patients in each treatment group is not determined in advance but the trial design allows either continuous or intermittent assessment of the response, thereby allowing the trial to be stopped as soon as statistical difference between the groups is obtained or when such a result seems unlikely. Thus the trial can be terminated when the predetermined result is obtained (for example, a 50% reduction in the Hamilton Depression score in an antidepressant drug trial). In such a modified sequence design study, formal analysis of the data is undertaken at several predetermined intervals. Such interim analyses may reduce the power of the statistical analysis however. Large, definitive clinical trials of the type that have been used for Phase 3 studies are difficult to organize, prolonged, very expensive to perform and often yield inconclusive results. This has led to the design of smaller, controlled trials which, while of more limited statistical power, are subject to meta-analyses. Where numerous controlled trials on a drug have been undertaken and the outcome varies, the data can be collected in a systematic review and the accumulated results analysed by appropriate statistical methods. The resultant meta ("overall") analysis must meet the criteria for a good scientific study. Meta-analyses can involve 100 000 patients, or more, but problems may arise in identifying all the suitable trials of a new drug (and in assessing their standards from the published literature), added to which is the bias due to the fact that only positive results are usually published.

Cost of treatment with psychotropic drugs

It is self-evident that any new psychotropic drug is likely to be expensive. This situation also applied to the drugs used to treat other chronic illnesses such as cardiovascular disease, rheumatoid arthritis and diabetes. However, the cost of treatment implies more than the price of the drug. As most psychiatric disorders are chronic, costs must take into account the acute, maintenance and prophylactic phases of treatment. Thus in assessing the true cost, it is necessary to consider the ancillary procedures needed to monitor the patients' response to treatment (laboratory tests, etc.), managing any adverse effects of the medication, the relative costs of in-patient versus out-patient treatment, costs saved to the social and health services as a result of improved compliance and better response to treatment and the comparative costs of alternative treatments. It has been estimated that the cost of a new psychotropic drug for the treatment of depression, bipolar disorder or schizophrenia is approximately 10–15% of the total cost of treatment. It is also necessary to take into account the costs of not providing adequate treatment. These factors include the risks of premature death, and the increased morbidity, including the loss of productivity and the adverse effect of the illness on the social life of the patient.

Thus despite the much higher cost of a new psychotropic drug, Quality of Life assessments, which take into account the true cost of treatment, consistently show that new antidepressants and antipsychotics are superior to the older, and cheaper, medications. Most importantly, when optimal total care is provided for the patient, the quality of life is substantially improved which surely must be the aim of clinical psychopharmacology.

The limitation of pre-clinical studies on the development of novel psychotropic drugs

Serendipity has played a major role in the discovery of most classes of psychotropic drugs. For example, the observation that the first anti-depressants, the tricyclic antidepressants and the monoamine oxidase inhibitors, impeded the reuptake of biogenic amines into brain slices, or inhibited their metabolism, following their acute administration to rats, provided the experimenter with a mechanism that could be easily investigated *in vitro*. Such methods led to the development of numerous antidepressants that differed in their potency, and to some extent in their side effects (for example, the selective serotonin reuptake inhibitors) but did little to further the development of novel antidepressants showing greater therapeutic efficacy. The accidental discovery of atypical antidepressants such as mianserin led to the broadening of the basis of the animal models used to detect potential antidepressants with greater emphasis being placed on the chronic effects of the drugs *in vivo*. However, with few exceptions, all the *in vitro* and *in vivo* models in current use are based on the acute effects of novel compounds. Recently, with the impact of high-throughput screening methods based on the activity of compounds on multiple neurotransmitter receptors *in vitro*, even acute *in vivo* methods have been reduced in an attempt to decrease the time taken to proceed to the initial clinical assessment. Only time will tell whether the extensive use of genomics, microarray screens and receptor profiles of novel compounds will lead to genuinely novel psychotropic drugs. So far, there appears to be little advance in the therapeutic potential of the psychotropic drugs in development.

A comment on the limitation of clinical trials of new psychotropic drugs

A typical placebo controlled trial consists of 50–60 patients including a reference drug. Trials of new psychotropic drugs usually last for 6–8 weeks; the recommended duration of treatment in clinical practice is usually about 6 months. Most clinical protocols do not provide justification for the sample size used, or even specify the statistical power of the data obtained. As the proportion of non-responders for many psychotropic drugs may range from 20–30%, it can be argued that such limited trials (with a statistical power that is too low to show differences between treatments, conducted over too short a period in comparison with clinical practice and often excluding non-compliant patients from the final analysis) are unlikely to show any difference between a new and standard drug. This means that few studies are able to demonstrate an improved efficacy of a new drug over a standard drug. It has been calculated that the sample size that would be required to show a difference of 5% between two psychotropic drugs, assuming that approximately 20% will be non-responders or partial responders, would be between 1250 and 2380 patients per arm of the trial. The expense of such trials would, of course, be prohibitive! This does show that the apparent limited efficacy of most classes of psychotropic drugs is a reflection of the limitation of the clinical trial rather than their real potential differences, which could only be determined by using much larger numbers of patients in trials that last for several months.

Decision-making in the choice of a psychotropic drug

Despite the considerable advances that have been made in psycho-pharmacological research, there are many areas in which objective decisions based on scientific evidence with regard to the choice of the appropriate drug are sparse. In an attempt to overcome this problem, several authors have recently produced prescribing guidelines based on the evidence of the most appropriate drug to use. Such evidence extends from studies that are supported by randomized control trials (highest category), those which are supported by limited controlled trials (alternative category if drugs of the first category are ineffective) to those based on uncontrolled or anecdotal evidence (lowest category, unproven usefulness). A summary of the treatment options for the major psychiatric disorders and for Alzheimer's disease is found at the end of the appropriate chapter.

General principles of prescribing psychotropic drugs

The decision to use a psychotropic drug must take into account the potential risks and benefits. This should be discussed with the patient and/or carer. Before prescribing, a full evaluation of the symptoms should be made and the diagnosis confirmed. Polypharmacy should be avoided. If a drug combination is necessary, the pharmacodynamic and pharmacokinetic interactions should be considered.

In general, the lowest effective dose of the drug should be used, particularly in elderly patients. Dose titration should be undertaken slowly. Similarly, on discontinuation of a drug, the dose should be reduced slowly, the rate of decrease being decided by the elimination half-life of the drug. Some psychotropic drugs produce a discontinuation syndrome that can usually be avoided by slow withdrawal. In particular, sedatives, anxiolytics and antidepressants can cause withdrawal effects.

In switching drugs, the half-life of elimination that is being stopped should be considered if drug interactions are to be avoided. The time taken for the withdrawal of a drug depends on the duration of treatment; sedatives, antiepileptics and anxiolytics may take several weeks to withdraw.

5 Molecular Genetics and Psychopharmacology

In recent years the psychopharmacologist has paid increasing attention to the examination of brain proteins with which psychotropic drugs react, and also the molecular mechanisms that control the synthesis and cellular function of these proteins. For this reason, any understanding of psychopharmacology requires some knowledge of the basic techniques of molecular genetics.

Genes are composed of deoxyribonucleic acid (DNA) which is a long polymer composed of deoxyribonucleotides. Each deoxyribose nucleotide has one of the following purine or pyrimidine bases, namely adenosine, guanine, thymine or cystosine. A single gene may contain from a few thousand to several hundred thousand bases that are arranged in a specific sequence according to the information contained in the gene. It is this sequence of bases which determines the structure of the gene product which is a protein. In addition, the gene also contains information regarding the way in which the gene is expressed during development and in response to environmental stimuli.

The role of DNA in storing and transferring genetic material is dependent on the properties of the four bases. These *bases are complementary* in that guanine is always associated with cytosine, and adenosine with thymine. Watson and Crick, some 40 years ago, showed that the stability of DNA is due to the double helix structure of the molecule that protects it from major perturbations. Information is ultimately transferred by separating these strands which then act as templates for the synthesis of new nucleic acid molecules.

There are two ways in which DNA molecules may act as templates. Firstly, DNA is used as a template for replicating additional copies during cell division. This occurs by free deoxyribonucleotides binding to the complementary bases of the exposed DNA strand and then being linked by the enzyme DNA polymerase to form a new DNA double helix. Secondly, small sections of the DNA molecule are used as a template for the synthesis of *messenger ribonucleotides* (mRNAs) which are responsible

Fundamentals of Psychopharmacology. Third Edition. By Brian E. Leonard
© 2003 John Wiley & Sons, Ltd. ISBN 0 471 52178 7

for carrying the message for the synthesis of specific proteins. mRNAs differ from DNA in that they are much shorter (generally 7000 base pairs in length) and are single stranded. mRNAs contain the information necessary for the synthesis of a specific protein and also contain the pentose sugar moiety ribose instead of deoxyribose found in DNA. In addition, thymine is replaced by the pyrimidine base uracil which, like thymine, is complementary to adenine.

The human genome contains approximately 100 000 genes which are distributed with a total DNA sequence of 3 billion nucleotides. The DNA of the human genome is divided into 24 exceptionally large molecules each of which is a constituent of a particular chromosome, of which 22 are autosomes and two are sex chromosomes (X and Y chromosomes).

Translation of the information encoded in DNA, expressed as a particular nucleotide sequence, into a protein, expressed as an amino acid sequence, depends on the genetic code. In this code, sequences of three nucleotides (termed a *codon*) represent one of the 20 amino acids that compose the protein molecule. Because there are 64 codons which can be constructed for the four different bases, and only 20 different amino acids that are coded for, several amino acids may be coded for by more than one codon. There are also three codons, called *stop codons*, that terminate the transfer of information. Furthermore, although all cells contain the same complement of genes, certain cells (for example, the neurons) have specialized genes that encode specific proteins for the synthesis of specific transmitters. The expression of such genes is under the control of regulatory proteins called transcription factors which control the transcription of mRNAs from the genes they control.

The expression of enzymes that control neurotransmitter systems is controlled not only by factors operating during embryonic development, but also by the degree of neuronal activity. Thus the more active the nervous system, the greater the genetically controlled synthesis of the neurotransmitters which clearly play an important role in the behaviour of the organism. Regulation of the genes also determines the response of the brain to drugs, hence the importance of molecular genetics to psychopharmacology.

One of the most important areas of molecular genetics concerns the role of specific base sequences, called *regulatory sequences*, that surrounded the sections of the gene that encode the amino acid sequence of a protein. These regulatory sequences are activated or inactivated by specific transcription factors and it is the complex interaction of regulatory sequences and transcription factors that underlies the adaptation of brain function to the effects of some psychotropic drugs. For example, it is well known that the optimal response to an antidepressant or neuroleptic drug requires several weeks of treatment. Such adaptive changes are probably a reflection of the molecular genetics of neurotransmitter function and may help to explain the lack of success in developing antidepressants or neuroleptics that have a rapid therapeutic action.

How may genes be manipulated?

One of the main goals of molecular genetics is to determine the base sequence of the human genome. This is the purpose of the Human Genome Project, an international collaborative research programme aimed at providing a complete analysis of the human genome within the next decade. The first step in such an analysis is to isolate the small sequences of bases in DNA that are transcribed into mRNAs. The information contained in the mRNAs can be isolated and amplified by a technique called *cDNA cloning*. In this technique, mRNAs from brain tissue, for example, are purified and then treated with reverse transcriptase which converts mRNAs into single complementary strands of DNA. This is called *complementary DNA* (cDNA). The cDNA provides a template for producing a second strand that is complementary to the first. This double-stranded cDNA is then incubated with bacterial plasmids to produce *recombination DNA plasmids*. Plasmids may be considered as bacterial viruses that can reproduce themselves when inserted into the appropriate bacteria so that during the process of bacterial cell division multiple copies of the cDNA that had been inserted in the plasmid are formed. As each bacterium is likely to be infected with a plasmid, containing a different type of cDNA, the resulting medium will contain a mixed population of cDNAs from the original brain tissue. This is called a *cDNA library*.

The individual components of the cDNA library may be obtained by grouping individual bacteria on a culture medium so that they reproduce to form identical clones. This enables a large quantity of specific cDNAs to be produced in a pure form. The cDNA within these plasmid-containing bacteria can then be removed, and the precise nucleotide sequence determined by standard automated analytical procedures.

Since the brain expresses many mRNAs that are also found in non-nervous tissue and are therefore of little interest to the psycho-pharmacologist, it is necessary to isolate only those cDNAs that, for example, encode for a specific enzyme or receptor protein. Several techniques have been developed to achieve this. For example, a specific cDNA plasmid may be inserted into cultured mammalian cells such as fibroblasts that can express the specific receptor or enzyme. Once this has been expressed in the culture medium, the receptor or enzyme can be identified by adding a specific ligand or substrate. This enables those cells that expressed the specific macromolecule of interest to be identified and

Brain mRNAs

    Reverse transcriptase transcribes these different mRNAs into single complementary strands of DNA

$$\downarrow$$

Single-stranded brain cDNAs formed

    Single-stranded cDNAs form template for double-stranded DNA

$$\downarrow$$

Double-stranded brain cDNAs formed

    Double-stranded cDNAs added to bacterial plasmids that insert the cDNA into the plasmid

$$\downarrow$$

Recombinant DNA plasmid containing the brain DNA

    Recombinant DNA then inserted into bacteria which reproduce the brain DNA

$$\downarrow$$

cDNA library formed with each bacterium multiplying the specific cDNA it contains

$$\downarrow$$

Individual bacteria isolated and cultured to produce clones that yield specific cDNAs

    Specific cDNAs (for example a receptor) inserted in plasmid that transfects a mammalian cell (e.g. fibroblasts) in culture

$$\downarrow$$

Mammalian cell containing the specific cDNA then exposed in a culture medium to a toxin which destroys all non-transformed mammalian cells

    Add radioligand that identifies the receptor of the mammalian cell

$$\downarrow$$

Identification and isolation of transformed cells which can then be cultured to provide unlimited quantities of the receptor protein

Figure 5.1.   Summary of principal methods used in molecular genetics.

subsequently isolated. Once a particular cDNA has been isolated in this way it can be used to make unlimited quantities of the macromolecule whose sequence it encodes. As mammalian cells are generally used for this method of amplification, the amino acid sequence is the same as that used in the limbic brain. Furthermore, if, for example, the cDNA encodes a neurotransmitter receptor, it is likely that it will be integrated into the plasma membrane of the cell surface and therefore largely reflect the portion of the receptor in the neuron. This enables such receptor-containing cells to be used for screening the affinity of putative psychotropic drugs on receptors that were derived from human brain. This method is now commonly used in the pharmaceutical industry to screen numerous compounds for their potential therapeutic application: for example, screening compounds for their affinity for the human D_4 receptor as potential atypical neuroleptics.

Another important application of cDNAs is to identify specific proteins in a tissue homogenate or tissue section. Since cDNAs undergo complementary base pairing, adding a radioactively labelled cDNA to a homogenate or tissue slice will bind it to the complementary sequence by a process of *hybridization*. Thus the amount of radioactive cDNA that hybridizes to the tissue or tissue extract is a measure of the amount of mRNA that is complementary to it. When this procedure is undertaken on slices of brain, it is known as *in situ hybridization*. In this way it is possible to determine the distribution of specific receptors in a tissue by accurately determining the distribution of mRNA that encodes for the receptor protein. This is a particularly valuable technique for the administration of psychotropic drugs.

A variety of techniques have now been developed to manipulate gene expression using cDNAs. For example, it is possible to introduce copies of a new gene (in the form of cDNAs) into a cultured cell line by a process of *transfection*. This is achieved by means of plasmids that transfect the human or mammalian cells in culture. Those cells that have had the DNA sequence integrated into their chromosomes can then be separated from those cells in which integration has not occurred by incubating the mixed cell population with a toxin to which the engineered cells are resistant whereas the normal cells are not. In this way clones of cells that contain the new genetic material can eventually be isolated.

A major advance in this technique has arisen through the development of *transgenic mice*. This technique involves injecting foreign DNA into the genome of the mouse embryo. As a consequence, the foreign DNA can give rise to a line of mice that contain the foreign DNA. Using this technique, mice have now been produced whose brains express the A4 protein – a marker for Alzheimer's disease. A variant of this technique is to replace a normal gene with a foreign gene in the chromosome, thereby giving rise to a progeny that lack both the normal gene and its function. Sibling mating then gives rise to offspring which have two defective genes. This method has so far largely been confined to mice which are termed "knock-out" mice. This method could prove to be particularly useful for determining the physiological role of specific neurotransmitter receptors.

Pharmacogenetics and psychopharmacology

For more than 40 years, epidemiological studies have clearly demonstrated a tendency for diseases such as schizophrenia, bipolar disorder and autism to run in families. Thus it has been shown that such disorders are much more frequent in close relatives of patients than in the general population. For example, estimates of the increased risk of suffering from the disorder if the patient has a sibling with the disorder range from nine- to eleven-fold for schizophrenia and about sevenfold for those with bipolar disorder. These major psychiatric disorders show a significantly greater concordance rate in genetically identical twins. Thus the concordance rate for monozygotic twins in schizophrenia is approximately three times that observed in dizygotic twins. In bipolar disorder, the corresponding concordance rate is approximately eight times greater in monozygotic than in dizygotic twins. From such studies it has been calculated that between 60 and 80% of the liability of these two disorders is genetic in origin. However, it must be emphasized that these calculations do not identify specific genetic causes for the conditions but they do demonstrate that the genetic, as well as environmental components, play a significant role.

The question arises regarding how the genes that contribute to major psychiatric disorders can be identified. Many of the medical conditions for which a genetic component has been identified follow a genetic pattern that clearly follows classical Mendelian inheritance. For example, in cases of Huntington's disease and cystic fibrosis, the two parents who carry the recessive gene give rise to offspring in the ratio of 1:2:1, one expressing the disease, two not showing the symptoms but carrying the gene and one not carrying the gene for the disorder. Such conditions follow the Mendelian pattern of inheritance because the condition is caused by a mutation of a single gene. While the locating of the underlying gene in such situations is often difficult and time-consuming, the techniques of classical molecular genetic analysis, and linkage studies followed by positional cloning, are now well established. For monogenic diseases such as Huntington's, a common pattern emerges in which a single gene, or small number of genes, that may harbour a number of rare mutations can be identified. Each mutation alone is then sufficient to produce a phenotype of the disease.

Regarding bipolar disorder and schizophrenia, while there is some evidence that some families transmit the risk of the disease in a Mendelian fashion, the overall pattern of disease transmission is complex and it is unlikely that these conditions are due to a single gene. This suggests that there may be multiple genes involved, either many genes with strong alleles or common variants in many genes, each of which increases the risk of the disease in a modest way. An example of this would be Alzheimer's disease, in which significant associations have been demonstrated between apolipoprotein (APO) E_4 and the occurrence of the disease. An account of the genetic basis of Alzheimer's disease can provide a useful example of the relationship between the genetic basis and the expression of the disease.

Alzheimer's disease exists in two major forms, the so-called early and late onset types. The former follows typical Mendelian inheritance while the latter shows a more complex, non-Mendelian, pattern of inheritance. The early onset form of the disease has permitted the identification of several genes which are causally related to the condition.

In the elderly, in which Alzheimer's disease has been estimated to occur in up to 20% of those aged 80 years, it has been shown that one allelic form of APO E is associated with an increased risk for developing the disease. Of the three APO E allelic forms in man, APO E_4 is associated with the late onset form of the disease; this may account for up to 50% of the genetic risk for the late onset form whereas those carrying the less frequent E_2 allele appear to be protected from the disease.

In the early onset familial form of the disease, affecting approximately 5% of cases, there is a clear autosomal dominant pattern of inheritance. Mutations in three genes have been identified involving the beta amyloid precursor protein, presenilin-1 and presenilin-2. The function of these proteins is described in more detail in the chapter on the dementias (Chapter 14). It has been estimated that mutations in these genes account for approximately 50% of the cases of the early onset disease.

Summary of methods used to detect possible genetic defects in psychiatric disorders

The genetic basis of late onset Alzheimer's disease conforms to the common disease–common variant hypothesis which states that genetic susceptibility is attributable to common variants present in the population at a high frequency. Significant associations have been demonstrated between several common polymorphisms such as APO E_4 and Alzheimer's disease, already referred to. Individuals differ from each other at many positions across the genome and a variation at a particular nucleotide is called a polymorphism. It has been calculated that approximately one nucleotide base in every 1000–2000 nucleotides differs between chromosomes. If, as seems likely, the common disease–common variant hypothesis applies to schizophrenia and bipolar disorder then it may be essential to undertake association studies which follow the inheritance of a gene within a population rather than within families. Association studies test if a polymorphism is more frequently found in those with the disease (called "cases") than in normal individuals (controls). In such tests, the transmission of a polymorphism from a heterozygous parent to an affected offspring is followed. If the polymorphisms are not associated with the disease, then the rate of transmission from parent to affected offspring in a population will be 50%. Significant deviations from this predicted transmission rate indicate a possible association with the disease. Such studies are an attractive means to understanding complex psychiatric diseases because they have the power to identify causal associations between a particular allele and a heterogeneous disease and do not require the collection of large pedigrees containing multiple affected individuals. However, for such a method to be applied, the polymorphisms used in the assessments must have been identified. This necessitates the collection of a large group of polymorphisms to form a library of potential disease-causing alleles. Traditionally techniques for the detection of polymorphisms have involved gel-based screening methods or direct DNA sequencing of numerous individuals. Such methods are laborious and time-consuming. Microarray technology has revolutionized the approach by developing DNA microchips that contain a high density of oligonucleotides which are capable of rapidly detecting variations in nucleotide sequences. Micro-arrays consist of microchips of DNA attached to the surface of a solid support that may vary according to the density and the form, or size, of the DNA on the surface. There are different commercially available forms of microarray chips and the presence of many independent DNA molecules on the chip surface allows hybridization of many different species simultaneously and for the results to be similarly detected on a microscope slide. By labelling the final products formed with a fluorescent dye, the resulting hybridization pattern can be detected by a confocal microscope.

The major question which arises now that the technology for rapid screening has become available is which genes should be chosen? If the possible cause of the disease is known then the answer is clear. However, for most of the major psychiatric disorders the causes are unknown although neurochemical, neurodevelopmental, autoimmune and environ-mental factors are probably involved. For this reason, association studies in schizophrenia and bipolar disorder have focused on genes related to the dopaminergic and serotonergic systems. Unfortunately, polymorphisms related to these genes have not convincingly been found to be associated with schizophrenia or bipolar disorder. However, several other lines of evidence suggest that schizophrenia may be a neurodevelopmental disorder in which the frontal association cortex, an area responsible for several important high-level functions, has been shown to be malfunctional. Thus schizophrenia may result from a disorder of neuronal migration. If so, the discovery of polymorphisms in genes that regulate cortical development could prove to be a useful area of investigation. This approach has already identified the gene *dsh* (dishevelled, named after a gene identified in the fruit fly, Drosophila) in the mouse which, when absent, leads to a reduction in the startle response. Prepulse inhibition, the reduction in the startle that the animal shows to a previous stimulus, has been shown to be diminished in patients with schizophrenia. While it is premature to propose that *dsh* deficient mice are a model for schizophrenia, such findings do suggest that such genes may play an important role in the early differentiation of the brain. During the normal development of the brain, a large number of genes are activated and become involved at different times and have different functions. In the early pattern formation of the brain, during the development of the neural tube, the homeotic genes (the so-called *hox* family genes) encode for transcriptional factors that bind to DNA and thereby regulate the expression of other genes. This process is believed to convey information on dorsoventral positioning to the cells of the developing neural tube. However, there is evidence that a mutation in a homeobox gene is associated with gross brain defects which makes it unlikely that a mutation in the early genes could be responsible for the subtle changes found in schizophrenia.

There is evidence that the cortex of the brain of schizophrenic patients contains neurons that are in abnormal positions when compared to non-schizophrenic individuals. This suggests that the migration of neurons may be abnormal during the developmental period. The neuronal cell adhesion molecule (NCAM) is an immunoglobulin that mediates adhesion between neurons, thereby exerting a key role in morphogenesis, differentiation and the migration of neurons. NCAM is encoded by a single gene that undergoes alternative splicing to generate several alleles which exhibit different spatial and temporal patterns of expression in vertebrates. The NCAM gene is located on chromosome 11 and two polymorphisms are known to occur in the NCAM gene region. However linkage analysis of 71 families has failed to confirm that an abnormality in the NCAM gene occurs in schizophrenia.

During brain development, neurons send out numerous dendrites in which growth factors play a prominent part. The neurotrophins comprise a family of structurally and functionally related growth factors that include nerve growth factor (NGF), brain derived neurotrophic factor (BDNF) and the neurotrophins 3 and 4/5. These peptides cause neuronal growth, increase the size of the body of the neuron and maintain the survival of the neurons of the dopaminergic, serotonergic and glutaminergic systems. As a decrease of 20–30% in BDNF mRNA has been reported to occur in the hippocampi of schizophrenic patients, it seems possible that a defect in this growth factor could be responsible for the occurrence of smaller neurons in these patients. The BDNF gene is located on chromosome 11 and preliminary findings from 72 nuclear families suggest that the frequency of the A2 allele is significantly higher, and that of the A1 allele significantly lower, in schizophrenic patients. The NT-3 gene, located on chromosome 12, and the promoter region of this gene contain a highly polymorphic marker yielding at least 11 dinucleotide repeat alleles. Of the case-controlled association studies undertaken so far, abnormal alleles have been reported in two of the five studies.

Lastly, studies on the different polymorphic forms of the synapsins, that organize the mobilization of neurotransmitter vesicles thereby regulating neurotransmitter release, could account for some of the subtle changes in neurotransmission that occur in schizophrenia. However, to date linkage analysis studies have failed to reveal any positive associations between the various polymorphisms of the synapsin gene and schizophrenia.

The genetic basis of obsessive–compulsive disorder (OCD)

There have been over 18 family studies of OCD during the past 70 years but, due to methodological differences, the familial aspects of the disorder remain controversial. Family studies look for the prevalence of the disorder among the biological relatives of the probands (i.e. individuals who are affected by OCD) and the prevalence is then compared with that seen in the general population or in a control group. The latter are usually unaffected subjects or relatives of those with OCD. Despite the limitations of the studies, most have found a significant increase in the rates of OCD among the first-degree relatives of the probands when compared with the general population. Similarly, there is evidence from family studies of patients with chronic motor tics and Tourette syndrome that the rates of these conditions, and OCD, are higher among the relatives of patients with Tourette syndrome. More recent studies have suggested that some of these cases are familial but unrelated to tics while in other cases there appears to be no family history of either OCD or tics.

Twin studies comparing mono- and dizygotic twins have shown concordance rates of between 25 and 87%, depending on the study. Since none of the studies show a concordance rate of 100%, it is clear that non-genetic factors must influence the expression of OCD.

Linkage analysis studies, in which the OCD is linked to a known polymorphic marker, are used to determine if there is a single gene locus causing susceptibility for the disorder. Using such an approach for a battery of candidate genes coding for receptors and enzymes involved in dopaminergic and serotonergic transmission (i.e. for the two neurotrans-mitters most likely to be involved in OCD), no evidence was found for a link.

Association studies have proven to be more fruitful. In such studies, the allelic frequencies for specific marker genes are compared with a control population. When OCD patients were investigated for the association of tics with the dopamine receptor 2 marker it was shown that there was an increased frequency of homozygosity for the allele A2 of TaqIA at the D_2 receptor locus. Not all investigators could replicate this finding however. No positive associations have been found between OCD and the D_3 gene while there was some association found between OCD with tics and the D_4

gene. Two other catecholaminergic markers have been investigated in patients with OCD. Thus a positive association has been reported between the low activity allele of catechol-O-methyl transferase in male patients and a higher frequency of the low activity allele of monoamine oxidase type A gene in female patients. There is also evidence that the serotonin transporter gene is abnormal. In conclusion, evidence from genetic studies lends support to the view that a single gene defect occurs in patients with OCD while association studies of candidate genes, in spite of methodological difficulties, have highlighted the loci for D_2 and D_4 receptor genes together with those for catechol-O-methyl-transferase and monoamine oxidase A.

Genetics of panic disorder

Studies assessing the diagnosis of panic disorder by the direct interview of family members, a method commonly employed in the 1980s, showed that the risk of developing the disorder is higher in the first-degree probands. This has been estimated to be 17% for first-degree relatives compared to 2% for the control population. In addition, relatives of probands had a higher prevalence of generalized anxiety disorder and major depression. This was confirmed in another study of anxiety disorders in female relatives and showed a morbidity risk for all anxiety disorders to be 32% among first-degree relatives of agoraphobic patients with panic attacks and 33% in those with panic disorder. The risk was found to be even greater in the offspring when both had anxiety disorders. Overall, family studies have shown that first-degree relatives of probands with panic disorder have a three- to 21-fold higher risk of developing panic disorder than first-degree relatives of healthy probands.

The relationships between panic disorder and other types of anxiety disorder have also been the subject of study. Thus some investigators have reported that relatives of those with agoraphobia have a higher risk for the disorder than relatives of patients with panic disorder, leading to the suggestion that agoraphobia should be considered a more severe form of panic disorder which has an independent genetic transmission. Other studies, however, have found that the diagnosis of separation anxiety and agoraphobia in probands increased the risk of both panic disorder and agoraphobia in the relatives of the patients. Such observations support the hypothesis that panic disorder and agoraphobia are two phenotypic expressions of the same condition due to a different degree of genetic penetrance.

The analysis of the relationship between panic disorder and major depression has produced conflicting results. The possible link between these disorders has been provided by the frequent occurrence of major depression in patients with panic disorder and agoraphobia, both conditions responding to antidepressant treatments. Whereas most of the genetic analyses available suggest that there is an independent genetic basis for these conditions, it is noteworthy that relatives of patients with both panic disorder and agoraphobia are more likely to develop depression, phobias and alcoholism when compared with relatives of probands with panic disorder alone. There does not appear to be an association between generalized anxiety disorder and panic disorder, suggesting that they are separate entities. Generalized anxiety disorder appears to be more prevalent (approximately 20%) in relatives of probands with the disorder than in those of relatives with panic disorder (5%) or agoraphobia (4%).

Twin studies have demonstrated only a moderate concordance in monozygotic versus dizygotic pairs. Using the hypersensitivity to carbon dioxide as a challenge test, it has been shown that there is a significantly higher concordance rate in monozygotic (56%) than in dizygotic (13%) twins.

In recent years, emphasis has tended to switch from family and twin studies to molecular genetics. Linkage analysis in families with a psychiatric disorder has often proven to be a fruitful method to determine the degree of inheritance of a disorder. The method of parametric linkage estimates the likelihood of the distribution of genetic markers of an illness by a predetermined model and expressed as the logarithm of the odds score (the so-called lod score). For simple Mendelian inheritance of a disease, a lod score of 3.0 or greater, obtained by scanning the genome for markers of the disease, is considered to be a statistically significant linkage. However, most psychiatric disorders do not follow classical Mendelian genetics so such an approach is of limited value. For this reason, other linkage methods have been developed. For example, the allelic-sharing method is based on detecting the frequency of the inheritance of the same genetic marker from each parent. The presence of a gene that causes the disorder is revealed when the allele that is shared between the siblings is greater than 50%. To date, all the linkage studies in panic disorder have been inconclusive. Neither has the search for candidate genes for neurotransmitters (for example, GABA, tyrosine hydroxylase, serotonin receptors, dopamine receptors, adrenoceptors, opioid receptors) proven to be any more fruitful. However, there is some preliminary evidence for an association between the cholecytokinin (CCK) promoter gene and panic disorder which, if replicated, would support the hypothesis that the CCK-B receptor is hypersensitive in panic disorder. This is discussed in more detail in Chapter 9.

Genetics of attention deficit/hyperactivity disorder (ADHD)

ADHD is the most common psychiatric disorder with onset in childhood. The condition is characterized by inattention and/or hyperactivity and impulsivity which is associated with cognitive, social and academic impairments. It has been estimated that in up to 60% of patients, these impairments persist into adulthood. Males are affected more than females (4:1).

ADHD is a familial disorder with a population-based prevalence of about 10% and a prevalence rate in siblings of approximately 25%. Detailed studies of the disorder suggest that there is a five- to sixfold increase in first-degree relatives of affected persons. However, as with other psychiatric disorders, the finding of familial aggregation alone does not necessarily lead to the conclusion that the disorder is of genetic origin as such studies do not separate genetic from environmental factors.

Twin studies have been useful in discriminating the genetic from environmental factors. The concordance rate for monozygotic versus dizygotic twins has been estimated at 51% and 33% respectively, and it has been estimated that approximately half the variance in the trait factors of hyperactivity and inattentiveness are accounted for by the genetic basis of the disorder. There is evidence that, in ADHD, there is an incompletely penetrant autosomal-dominant gene; the penetrance of the gene being calculated as 46% in boys and 31% in girls.

Molecular genetic studies have been particularly fruitful in evaluating the neurochemical basis of the disorder. Genes involved in the dopaminergic system were considered to be important as the most effective symptomatic treatment of the condition has been methylphenidate and dextroamphetamine, drugs which potentiate the release, and inhibit the reuptake, of dopamine. In addition, the involvement of dopamine in ADHD is further implicated by the increased vulnerability of these patients to drug abuse. As discussed in Chapter 15, the dopaminergic system has been implicated in reward mechanisms so the search for abnormalities in the genes encoding for different aspects of them seems a reasonable start.

Of the genes for the dopamine receptors which have been studied, the candidate gene for the dopamine D_4 receptor has been shown to be positively associated with ADHD. However, not all investigators have verified this finding.

One of the major limitations in studies of the genetics of behavioural disorders in children arises from the overlap with other conditions. For example, nearly 50% of the patients with ADHD also have co-morbid conduct disorders. In addition, a subtype of the disorder may exist in those children in which the disorder persists into adulthood. An additional problem arises from the overlap between ADHD and bipolar disorder; this has been estimated to be as high as 16%.

In CONCLUSION, although positive genetic studies have been reported and subsequently replicated, the results must be treated with caution as they are based on small sample sizes with restricted statistical power and complicated by co-morbid illnesses. Nevertheless, preliminary evidence suggests that ADHD, like many major psychiatric disorders, does have a genetic basis.

The impact of molecular neurobiology on psychopharmacology: from genes to drugs

About 150 years ago, Charles Darwin observed that "those who make many species are the 'splitters', and those who make few are the 'lumpers'''. Today, the "splitters" dominate research in the life sciences. Such researchers can generate massive quantities of data on genes and their networks, proteins and their pathways and the numerous cascades of messenger molecules that ultimately result in a physiological response. Technological progress in recent years has enabled the genome of species as diverse as the nematode worm *Caenorhabditis elegans* and the fruit fly *Drosophila melanogaster* to the mouse and man to be unravelled, thereby opening up the possibility not only of identifying genes that are responsible for physiological processes but also those that are aberrant and cause genetically based diseases.

Few would deny the importance of such research, but the very success of the "splitters" has had a seriously detrimental effect on the equally important role of the "lumpers", who attempt to integrate the molecular/cellular approach with the behavioural/psychological consequences. As a consequence, the "lumpers" are becoming a threatened species of researchers. There are several reasons for this, not the least of which is the widespread opposition to vivisection and the lack of training in behavioural pharmacology in university courses. As a consequence, research (and funding for behavioural research) has declined in prestige. This has had an adverse impact not only in areas of basic life science research but also in the pharmaceutical industry where the ultimate validation of the therapeutic potential of a new molecule depends on behavioural pharmacology. As a senior neuropharmacologist has recently remarked "Many can genotype but few can phenotype".

Despite this unfortunate disparity between molecular neurobiology and behavioural pharmacology, it is essential that the neuropharmacologist and biological psychiatrist are fully conversant with the basic concepts of the subject in order to appreciate both its success and limitations.

An outline of the terminology

Pick up any intelligent newspaper or magazine, view any television programme dealing with the life sciences or medicine, and the impact of cloning is likely to be discussed. To understand the basis of cloning, it is necessary to consider how bacteria have evolved to resist infection by external sources of genetic material. It has long been recognized that if a virus could infect one strain of bacteria, it could then also infect other bacteria of the same strain but not those of a different strain. Thus virus infection was shown to be restricted to a particular strain, a restriction now known to be due to two classes of enzyme, namely the methylases, which modify bacterial DNA marking them as "self", and the destruction enzymes, which act as molecular "scissors" and can destroy foreign DNA.

Restriction enzymes are sequence-specific in that they cut DNA at specific locations along the nucleotide chain. While some of these enzymes yield "blunt" ends to the resulting DNA fragment, others make staggered cuts in the DNA chain to produce "sticky" ends. Over 250 restriction enzymes are now commercially available.

Cloning would not be possible without restriction enzymes. DNA chains with a "sticky" end act like molecular "Velcro", thereby enabling two pieces of DNA with complementary nucleotide sequences to be joined together. The linking of the DNA strands is brought about by the enzyme DNAligase which permanently joins the assembled DNA sequences with covalent bonds, thereby producing a recombinant DNA molecule.

The next stage is to ensure that the recombinant DNA molecule is copied by the enzymes which synthesize nucleic acids. These DNA and RNA polymerases synthesize an exact copy of either DNA or RNA from a pre-existing molecule. In this way the DNA polymerase duplicates the chromosome before each cell division such that each daughter cell will have a complete set of genetic instructions which are then passed to the newly formed RNA by RNA polymerase. While both DNA and RNA polymerase require a preformed DNA template, some viruses (such as HIV) have an RNA genome. To duplicate that genome, and incorporate it into a bacterial or mammalian cell, the viruses encode a reverse transcriptase enzyme which produces a DNA copy from an RNA template.

Thermostable DNA polymerases have now been produced for polymerase chain reaction (PCR) studies in which specific segments of the DNA molecule can be mass produced from minute quantities of material. RNA polymerases are then used to create RNA transcripts from cloned genes in vitro. Reverse transcriptases have their specific uses in molecular biology. These enzymes are used to form "cDNA libraries" which are batteries of molecules each one representing a single gene expression. Such DNA libraries can then be analysed to determine which genes are active under different conditions and in different tissues. cDNA libraries are now used experimentally in microarray assemblies to detect gene changes following drug treatment. This will be discussed further later in this chapter.

In a typical experimental situation, the gene of interest is incorporated into a plasmid, which is a natural vector used by either a bacterium or other cell type. To transfer the DNA fragment of a gene, the plasmids are digested with one or two restriction enzymes and the desired fragment joined into a single DNA recombinant molecule using DNA ligase. To express the new gene *in vitro*, the plasmid containing the recombinant DNA is then incubated with an RNA polymerase to form new RNA which is then used to programme an *in vitro* system which translates the information necessary for the synthesis of a new protein.

The foregoing is only intended to give a brief overview of the mechanisms behind cloning. So far, the impact on diseases in man has been limited to experimental approaches to the treatment of cystic fibrosis and rare conditions in which a recessive gene is responsible. However, cloning techniques have provided important information in producing animals, usually mice, which have been manipulated to express or remove genes that are implicated in psychiatric disorders. Such "knock-out" and "knock-in" mice now provide important information in which specific genes can be studied for their effects on behaviour, which may ultimately be an important contribution to understanding the genetic basis of psychiatric and neurological diseases.

Genetically modified mice and their importance in psychopharmacology

Just as adding genes from a complex to a simpler organism (for example, from man to a fruit fly) may be helpful in understanding the function of a gene, so it may help to understand how a gene functions by eliminating it. To date, most gene "knock-out" studies have been undertaken in mice because of:

(a) the relative ease with which genes can be manipulated and eliminated;
(b) the relatively rapid rate at which mice breed;
(c) their well established and relatively complex behaviour.

The success, and also the limitations of the gene elimination strategy can be illustrated by studies on the molecular basis of memory and learning. In the early 1980s it had been shown that the glutamate NMDA receptor was an essential component of memory formation, the term "long-term potentiation" (LTP) being applied to the molecular mechanism involved. The drugs which were then available were limited in their specificity for the NMDA receptor but by selectively deleting genes thought to be involved in memory it was possible to identify the precise components of the NMDA-linked messenger complex located in the hippocampus. Further studies enabled genes ranging from those encoding neurotransmitter receptors, protein kinases and transcription factors to be identified. However, there are limitations to these techniques which should be considered.

A major problem with "knock-out" technology relates to the need to delete the gene at the very early stage of embryonic development. Often this results in the death of the neonate. Even if the gene is not essential for survival, it could have a key role to play in development that is unrelated to neuronal plasticity. Thus the deficits in learning and memory seen in the mature mouse could be the result of a developmental defect rather than a specific abnormality in the NMDA receptor complex. Alternatively, the deletion of a gene that from experimental studies might be expected to have a major effect on learning and memory in practice may have no apparent effect. This is due to the mechanism of compensation whereby other genes take over the function of the deleted gene.

Thus developing "knock-out" mice to understand the function of a particular gene gives little information on the timing when the gene becomes active. Nor does it necessarily reflect the location of the gene in the intact (wild-type) mouse or indeed, the long-term effect of the nervous system on its function. Nevertheless, these are largely technical drawbacks that will undoubtedly shortly be solved. In principle, studying the actions of psychotropic drugs on genetically modified animals will allow the detrimental effects of a deleted gene on the general health of the animal to be avoided. Such an approach will also allow investigations of the interactions between neuronal signalling pathways by assessing the synergistic interactions between the behavioural and other biological effects of the deleted gene and drugs.

The importance of genomics to psychopharmacology

Virtually every physical and psychiatric disorder has a genetic component. However, the vast majority of these diseases have a complex pattern of inheritance and there is no evidence that a single genetic locus is responsible for any of the major psychiatric disorders. Rather it appears that multiple alleles (gene products) occurring at multiple sites within the genome interact to produce a vulnerability to the disorder. The enthusiastic reception for the unravelling of the human genome rests largely on the promise that it will soon lead to an understanding of the pathological basis of most diseases which, in turn, will aid the development of more effective therapeutic treatments.

Following the sequencing of the human genome it was found that there were between 30 000 and 40 000 genes that code for proteins, only twice as many as occur in the fruit fly or the nematode worm! However, it does appear that human genes are more complex than those of flies and worms in that they generate a large number of proteins due to the alternative ways of splicing the molecules. Hopefully knowledge of the human genome will enable genes to be identified that convey a risk for psychiatric diseases in addition to those genes which are linked to a therapeutic response to drug treatment. Knowledge of the latter forms the basis of pharmacogenomics which, hopefully, will eventually lead to the development of specific treatments for the individual patient.

The potential value of pharmacogenomics can be illustrated by two examples involving the response of individual patients to antidepressants. In this approach, the potential importance of the cDNA microarray technique for identifying changes in thousands of individual genes that are expressed in the mouse brain is now widely accepted. Experimental studies have indicated that different antidepressants exert distinct effects on gene expression in the mouse brain, these differences becoming more marked as the duration of the treatment increased. Such findings may eventually lead to an individualized treatment strategy for depressed patients based upon their cDNA analysis.

At the practical clinical level, individual differences in the pharmaco-kinetic characteristics of antidepressant drugs have been more successful. It is well established that the enzymatic activity of different allelic forms of the cytochrome P450 oxidase system in the liver is particularly important in the metabolism of many psychotropic and non-psychotropic drugs (see pp. 91–94). Of the major forms of cytochrome P450 in man, the 2D6 isozyme is particularly important in the metabolism of antidepressants and a potential cause of drug interactions. Three of the five commonly available SSRI antidepressants (fluoxetine, paroxetine and sertraline) undergo autoinhibition of this isozyme and can therefore increase the tissue concentration of a more toxic drug (for example, an antiarrhythmic or beta-blocker) should it be given concurrently.

Over 50 allelic variants of the cytochrome P450 2D6 gene have been identified, including individuals who lack the gene and others who have multiple copies of the gene. This means that an individual (the functional genotype) can either be normal, a slow or an ultra-fast metabolizer of a drug that passes through the 2D6 pathway in the liver. Slow metabolizers will therefore be at an increased risk for adverse effects while the rapid metabolizers will have little benefit from the normal doses. Thus genotyping the enzymes that metabolize the commonly used psychotropic drugs could help to optimize the response, and to indicate the potential for adverse drug effects, of the individual patient.

A new term has recently been introduced to cover the application of pharmacogenomics to the design of drugs for the individual patient, namely theranostics (from therapeutics+diagnostics). This approach involves creating tests that can identify which patients are most suited to a particular therapy and also to provide information on how effective this drug is in optimizing the treatment. Theranostics is said to adopt a broad dynamic and integrated approach to therapeutics which may be of practical relevance in differentiating diseases which are closely associated diagnostically (for example, Alzheimer's disease and Lewy body dementia) by applying a combination of immunoassays that enhance the differential diagnosis. Several biotechnological companies now specialize in designing immunoassays for application to infectious diseases such as hepatitis by genotyping the hepatitis C virus for example. There are six genotypes of the virus known: genotype 1 is more resistant to standard therapy (requiring at least one year of continuous therapy) whereas the other genotypes usually respond to treatment within 6 months. Clearly a knowledge of which viral genotype is present is important in determining the duration of treatment in the individual patient and hopefully it will soon be possible to extend such approaches to the drug treatment of central nervous system disorders.

Applying pharmacogenomics to the pharmacodynamic aspects of psychopharmacology is still at a very early stage of development, largely because so little is known of the psychopathological basis of the major psychiatric disorders or of the mechanisms whereby psychotropic drugs work. In depression, for example, it is widely assumed that the inhibition of the serotonin transporter on the neuronal membrane is ultimately responsible for the enhanced serotonin function caused by the SSRI antidepressants. The serotonin transporter is structurally complex. The promoter region of the transporter, to which serotonin is linked before it is transported back into the neuron following its release into the synaptic cleft, exists in several polymorphic forms which are broadly categorized into the long and short forms. It is known that when the polymorphic form occurs in which an additional 44 pairs of nucleotide bases are inserted, there is a higher transcription rate and a greater degree of binding of serotonin to the promoter region. The practical importance of this finding is that depressed patients with the long form of the transporter show a better response to SSRIs than those with the short form. In bipolar patients, there is an indication that the short form of the promoter is more likely to result in the precipitation of a manic episode if given an SSRI during the depressive phase of the disorder. There is also some evidence that the short and long forms of the transporter may be correlated with the frequency of extrapyramidal side effects and akathisia, which is sometimes caused by SSRIs.

There are two caveats that should be taken into account with regard to the application of pharmacogenomics. Drug response is as complex as the underlying genetic basis of the disease due not only to the genotypic variation taking place at mostly unknown chromosomal loci, but also from variations in gene expression, post-translational modification of proteins, pharmacokinetic features of the drugs, the effect of diet, drug interactions, etc. One would therefore anticipate that the effects of individual genes on the drug response are relatively slight. Thus it has been shown in studies of pharmacogenetic markers that they only confer a twofold increased likelihood of predicting drug response. However, the widespread application of microarray technology, whereby information on thousands of genes can be determined simultaneously, may help to overcome the limitations of the candidate gene approach, the method which until now has been used to obtain information on a few genes presumed to be involved in the underlying pathology of a disease or its response to drug treatment.

Another aspect requiring attention concerns the statistical evaluation of the results. For example, recently it has been shown that in a study of asthma one genotype had a 100% positive predictive value for non-response to a drug. However, because the susceptibility genotype only occurs in less than 9% of patients, in practice less than 10% of the non-response to treatment can be attributed to this abnormal genotype. In this case, it has been calculated that avoidance of the drug as a result of pharmacogenomic profiling would only improve its efficacy from 46% to 51%. Thus the reliance on candidate gene variation, which ranges from 2% to 7%, is currently not in the range for practical application.

In CONCLUSION, molecular genetics is providing important tools that enable the physiological role of specific receptors and enzymes to be elucidated. *In situ* hybridization is a powerful technique for locating receptors in specific brain regions and in studying the influence of drug treatment on these receptors. The accuracy, specificity and sensitivity of such a technique is substantially greater than any other available technique. Transgenic mice and "knock-out" mice are also providing valuable models of human disease that have not been obtained by other methods. With regard to psychiatric illnesses, molecular genetic techniques are being used in human genome screening which are designed to locate those genes that may be responsible for bipolar disorder and schizophrenia. By collecting cell lines from family pedigrees, it may be possible to determine the genes that contribute to alcoholism and Alzheimer's disease in addition to those involved in schizophrenia and the affective disorders. This may eventually lead to the identification of new methods for the pharmacotherapy of such conditions.

6 Psychotropic Drugs that Modify the Serotonergic System

Over a century ago, a substance was recognized in clotted blood which was found to cause vasoconstriction. This substance was still present following adrenalectomy therapy suggesting that it differed from adrenaline and noradrenaline. Eventually, Rapaport, Green and Page in 1947, purified the vasoconstrictor factor from serum and identified it as serotonin ("serum tonic"). Independently of the American investigators, Erspamer and colleagues in Italy had identified a substance they termed "enteramine" from the intestine. "Enteramine" was subsequently found to be identical to serotonin and was subsequently synthesized by Hamlin and Fisher in 1951. Chemically, serotonin or enteramine is the indoleamine 5-hydroxytryptamine (5-HT).

Following the isolation and synthesis of serotonin in the early 1950s, there has been increasing interest in the physiological function of this amine. Initially, it was assumed that its main function was that of a peripheral hormone because of the relatively high concentrations that were found in the gastrointestinal tract and blood. Twarog and Page soon showed, however, that it was also present in the mammalian brain thereby suggesting that it may have a neurotransmitter role there. Interest in the physiological role of serotonin in the central nervous system has preoccupied neurobiologists since that time.

The detection of serotonin in nervous and non-nervous tissue was aided by the development of the Falck–Hillarp histochemical technique, a method whereby freeze-dried sections of tissue, when exposed to formaldehyde vapour cause indoleamines to emit a yellow fluorescence. Dahlstrom and Fuxe used this technique to show that the highest concentration of serotonin in the brain is located in the raphé nuclei, projections from these cell bodies ascending to the forebrain via the medial forebrain bundle. Descending fibres were also shown to project to the dorsal and lateral horns and the intermediolateral column of the spinal cord. Detailed observation of the distribution of the serotonergic system in the brain became possible with

Fundamentals of Psychopharmacology. Third Edition. By Brian E. Leonard
© 2003 John Wiley & Sons, Ltd. ISBN 0 471 52178 7

the development of specific antibodies to the amine and the introduction of autoradiographic methods for both the human and rodent brain.

For serotonin to be considered as a neurotransmitter, it was essential to establish that it produced its physiological effects by activating specific receptors located on the intestinal wall, platelet membrane or on nerve cells. A major development occurred in 1957 when Gaddum and Picarelli showed that the action of serotonin on the guinea-pig ileum could be blocked by either phenoxybenzamine (dibenzyline) or morphine. These investigators termed the two types of serotonin receptors on the intestinal wall "D" (for dibenzyline) or "M" (for morphine) receptors, the "M" type receptors being associated with the nerves supplying the intestine that produced contraction of the smooth muscle by facilitating acetylcholine release, while the "D" receptors were located on the smooth muscle wall. More recently, it has been realized that the "D" receptors are widely distributed in the body and coincide with 5-HT$_2$ receptors which, when activated by selective agonists, contract smooth muscle and aggregate platelets. They also occur in synaptosomal membranes where they are possibly associated with postsynaptic membrane structures. By contrast, the "M" receptor has not been unequivocally identified in neuronal membranes. However, increasing evidence now suggests that the peripheral "M" receptor is identical to the 5-HT$_3$ receptor in the brain. Thus in a period of some 20 years, the distribution of serotonin in both nervous and non-nervous tissue has been determined, many of its physiological properties explained and the types of receptors upon which it acts to produce its diverse physiological effects evaluated. The main serotonergic pathways in the human brain are illustrated in Figure 6.1.

5-HT receptor subtypes

Current knowledge of 5-HT receptors has been derived from advances in medicinal chemistry, from the synthesis of ligands that show considerable specificity for subpopulations of 5-HT receptors. The application of such ligands to our understanding of the distribution of the 5-HT receptor subtypes has been largely due to quantitative *in vitro* autoradiographic techniques and the application of such imaging techniques as positron emission tomography. Functional studies undoubtedly lag behind but the development of sophisticated electrophysiological techniques and studies of changes in secondary messenger systems which respond to the binding of selective ligands to the 5-HT receptor subtypes have opened up the probability that the physiological importance of the numerous receptor subtypes will soon be clarified.

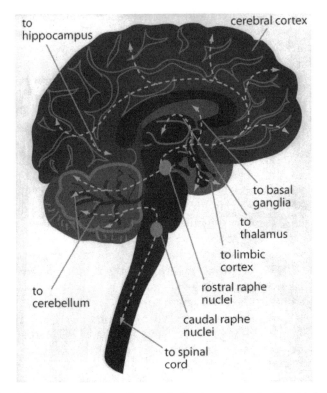

Figure 6.1. Main serotonergic pathways in the human brain. The higher centres of the brain are innervated by the serotonergic tracts originating from the rostral raphé nuclei while the cerebellum and spinal cord are innervated from tracts originating from the caudal raphé.

As a consequence of the application of these various techniques, the International Union of Pharmacological Societies (IUPHAR) Commission on serotonin nomenclature has published two major reports which attempt to classify the various receptor subtypes according to their ligand binding properties and secondary messenger systems. The first report classified 5-HT receptors into 5-HT$_1$-like (comprising 5-HT$_{1A, 1B, 1C}$ and $_{1D}$), 5-HT$_2$ (formerly the 5-HT-D receptor) and 5-HT$_2$ (formerly the 5-HT-M receptor). The detection of a novel 5-HT receptor, that could not be classified as 5-HT$_1$, 5-HT$_2$ or 5-HT$_3$, in both the peripheral and central nervous systems, extended the receptor types to 5-HT$_4$. The application of molecular biology techniques has led to the cloning and sequencing of at least six different 5-HT receptors, namely 5-HT$_{1A}$, 5-HT$_{1B}$, 5-HT$_{1C}$, 5-HT$_{1D}$, 5-HT$_2$ and 5-HT$_3$. Further studies of the second messenger systems to which these receptor subtypes are attached have shown that the 5-HT$_1$-like, 5-HT$_2$ and 5-HT$_4$

receptors belong to the G protein coupled receptor superfamily, whereas the 5-HT$_3$ receptor belongs to the same family as the nicotinic, gamma-aminobutyric acid-A (GABA-A) and glycine receptors which are ion gated channel receptors.

The most recent publication of the IUPHAR Commission has redefined the 5-HT receptor subtypes according to their second messenger associations and thereby helped to stress the functional role of the receptor subtypes rather than relying primarily on the specificities of ligands that bind to them. This approach has led to the classification of 5-HT receptors into those linked to adenylate cyclase (5-HT$_{1A}$, 5-HT$_{1B}$, 5-HT$_{1D}$, 5-HT$_4$), those linked to the phosphatidyl inositol system (5-HT$_{2A}$, 5-HT$_{2B}$ and 5-HT$_{2C}$), and those linked directly to ion channels (5-HT$_3$). Table 6.1 summarizes the accepted classification of the 5-HT receptor subtypes, all of which occur in the brain, together with the most specific agonists and antagonists which have been developed. The structures of the seven subtypes of the serotonin receptor have now been determined. Apart from the ionotropic 5-HT$_3$ receptors (Figure 6.2), the other receptors are of the metabotropic type (Figure 6.3, 5-HT$_2$ receptor). Figure 6.4 illustrates the molecular structure of the 5-HT$_4$ receptor.

More recently, the family of 5-HT receptors has been dramatically increased to include 5-HT$_4$, 5-HT$_{5A}$ and 5-HT$_{5B}$, 5-HT$_6$ and 5-HT$_7$. The 5-HT$_6$ and 5-HT$_7$ receptors are positively linked to adenylate cyclase. Of these, only the 5-HT$_4$ receptor has so far not been cloned. Of these newly discovered receptors, only the 5-HT$_4$ receptor has been investigated in some detail. This receptor is quite widely distributed in the brain and peripheral tissues where they are positively coupled to adenylate cyclase. In the brain, the 5-HT$_4$ receptors facilitate acetylcholine release and may play a role in peristalsis. It has been hypothesized that in the brain 5-HT$_4$ receptors may also play a role in facilitating cholinergic transmission and thereby have a potential role to play in preventing cognitive deficits which are associated with cortical cholinergic malfunction. The possible clinical significance of 5-HT$_4$ receptors must await the development of specific agonists and antagonists. So far, such compounds have not been developed. Figures 6.5, 6.6 and 6.7 illustrate the distribution of 5-HT$_3$, 5-HT$_4$, 5-HT$_6$ and 5-HT$_7$ receptors in the human brain.

Despite the dramatic advances which have taken place in the identification and characterization of 5-HT receptor subtypes, it is evident that many of the ligands used to characterize these receptor subtypes are not completely selective. It must also be emphasized that receptors are the products of genes and are therefore subject to genetic changes and, as a consequence, variability in physiological and pharmacological responsiveness. Thus affinity, potency and intrinsic activity of a drug at one receptor may vary depending on the time, species and receptor–effector coupling. It

Table 6.1. Distribution and selectivity of drugs for 5-HT receptor subtypes

---

$5\text{-}HT_{1A}$ *receptors*
  Hippocampus, septum, amygdala, cortical limbic area
  Agonists: buspirone, gepirone, ipsapirone, flesinoxan
  Antagonists: WAY 100135, BMY 7378, NAN-190
  Possible clinical use of agonists: anxiolytics, antidepressants
$5\text{-}HT_{1B}$ *receptors*
  Substantia nigra, globus pallidus, dorsal subiculum, superior colliculi
  Non-selective: pinodol, propanolol
  ? *selective partial agonists*: CP-93, 129
  Possible clinical use of antagonists: antidepressants
$5\text{-}HT_{1D}$ *receptors*
  Caudate nucleus but widely distributed in human dry and GP brain, similar to
  $5\text{-}HT_{1B}$ of rat brain
  Non-selective: rauwolscine, yohimbine
  ? *selective*: L-694, 247
  Possible clinical use of antagonists: antidepressants
$5\text{-}HT_{1E}$ *receptor*
  In mammalian brain
  Possible clinical use: ?
$5\text{-}HT_{2A}$
  Neocortex but widely distributed in the mammalian brain
  Agonists: DOI, DOB
  Non-selective antagonists: ketanserin, ritanserin
  Possible clinical use of antagonists: antidepressants, anxiolytics, ? neuroleptics
$5\text{-}HT_{2B}$
  In mammalian brain
  Possible clinical use: ?
$5\text{-}HT_{2C}$
  Choroid plexus
  Non-selective antagonists: spiperone, amperozide, pimozide
  Possible clinical use of antagonists: neuroleptics
$5\text{-}HT_3$
  Area postrema, entorhinal and frontal cortex, hippocampus
  Agonists: ondansetron, granisetron, zacopride
  Possible clinical use of antagonists: antiemetics, anxiolytics, ? antidementia
$5\text{-}HT_4$
  Collicular and hippocampal neurons
  Antagonists SC-205-557, SC-53606
  Agonist: SC-49518
  Possible clinical use: ?

8-OHDPAT = Dipropylamino-8-hydroxy-1,2,3,4-tetrahydronaphthylene
RU-24969 = 5-methoxy-3-(1,2,3,6-tetrahydropyridin-4-yl) 1H indol
mCPP   = 1-(3 chlorophenyl) piperazine
TFMPP   = 1-(m-trifluoromethylphenyl) piperazine
DOI   = 1-(2,5-dimethoxy-1-iodophenyl) 2-aminopropane
MDL 73005 = 8,2 (2,3-dihydro-1,4-benzodioxin-2yl) methylamino-ethyl-8-azaspirol (4,5) decan-7,9-dione
NAN 190 = 1-(2-methoxyphenyl) 4-(4(2-phthalimido)entyl-piperazine)
5-CT   = 5-carboxamidotryptamine
ICI 169369 = (2-(2-dimethylamino-ethylthio-3-phenylquinoline))
ICS 205-930 = (3-tropanyl)-IH-indole-2-carboxylic acid ester
DOM   = 2,5-dimethoxy-4-dimethylbenzene ethamine

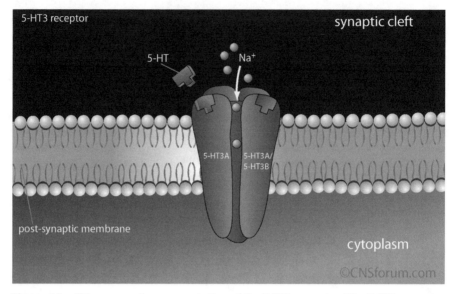

Figure 6.2. Diagrammatic representation of the 5-HT$_3$ receptor. The 5-HT$_3$ receptor is distinct from the other 5-HT receptor subtypes, in that it is a ligand gated ion channel that is permeable to sodium and potassium. The 5-HT$_3$ receptor is structurally similar to the nicotinic acetylcholine receptor and is composed of five sub-units. Two sub-units have been cloned, 5-HT$_{3A}$ and 5-HT$_{3B}$, and homomeric (5-HT$_{3A}$) and heteromeric (5-HT$_{3A}$/5-HT$_{3B}$) forms of the receptor have both been characterized.

is already known, for example, that ipsapirone, buspirone, spiroxatrine and lysergic acid diethylamide (LSD) may behave either as agonists or antagonists depending on the functional model being used to assess their activity. A similar problem arises with intrinsic activity which is usually assumed to be a direct reflection of the pharmacological properties of the drug. It seems possible that the affinity can also be influenced by the nature of the genetically determined receptor–effector coupling and is therefore tissue (and species) dependent. Such factors may help to explain why the identification and subclassification of 5-HT receptor subtypes is complex and often confusing.

This dilemma can be illustrated by the attempts being made to identify the functional role of 5-HT receptor subtypes using ligands which are believed to be specific in their binding properties. Such ligands may prove to be non-selective, more selective for an as yet unidentified 5-HT receptor subtype or more selective for a non-5-HT receptor site. Conversely several non-5-HT ligands are known to bind to 5-HT receptors with a high affinity. For example, the alpha$_1$ adrenoceptor antagonist WB4101, and the beta adrenoceptor antagonist pindolol, have a high affinity to 5-HT$_{1A}$ receptors.

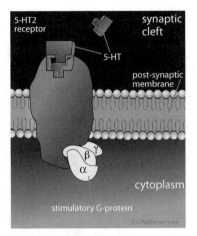

Figure 6.3. Diagrammatic representation of the 5-HT$_2$ receptor. The 5-HT$_2$ receptor consists of three subtypes (5-HT$_{2A,2B}$ and $_{2C}$). All are metabotropic in their action but have different physiological properties (see text for details).

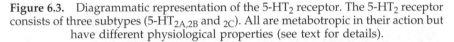

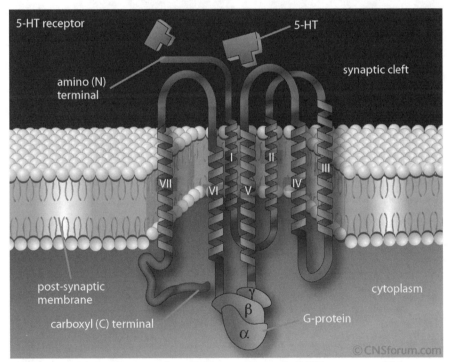

Figure 6.4. Molecular structure of the metabotropic 5-HT$_4$ receptor. This seven-membrane spanning structure is typical of most metabotropic neurotransmitter receptors.

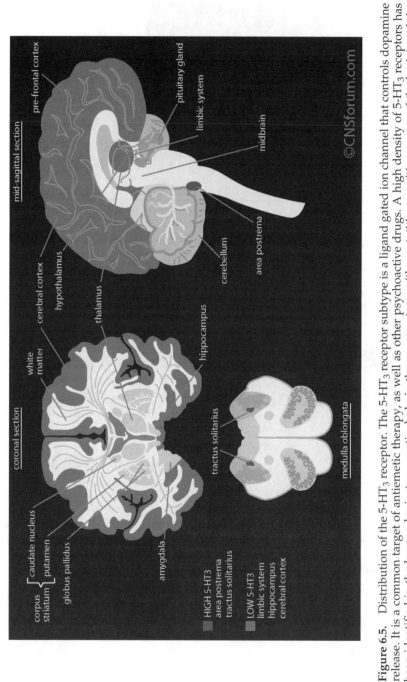
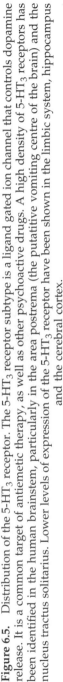

Figure 6.5. Distribution of the 5-HT$_3$ receptor. The 5-HT$_3$ receptor subtype is a ligand gated ion channel that controls dopamine release. It is a common target of antiemetic therapy, as well as other psychoactive drugs. A high density of 5-HT$_3$ receptors has been identified in the human brainstem, particularly in the area postrema (the putatitive vomiting centre of the brain) and the nucleus tractus solitarius. Lower levels of expression of the 5-HT$_3$ receptor have been shown in the limbic system, hippocampus and the cerebral cortex.

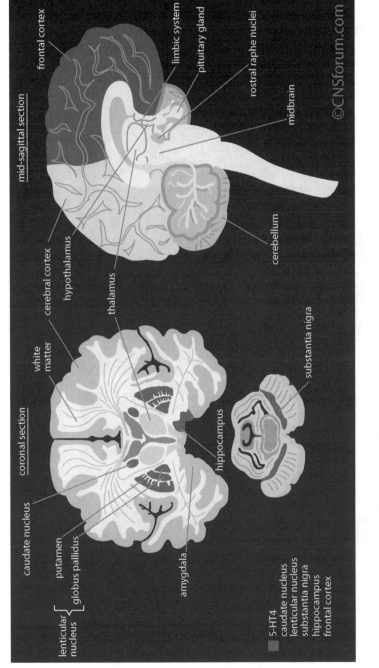

Figure 6.6. Distribution of 5-HT$_4$ receptors. The 5-HT$_4$ receptor subtype is coupled to a G protein that stimulates the intracellular messenger adenylate cyclase that, in turn, regulates neurotransmission. In the human brain, a high density of 5-HT$_4$ receptors has been identified in the striatonigral system, notably in the caudate nucleus, lenticular nucleus (putamen and globus pallidus) and the substantia nigra. Lower levels of expression of the 5-HT$_4$ receptor have been shown in the hippocampus and the frontal cortex.

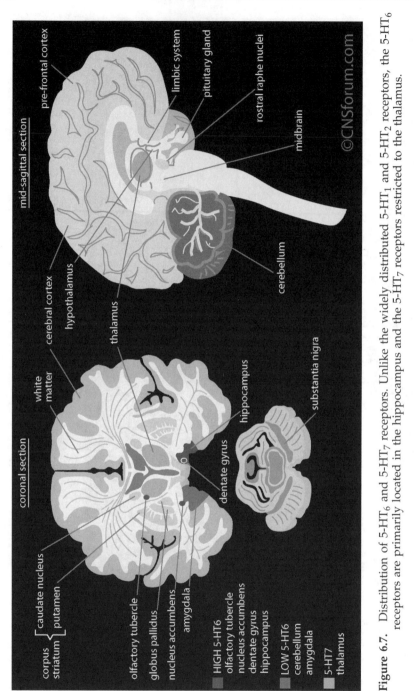

Figure 6.7. Distribution of 5-HT$_6$ and 5-HT$_7$ receptors. Unlike the widely distributed 5-HT$_1$ and 5-HT$_2$ receptors, the 5-HT$_6$ receptors are primarily located in the hippocampus and the 5-HT$_7$ receptors restricted to the thalamus.

Table 6.2. Serotonin receptor subtypes and disease states

Physiological or pathological condition	Serotonin receptor subtype implicated
Feeding behaviour	5-HT_{1A} agonists enhance food consumption in experimental animals $5\text{-HT}_{1B}/5\text{-HT}_{2C}$ agonists decrease food consumption in experimental animals
Thermoregulation	5-HT_{1A} agonists cause hypothermia in experimental animals 5-HT_{1B} and 5-HT_2 agonists cause hyperthermia in experimental animals
Sexual behaviour	5-HT_{1A} agonists both facilitate and inhibit sexual behaviour in male rats 5-HT_{1B} agonists inhibit sexual behaviour in the male but facilitate this behaviour in the female rat
Cardiovascular system	5-HT_1, 5-HT_2 and 5-HT_3 receptors may be involved in the complex action of serotonin on blood pressure 5-HT_2 agonists appear to be hypertensive agents whereas the antagonists are hypotensives
Sleep	5-HT_{1A} agonists delay the onset of REM sleep 5-HT_2 antagonists suppress REM sleep
Hallucinogenic activity	Most "classical" hallucinogens such as LSD and mescaline are antagonists at 5-HT_2 receptors
Antipsychotic activity	Many atypical neuroleptics (e.g. amperozide and risperidone) are 5-HT_2 receptor antagonists. In animals, 5-HT_3 antagonists have profiles similar to chronically active neuroleptics
Anxiolytic activity	Several novel anxiolytics (e.g. buspirone, ipsapirone) are 5-HT_{1A} partial agonists 5-HT_2 and 5-HT_3 antagonists have anxiolytic properties
Depression	5-HT_{1A} receptors are functionally sensitized by chronic antidepressant treatments in rats 5-HT_2 receptor numbers are increased and activity decreased, in depression; return to control values in response to treatment

Nevertheless, despite these cautions, there is a growing body of information which implicates different 5-HT receptor subtypes in a variety of physiological and pharmacological responses and these will be briefly reviewed (see Table 6.2).

Serotonin and sleep

It has been known for some years that the functional activity of 5-HT neurons in the brain changes dramatically during the sleep–wake arousal cycle. Thus from a stable, slow and regular discharge pattern during quiet wakening, neuronal activity gradually declines as the animal becomes drowsy and enters slow-wave sleep. During rapid eye movement (REM) sleep, 5-HT activity is totally suppressed but in anticipation of awakening the neuronal activity returns to its basal level several seconds before the end of the REM episode. During arousal or wakening, the 5-HT neuronal discharge pattern increases considerably above the quiet waking state.

Koella has reviewed the evidence implicating the involvement of serotonin in the sleep–wake cycle but the involvement of specific serotonin receptor subtypes in sleep mechanisms is unclear. Experimental evidence suggests that 5-HT_{1A} agonists delay the onset of REM sleep while 5-HT_2 antagonists suppress REM and have variable effects on non-REM sleep.

It must be emphasized that most studies of the relationship between the serotonergic system and sleep have been conducted in rats and therefore the relevance of such findings to man remains unproven. From such experimental studies, it has been shown that blockade of 5-HT_2 receptors increases the proportion of slow-wave sleep and decreases the quantity of REM sleep. Whether this effect of 5-HT_2 antagonists can be ascribed to a specific effect on slow-wave sleep is, however, a matter of conjecture as any increase in time spent in one stage of sleep will be reflected in a decrease in the time spent in other stages of sleep. However, experimental evidence suggests that most drugs that alter serotonergic transmission reduce REM sleep. There is evidence that the 5-HT_2 antagonist ritanserin improves sleep quality in those suffering from "jet lag" which suggests that the 5-HT_2 receptors may be involved in adjusting the sleep–wake cycle to the photoperiod. Furthermore, experimental data suggest that activation of 5-HT_2 receptors may vary according to the sleep–wake cycle. Such findings suggest that 5-HT_2 receptors are involved in the regulation of circadian rhythms and the sleep–wake cycle. With regard to the overall role of 5-HT in sleep, Koella has postulated that serotonin may produce its various effects on sleep architecture by influencing cognition and vigilance.

Details of the effects of psychotropic drugs on the sleep profile are discussed in Chapter 10.

Serotonin and hallucinogenic activity

There is abundant experimental evidence to show that serotonin plays a major role in the mechanism of action of hallucinogens, but it is presently unclear whether the actions of hallucinogens can be explained by their agonistic or antagonistic actions. LSD, for example, may behave either as an agonist or antagonist depending on the particular tissue, concentration and experimental condition, whereas the tryptamine type of hallucinogens usually act as agonists. Experimental evidence nevertheless suggests that the behavioural effects of a number of indole alkylamine (e.g. LSD-like) and phenylalkylamine (e.g. mescaline-like) hallucinogens can be attenuated by 5-HT$_{2A}$ antagonists and that the potency of these classes of hallucinogens at 5-HT$_{2A}$ (and possibly 5-HT$_{2C}$) sites correlate with their hallucinogenic potency in man. It seems unlikely however that all hallucinogens owe their activity to their potency in stimulating 5-HT$_{2A}$ receptors; LSD and 5-methoxydimethyltryptamine for example interact with 5-HT$_{2C}$ sites, while phenyclidine may owe its hallucinogenic potency to an action on N-methyl-D-aspartate (NMDA) and a subclass of sigma receptors. Nevertheless, the balance of evidence suggests that most "classical" hallucinogens such as LSD, mescaline and psilocybin act as partial agonists on 5-HT$_{2A}$ receptors.

Details of the pharmacological properties of hallucinogenic drugs are discussed in Chapter 15.

Serotonin and drugs of abuse

The role of 5-HT in the control of alcohol intake has received considerable attention following the discovery that 5-HT reuptake inhibitors reduce alcohol intake in alcohol dependent rats. Similar effects have been found for intracerebroventricularly administered 5-HT or its precursor 5-HTP. Regarding the type of 5-HT receptor involved, there is experimental evidence that the 5-HT$_{1A}$ partial agonists buspirone and gepirone are effective. Differences were found between the effects of the 5-HT$_3$ antagonist ondansetron and the 5-HT$_{2A}$/5-HT$_{2C}$ antagonist ritanserin. Thus the 5-HT$_3$ antagonist ondansetron reduces alcohol intake without affecting the alcohol preference of rats, while ritanserin reduces both the alcohol preference and intake. This suggests that, at least in rats, different populations of 5-HT receptors may be involved in alcohol intake and preference.

Regarding other types of drugs of abuse, the 5-HT$_3$ antagonist MDL 72222 has been shown to block place preference conditioning induced in rodents by morphine or nicotine without affecting the preference for amphetamine. It is possible that these effects of 5-HT$_3$ antagonists are associated with the reduction in dopamine release as it is well established that the rewarding effects of many drugs of abuse are due to increased dopaminergic activity in limbic regions. On the strength of the experimental findings, it has been proposed that 5-HT$_3$ antagonists might be useful in treating drug abuse in man. Only appropriate placebo-controlled studies of 5-HT$_3$ antagonists will clarify the therapeutic value of such agents in different types of drug abuse.

A further discussion of the pharmacological properties of alcohol and other drugs of abuse is given in Chapter 15.

Serotonin and the antipsychotic activity of neuroleptics

Given the complexity of the serotonergic system and its interaction with multiple neurotransmitter systems in the mammalian brain, it is not surprising to find that 5-HT plays a role in the aetiology of schizophrenia. Meltzer has suggested that in schizophrenia a malfunction of the mechanism whereby 5-HT modulates the release of dopamine (for example, due to the decreased inhibition by 5-HT of the release of dopamine in the mesencephalon and frontal cortex) might contribute to the enhanced neocortical dopaminergic function which probably forms the biochemical basis of the disease. The antipsychotic activity of atypical neuroleptics such as clozapine and risperidone may therefore lie in the normalization of the relationship between the malfunctioning 5-HT and dopaminergic systems.

The novel antipsychotic drug clozapine has a very complicated neurochemical profile in that it has a high affinity for $5-HT_{2A}$, $5-HT_{2C}$, $5-HT_3$, $5-HT_6$ and $5-HT_7$ receptors in addition to its action on D_4 and D_3 receptors. Risperidone likewise has a high affinity for $5-HT_{2A}$ receptors as well as acting as an antagonist of D_2 receptors. Such drugs have received attention recently because of their reduced propensity to cause extrapyramidal side effects and for their efficacy in treating the negative symptoms of schizophrenia. These properties may partly reside in the antagonistic actions of the atypical neuroleptics on the various sub-populations of 5-HT receptors of which the $5-HT_{2A}$ receptor may be of primary importance.

In experimental studies, many clinically effective neuroleptics have been shown to act as $5-HT_{2A}$ receptor antagonists. Studies on post-mortem brain from schizophrenic patients have shown that the decrease in the number of $5-HT_{2A}$ receptors in the prefrontal cortex might be related to the disease process. It therefore seems unlikely that the antipsychotic activity of neuroleptics can be explained solely in terms of their action on $5-HT_{2A}$ receptors. Furthermore, no correlation exists between the average therapeutic doses of a neuroleptic and its affinity for $5-HT_{2A}$ receptors. It does seem possible, however, that several atypical neuroleptics such as amperozide, risperidone and possibly ritanserin do owe at least part of the pharmacological profile to their ability to inhibit $5-HT_{2A}$ receptors.

Following the discovery that selective $5-HT_3$ antagonists reduce the behavioural effects of the infusion of dopamine into the nucleus accumbens, there has been considerable interest in the possible role of $5-HT_3$ receptor antagonists as potential neuroleptic agents. While there is a growing body of evidence to suggest that $5-HT_3$ antagonists may be therapeutically valuable for the treatment of disorders of the gastrointestinal tract, as antiemetics and possibly anxiolytic agents, there is currently little evidence to suggest that such drugs are effective in the treatment of schizophrenia.

However, experimental studies of the 5-HT$_3$ antagonists on dopamine autoreceptors may eventually offer new leads to the development of novel antipsychotic drugs.

A more detailed discussion of the pharmacological properties of typical and atypical neuroleptics is given in Chapter 11.

Serotonin and anxiolytic activity

Although the benzodiazepine anxiolytics primarily interact with the GABA receptor complex, there is ample experimental evidence to show that secondary changes occur in the turnover, release and firing of 5-HT neurons as a consequence of the activation of the GABA-benzodiazepine receptor. Similar changes are observed in the raphé nuclei where a high density of 5-HT$_{1A}$ receptors occurs. Such findings suggest that 5-HT may play a key role in anxiety disorders.

Undoubtedly one of the most important advances implicating serotonin in anxiety has been the development of the azaspirodecanone derivatives buspirone, gepirone and ipsapirone as novel anxiolytics. All three agents produce a common metabolite, namely 1-(2-pyrimidinyl) piperazine or 1-PP, which may contribute to the anxiolytic activity of the parent compounds. It soon became apparent that these anxiolytic agents do not act via the benzodiazepine or GABA receptors but show a relatively high affinity for the 5-HT$_{1A}$ sites; the 1-PP metabolite however only possesses a very low affinity for the 5-HT$_{1A}$ site although it may contribute to the anxiolytic effect of the parent compound by acting as an alpha$_2$ adrenoceptor agonist. In experimental studies, these atypical anxiolytics have mixed actions, behaving as agonists in some situations and antagonists in others. For this reason they are considered to be partial agonists at 5-HT$_{1A}$ receptors, acting either as agonists on presynaptic 5-HT$_{1A}$ receptors or antagonists on postsynaptic 5-HT$_{1A}$ receptors.

In animal models of anxiety, 5-HT$_2$ receptor antagonists have been shown to be active. Ritanserin appears to exhibit both anxiolytic and anxiogenic activity in different animal models. Nevertheless, in man, preliminary evidence suggests that ritanserin is an effective anxiolytic agent, although a placebo-controlled trial of the 5-HT$_2$ antagonist ritanserin has shown no differences in the Hamilton Anxiety and the Clinical Global Impression scales between the drug-treated and placebo-treated patients.

The anxiolytic properties of 5-HT$_3$ receptor antagonists have been demonstrated in several animal models of anxiety. In these models, the 5-HT$_3$ antagonists mimic the anxiolytic effects of the benzodiazepines but differ from the latter in their lack of sedative, muscle relaxant and anticonvulsant action. These compounds appear to be extremely potent (acting in the ng–μg/kg range) and, providing the initial clinical finding of their anxiolytic activity is substantiated, this group of drugs could provide a valuable addition to the non-benzodiazepine anxiolytics. Thus experimental and clinical evidence suggests that 5-HT_{1A} receptor partial agonists and 5-HT_2 and 5-HT_3 antagonists may be useful and novel anxiolytic agents.

Serotonin and aggression, panic attack and related disorders

The possible overlap between anxiety, depression, panic attack, aggression and obsessive–compulsive disorders, and the involvement of serotonin in the symptoms of these disorders, has recently led to the investigation of various selective serotonin reuptake inhibitors (SSRIs) and selective 5-HT receptor agonists/antagonists in the treatment of these conditions. In experimental studies, there is evidence that drugs such as eltoprazine, which binds with high affinity to 5-HT_{1A}, 5-HT_{1B} and 5-HT_{2C} sites, are active antiaggressive agents, whereas selective 5-HT_{1A} agonists and 5-HT_2 and 5-HT_3 antagonists are inactive. There is also preliminary evidence to suggest that SSRIs such as fluoxetine reduce impulsive behaviour which may contribute to their therapeutic action in the treatment of obsessive–compulsive disorders and possibly in reducing suicidal attempts.

Zohar and Insel have suggested that the symptoms of obsessive–compulsive disorder are due to supersensitive 5-HT_1-type receptors and that the function of SSRIs such as clomipramine, fluoxetine and the non-selective 5-HT antagonist metergoline owe their efficacy to their ability to reduce the activity of these receptors.

It now seems generally accepted that the effects of anti-obsessional drugs may be mediated by serotonergic mechanisms. The apparent hypersensitivity of obsessive–compulsive patients to the trazodone metabolite m-chlorophenyl piperazine (mCPP, a non-selective 5-HT_{1B}, 5-HT_{2C} and 5-HT_2 agonist) suggests that a diverse group of 5-HT_1 and 5-HT_2 receptors are involved. The efficacy of buspirone, a partial agonist of 5-HT_{1A} receptors, in attenuating the obsessional symptoms further suggests that 5-HT_{1A} receptors are also involved. As the 5-HT reuptake inhibitors such as fluoxetine and fluvoxamine are particularly effective in attenuating the obsessive symptoms following several weeks of administration, it may be argued that the therapeutic effect of such drugs lies in their ability to desensitize the supersensitive 5-HT_1-type receptors. Which of the 5-HT_1 receptors is specifically involved is unclear, but neuroimaging studies on patients with obsessive–compulsive disorder implicate the striatum as the major brain region which is defective. The 5-HT receptors in the striatum are 5-HT_{1D} and 5-HT_2 in man which may implicate these receptor subtypes specifically in the aetiology of the condition.

With regard to generalized anxiety disorder, it has been postulated that an overactivity of the stimulatory 5-HT pathways occurs. Drugs such as buspirone and ipsapirone are effective in such conditions because they stimulate the inhibitory 5-HT_{1A} autoreceptors on the raphé nuclei and thereby reduce serotonergic function. It is noteworthy that the SSRIs often worsen anxiety initially because they temporarily enhance serotonergic function. Adaptive changes in the pre- and postsynaptic 5-HT receptors then occur leading to a reduction in the anxiety state.

A further discussion of the pharmacological properties of the anxiolytic drugs is given in Chapter 9.

Serotonin and its role in depression

Serotonin is believed to play a multifunctional role in depression which is to be anticipated from its involvement in the physiological processes of sleep, mood, vigilance, feeding and possibly sexual behaviour and learning, all of which are deranged to varying extents in severe depression. However, the involvement of precise serotonin receptor subtypes in depression, and in the action of antidepressants, is still far from clear. One approach to unravelling the changes in serotonin receptors in depression has been to study the effects of chronically administered antidepressants on serotonin receptor subtypes in rat brain. While there is evidence that most antidepressants show only a low affinity for the 5-HT_1 sites, there is experimental evidence to show that chronic antidepressant treatment results in a hypersensitivity of postsynaptic and a hyposensitivity of presynaptic 5-HT_{1A} receptors. In contrast to the 5-HT_{1A} receptors, many antidepressants from various chemical classes have a moderate affinity for 5-HT_2 receptors although there is no apparent correlation between the 5-HT_2 receptor affinity and the antidepressant potency.

Regarding the changes that occur in rat cortical 5-HT_2 receptor density following chronic antidepressant and lithium treatment, there is unequivocal evidence that the number of receptors increases in response to chronic drug treatment although it must be emphasized that chronic electroconvulsive shock results in a decrease in the receptor number. Similarly, in untreated depressed and panic patients, the density of 5-HT_2 receptors on the platelet membrane has been shown to be increased. The number of receptors normalizes on effective, but not ineffective, treatment. Using the serotonin-induced platelet aggregation response as a measure of the functional activity of 5-HT_2 receptors, it has been consistently shown that the 5-HT_2 receptor responsiveness is reduced in the untreated depressive but returns to control values following effective treatment irrespective of the nature of treatment. Thus changes in 5-HT_2 receptor density and

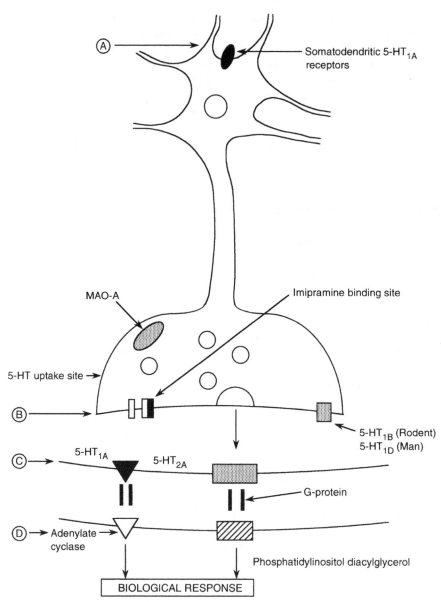

Figure 6.8. Changes that occur following the chronic administration of anti-depressants. Ⓐ SSRIs and MAOIs desensitize the inhibitory 5-HT$_{1A}$ somato dendritic receptors. Ⓑ SSRIs and MAOIs desensitize the inhibitory 5-HT$_{1B}$/5-HT$_{1D}$ inhibitory auto receptor on the presynaptic terminal. After acute administration, the TCAs and the SSRIs inhibit the uptake of 5-HT into the nerve terminal by binding to the

function appear to be disturbed in the depressed patient and return to control values only following effective treatment. The increase in the receptor number, and decrease in their responsiveness to serotonin, in the untreated depressed patient may suggest an abnormality in the coupling mechanism between the receptor site and the phosphatidylinositol second messenger system that brings about the platelet shape change underlying aggregation.

It has been hypothesized that depression could arise from a pathological enhancement of 5-HT$_2$ receptor function. This view would concur with the observations that the functional activity of 5-HT$_2$ receptors on the platelet membrane is enhanced in depression and the increase in the density of 5-HT$_2$ receptors in the frontal cortex of brains from suicide victims. It is possible that enhanced 5-HT$_2$ receptor function is associated primarily with anxiety, a common feature of depression, and that the increased activity of the 5-HT$_2$ receptors results in an attenuation of the functioning of 5-HT$_1$ receptors thereby resulting in the symptoms of depression. Whether this change in the activity of 5-HT$_1$ receptors is due to direct effects of the altered 5-HT$_2$ receptor function is uncertain. There is evidence that hypercortisolaemia, which is a characteristic feature of depression, reduces the activity of these receptors probably through central glucocorticoid type 2 receptors. Clearly further research is needed to determine the precise interaction between the 5-HT$_2$ and 5-HT$_1$ receptor types.

More recently, it has been speculated that the 5-HT$_{1B/1D}$ receptors may have a role to play in depression and in the mode of action of antidepressants. These receptors appear to be located presynaptically where they control the release of 5-HT; in experimental studies the non-selective 5-HT$_1$ antagonist methiothepin has antidepressant properties.

Figure 6.8. (*continued*) imipramine binding site (or its equivalent). 5-HT transport sites are also found on the cell body and axonal projection but their precise role in serotonergic transmission is unclear. Presumably the change in 5-HT is in the vicinity of the receptors. 5-HT$_{1B}$ and $_{1D}$ receptors appear to have a similar function but are structurally slightly different according to the species in which they are found. ©︎ TCAs, ECT and most non-SSRIs second generation antidepressants sensitize the postsynaptic 5-HT$_{1A}$ receptors thereby increasing serotonergic function. The density of 5-HT$_{2A}$ receptors is decreased by TCAs and SSRIs in rat brain following chronic treatment; in the depressed patient however the number of 5-HT$_{2A}$ receptors is increased and normalizes following effective treatment. ⓓ There is experimental evidence that the activity of the second messenger system associated with the 5-HT$_{2A}$ receptor is decreased following chronic antidepressant treatment. There is also circumstantial evidence that the G protein coupling mechanism between the 5-HT$_{2A}$ receptor and its second messenger is hypofunctional in depressed patients but normalizes following effective treatment. This suggests that some antidepressants may improve the receptor–second messenger G protein coupling mechanism.

Thus it may be speculated that the $5\text{-HT}_{1B/1D}$ receptors are supersensitive in depression, thereby leading to a reduced intersynaptic concentration of 5-HT with a consequent increase in the number of postsynaptic 5-HT_2 receptor sites. However, only the development of highly selective $5\text{-HT}_{1B/1D}$ antagonists will enable this hypothesis to be tested.

Although the precise mechanism whereby antidepressants produce their therapeutic effects is incompletely understood, there is a growing body of evidence to suggest that serotonin receptors, particularly of the 5-HT_{1A} and 5-HT_2 subtype, play a role in their actions. Only the 5-HT_{2A} receptor has, so far, been convincingly demonstrated to be malfunctional in depression and to be normalized following effective treatment. A further consideration of the pharmacological properties of the different classes of antidepressants is considered in Chapter 7. Figure 6.8 summarizes some of the proposed sites of action of different classes of antidepressants that modulate central serotonergic transmission.

In SUMMARY, it is evident that serotonin is involved in a variety of physiological processes and that disturbances of serotonergic function may be of importance in the aetiology of many gastrointestinal, cardiovascular and central nervous system diseases. The existence of subtypes of serotonin receptors and the impetus that this has given to the development of drugs with selective actions on these receptor subtypes is already leading to the development of new therapeutic agents. Evaluation of the functional status of serotonin receptor subtypes in psychiatric and neurological diseases may be of future importance in the diagnosis and assessment of treatment response in such patients. In this regard, the development of serotonin receptor probes coupled with such techniques as positron emission tomography may be of considerable importance in diagnosis in the future.

To date, at least four major subtypes of serotonin receptor have been described in detail and a major advance has been made with the isolation of genomic clones for these receptor subtypes. We now await the further development of selective ligands for all the serotonin receptor subtypes which may ultimately lead to a better understanding of the functional significance and clinical relevance of serotonin receptors in health and disease. Hopefully such a development will also result in the availability of more effective drugs to treat neurological and psychiatric diseases.

7 Drug Treatment of Depression

Introduction

The *Oxford Dictionary* defines depression as a state of "low spirits or vitality". Clearly, this state has been experienced by most people at some stage during their lives. However, the psychiatrist is seldom concerned with such a mood change unless it persists for such a long time that it incapacitates the individual. Should the depressed mood be associated with feelings of guilt, suicidal tendencies and disturbed bodily functions (such as weight loss, anorexia, loss of libido or a disturbed sleep pattern characterized by early morning wakening) and persist for weeks or even months, often with no initiatory cause, then psychiatric assistance is usually required. It is not proposed to discuss the various types of depression that have been identified because the drug treatment is essentially similar irrespective of whether or not there appears to be an initiatory cause. For example, bereavement is often associated with a severe depressive episode, particularly in the elderly, and while counselling may be of considerable assistance in enabling the patient to adjust to the changed circumstances the use of an antidepressant is often advisable.

Many psychiatrists still divide depression into the endogenous (i.e. no apparent external cause) and reactive (i.e. an identifiable external cause) types and, while such a division may be of some value regarding ancillary treatment, there is presently no evidence to suggest that the biochemical changes that may be causally linked to the illness differ nor is there any evidence that the way in which the patient should be assisted by drugs differs substantially. Other international classifications of depression are based on the mono- and bipolar dichotomy, a system of classification that separates those patients with depressive symptoms only from those that fluctuate between depression and mania (i.e. manic-depression) or have only manic symptoms. In such cases treatment strategies differ as specific and antimanic drugs such as lithium or the neuroleptics would be used to abort an acute attack of mania, while antidepressants are the drugs of choice

Fundamentals of Psychopharmacology. Third Edition. By Brian E. Leonard
2003 John Wiley & Sons, Ltd. ISBN 0 471 52178 7

to treat the depressive episodes and anxiety associated with depression. Readers are referred to the various classification manuals, such as the *Diagnostic and Statistical Manual of Mental Disorders* of the American Psychiatric Association (DSM-IV) or the *International Classification of Diseases*, 10th Revision (ICD10), for further details.

Historical development of antidepressants

The use of cocaine, extracted in a crude form from the leaves of the Andean coca plant, has been used for centuries in South America to alleviate fatigue and elevate the mood. It was only relatively recently, however, that the same pharmacological effect was discovered when the amphetamines were introduced into Western medicine as anorexiants with stimulant properties. Opiates, generally as a galenical mixture, were also widely used for centuries for their mood-elevating effects throughout the world. It is not without interest that while such drugs would never now be used as antidepressants, there is evidence that most antidepressants do modulate the pain threshold, possibly via the enkephalins and endorphins. This may help to explain the use of antidepressants in the treatment of atypical pain syndromes and as an adjunct to the treatment of terminal cancer pain. Finally, alcohol in its various forms has been used to alleviate anguish and sorrow since antiquity. Whilst the opiates, alcohol and the stimulants offer some temporary relief to the patient, their long-term use inevitably leads to dependence and even to an exacerbation of the symptoms they were designed to cure.

The development of specific drugs for the treatment of depression only occurred in the early 1950s with the accidental discovery of the monoamine oxidase inhibitors (MAOIs) and the tricyclic antidepressants (TCAs). This period marked the beginning of the era of pharmacopsychiatry.

Although the iminodibenzyl structure, which forms the chemical basis of the TCA series, was first synthesized in 1889, its biological activity was only evaluated in the early 1950s following the accidental discovery that the tricyclic compound chlorpromazine had antipsychotic properties. Imipramine is also chemically similar in structure to chlorpromazine, but was found to lack its antipsychotic effects. It was largely due to the persistence of the Swiss psychiatrist Kuhn that imipramine was not discarded and was shown to have specific antidepressant effects. It is not without interest that the first report of the antidepressant effects of imipramine was presented to an audience of 12 as part of the proceedings of the Second World Congress of Psychiatry in Zurich in 1957!

The introduction of the first MAOI in the early 1950s was equally inauspicious. Iproniazid had been developed as an effective hydrazide antitubercular drug, but was subsequently found to exhibit mood-elevating effects. This was shown to be due to its ability to inhibit MAO activity and was unconnected with its antitubercular action. Thus by the late 1950s, psychiatrists had at their disposal two effective treatments for depression, a TCA and an MAOI. But it was only in attempting to discover how these drugs may work, together with the evidence that the recently introduced antipsychotic drug resperine caused depression in a small number of patients, that the hypothesis was developed that depression was due to a relative deficit of biogenic amine neurotransmitters in the synaptic cleft and that antidepressants reversed this deficit by preventing their inactivation. While this hypothesis has been drastically revised in the light of research into the biochemical nature of depression, at that time it had the advantage of unifying a number of disparate clinical and experimental observations and in laying the basis for subsequent drug development.

Aspects of the biochemical basis of depression

Research into the chemical pathology of depression has mainly concentrated on four major areas:

1. Changes in biogenic amine neurotransmitters in post-mortem brains from suicide victims.
2. Changes in cerebrospinal fluid (CSF) concentrations of amine metabolites from patients with depression.
3. Endocrine disturbances which appear to be coincidentally related to the onset of the illness.
4. Changes in neurotransmitter receptor function and density on platelets and lymphocytes from patients before and following effective treatment.

Approximately 30 years ago, Schildkraut postulated that noradrenaline may play a pivotal role in the aetiology of depression. Evidence in favour of this hypothesis was provided by the observation that the antihypertensive drug reserpine, which depletes both the central and peripheral vesicular stores of catecholamines such as noradrenaline, is likely to precipitate depression in patients in remission. The experimental drug alpha-methyl-paratyrosine that blocks the synthesis of noradrenaline by inhibiting the rate-limiting enzyme tyrosine hydroxylase was also shown to precipitate depression in patients during remission. While such findings are only indirect indicators that noradrenaline plays an important role in human behaviour, and may be defective in depression, more direct evidence is needed to substantiate the hypothesis. The most obvious approach would be to determine the concentration of noradrenaline and/or its major central metabolite 3-methoxy-4-hydroxyphenylglycol (MHPG) in the brains of suicide victims. The problem with such post-mortem studies is that (a) the precise diagnosis may be uncertain, (b) there is usually a considerable post-mortem delay before the brain is removed at autopsy and (c) suicide is often committed by taking an overdose of alcohol together with drugs which grossly affect central monoamine neurotransmitter function. Unless these variables are carefully controlled, the value of the results obtained from such analyses is uncertain. Nevertheless, there is evidence that the neurotransmitter receptors in post-mortem brain are less labile than the neurotransmitters that act upon them. The finding that the density of beta adrenoceptors is increased in cortical regions of the brains from suicide victims who had suffered from depression is evidence of disturbed noradrenergic function which is associated with some of the symptoms of the illness. Such observations are further supported by the increase in the density of beta adrenoceptors on the lymphocytes of untreated depressed patients. As the density of these receptors is normalized by effective antidepressant treatment, it has been postulated that changes in the beta receptor density may be a state marker of the condition (Table 7.1).

Other studies have shown that the elevation of growth hormone in the plasma following the administration of the alpha-2 adrenoceptor agonist clonidine is diminished in depressed patients, which suggests that central postsynaptic alpha-2 adrenoceptors are also subfunctional in such patients. This is perhaps the most consistent finding to have emerged in studies of the hypothalamic–pituitary axis in depression. As the clonidine response does not return to normal after effective antidepressant treatment, this is possibly a trait marker of depression. It should be emphasized that the reduced growth hormone response to clonidine cannot be accounted for by drug treatment, age or gender of the patient, which supports the view that the noradrenergic system is dysregulated in depression. Lastly, determination of the urine or plasma concentrations of MHPG (an indicator of central noradrenergic activity) suggests that central noradrenergic function is suboptimal in depression. Taken together, these results suggest that central noradrenergic function is decreased in depression, an event leading to the increase in the density of the postsynaptic beta adrenoceptors that show

Table 7.1. Changes in brain and tissue amine neurotransmitters in depressed patients which may be indicative of the mechanism of action of antidepressants

---

Evidence from the brains of depressed patients who committed suicide
- Increased density of beta adrenoceptors in cortical regions
- Increased density of $5\text{-}HT_{2A}$ receptors in limbic regions
- Decreased concentration of 5-HIAA in several brain regions
- Increased muscarinic receptor density in limbic regions

---

adaptive changes in response to the diminished synaptic concentration of the transmitter. It should be emphasized however that none of the studies of noradrenergic function in post-mortem material or tissues from depressed patients are entirely satisfactory. Many of the findings cannot be replicated, the number of patients studied is relatively small and the tritiated ligands used to determine the receptor density for example vary in their selectivity.

There is also evidence that the density of muscarinic receptors is increased in limbic regions of depressed patients who have committed suicide. If it is assumed that such a change reflects an increased activity of the cholinergic system, it could help to explain the reduced noradrenergic function as there is both clinical and experimental evidence to suggest that increased central cholinergic activity can precipitate depression and reduce noradrenergic activity.

The role of serotonin (5-hydroxytryptamine, 5-HT) has also been extensively studied in depressed patients. Whereas the overall psycho-physiological effects of noradrenaline in the CNS appear to be linked to drive and motivation, 5-HT is primarily involved in the expression of mood. It is not surprising therefore to find that the serotonergic system is abnormal in depression. This is indicated by a reduction in the main 5-HT metabolite, 5-hydroxyindole acetic acid (5-HIAA), in the cerebrospinal fluid of severely depressed patients and a reduction in 5-HT and 5-HIAA in the limbic regions of the brain of suicide victims. The 5-HT receptor function also appears to be abnormal in depression. This is indicated by an increase in the density of cortical 5-HT_{2A} receptors in the brains of suicide victims and also on the platelet membrane of depressed patients. Platelets may be considered as accessible models of the nerve terminal.

Thus platelets are, like neurons, of ectodermal origin and contain enzymes such as enolase that are otherwise restricted to neurons. In addition, platelets contain storage vesicles for 5-HT from which the amine is released by a calcium-dependent mechanism. An energy-dependent transport site for 5-HT also occurs on the platelet membrane, the structure of which is identical to that found on neurons in the brain. Furthermore, the platelet membrane contains 5-HT_{2A} and alpha-2 adrenergic receptors that are functionally involved in platelet aggregation; there is evidence that the densities of these receptors are increased in depressed patients and largely normalized following effective treatment. Thus a number of important biochemical parameters may be determined from a platelet-rich plasma sample. It has been found, for example, that the transport of 3H-5-HT into the platelet is significantly reduced in the untreated depressed patient but largely returns to normal following effective treatment. This change occurs irrespective of the nature of the antidepressant used to treat the patient and may therefore be considered as a state marker of the illness.

The function of the 5-HT_{2A} receptor also appears to be subnormal in the untreated patient as shown by diminished aggregatory response to the addition of 5-HT *in vitro*, but normalizes when the patient recovers. As the number of 5-HT_{2A} receptors on the platelet membrane of depressed patients is increased (as shown by the increased binding of a specific ligand such as 3H-ketanserin) this finding suggests that the G protein transducer mechanism, which links the receptor to the second messenger phosphatidyl inositol system within the platelet, is possibly defective in depression. There is also evidence that the modulatory site on the 5-HT transporter, the imipramine binding site, is decreased in depression, but unlike the changes in 5-HT uptake, remains unchanged by effective treatment. This suggests that the number of imipramine binding sites on the platelet membrane is a trait marker of the condition. However, the precise relevance of this finding is uncertain as the binding of the more specific ligand, 3H-paroxetine, is unchanged in depression. These studies of platelet function before, during and following treatment can give important information of the biochemical processes which may be causally related to depression. However, it is still uncertain how the changes in platelet function precisely reflect those occurring in the brain. Platelets are unconnected with the nervous system and therefore the changes observed could be a reflection of the hormonal changes (for example, glucocorticoids) that occur in depression. There is also evidence that some of the alterations in platelet function are a consequence of low molecular weight plasma factors that occur in the depressed patient and which are absent following effective antidepressant treatment (Table 7.2).

More recently, several studies in both the United States and the UK have shown that patients undergoing treatment with an SSRI will rapidly relapse when given an amino acid-containing drink that is deficient in tryptophan. The onset of the symptoms of depression is rapid (less than 24 hours); there is clinical and experimental evidence that the reduction in brain serotonin

Table 7.2. Other clinical studies implicating an abnormal biogenic amine function in depression

- Decreased 5-HIAA concentration in CSF
- Decreased HVA (main dopamine metabolite) in CSF
- Decreased urinary excretion of the main central noradrenaline metabolite MHPG (?)
- Rapid relapse following administration of a tryptophan-free amino acid drink to depressed patients being treated with an SSRI
- Rapid relapse following administration of the tyrosine hydroxylase inhibitor alpha-methyl-tyrosine to depressed patients who respond to a noradrenaline reuptake inhibitor such as desipramine

? These findings are equivocal.

as a consequence of the lack of tryptophan is the cause of the altered mood state. However, those depressed patients who responded to desipramine, which enhances noradrenergic function, did not relapse when given the tryptophan-free drink. Such studies provide further evidence to suggest that serotonin plays a crucial role in the aetiology of depression. They also raise the possibility that some depressed patients have a pronounced deficit in noradrenergic function rather than serotonergic function, which may account for the differential response of some depressed patients to antidepressants which augment the serotonergic or noradrenergic system (Table 7.3).

While there has been considerable attention devoted to changes in noradrenergic and serotonergic function in depression, less attention has been paid to the possible involvement of dopamine in this disorder. This is surprising as anhedonia is a characteristic feature of major depression and a defect in dopaminergic function is thought to be causally involved in this symptom. Several studies have shown that the concentration of the main dopamine metabolite, homovanillic acid (HVA), is decreased in the CSF of depressed patients, particularly those with psychomotor retardation. These depressed patients who attempted suicide were also found to have a decreased urinary excretion of HVA and the second major dopamine metabolite, dihydroxyphenylacetic acid (DOPAC). It is of course possible that the dopamine deficit is more a reflection of the degree of retardation rather than the psychological state as similar changes in CSF HVA concentrations have been reported to occur in patients with Parkinson's disease. This implies that the changes in the basal ganglia probably overshadow any changes in the mesolimbic dopaminergic system as the contribution of this area is relatively minor.

With regard to the specific action of antidepressants on the dopaminergic system, there is evidence that buproprion (not marketed in most countries in Western Europe as an antidepressant but available in North America), amineptine and nomifensin (withdrawn because of the rare occurrence of haemolysis) owed their antidepressant efficacy to their ability to increase central dopaminergic function. There are also open label studies to suggest

Table 7.3. Evidence from depressed patients

- Increased density of 5-HT$_{2A}$ receptors on the platelet membrane
- Decreased uptake of 3H-5-HT into platelet
- Increased beta adrenoceptor density on lymphocyte membrane
- Increased density of alpha-2 adrenoceptors on platelet membranes (*)
- Blunted growth hormone response to a clonidine challenge
- Blunted prolactin response to a fenfluramine challenge

* These findings are equivocal.

that the novel dopamine receptor agonist roxindole and the selective dopamine uptake inhibitor pramipexole may have antidepressant action.

Thus when the results of the studies on platelets, lymphocytes, changes in cerebrospinal fluid metabolites of brain monoamines and the post-mortem studies are taken into account it may be concluded that a major abnormality in both noradrenergic and serotonergic function occurs in depression, and that such changes could be causally related to the disease process.

Circadian changes in neurotransmitter function in depression

Both clinical and experimental studies have shown that a number of transmitter receptors and amine transport processes show circadian changes. It is well established that depression is associated with a disruption of the circadian rhythm as shown by changes in a number of behavioural, autonomic and neuroendocrine aspects. One of the main consequences of effective treatment is a return of the circadian rhythm to normality. For example, it has been shown that the 5-HT uptake into the platelets of depressed patients is largely unchanged between 0600 and 1200 hours, whereas the 5-HT transport in control subjects shows a significant decrease over this period. The normal rhythm in 5-HT transport is only re-established when the depressed patient responds to treatment. Thus it may be hypothesized that the mode of action of antidepressants is to normalize disrupted circadian rhythms. Only when the circadian rhythm has returned to normal can full clinical recovery be established.

Chronobiological studies have shown that circadian rhythms occur in the responsivity of animals to light, dark and psychotropic drugs. This implies that the timing of drug administration so that the drug reaches the target organ at its optimum sensitivity could help to improve its therapeutic efficiency. The results of experimental studies suggest that most antidepressants delay the circadian phase and lengthen the circadian period. These changes could be due to the drugs acting on the circadian pacemaker in the superchiasmatic nucleus. However, other brain regions could also be responsible together with antidepressant-induced changes in the retina which would lead to a modification of the processing of light stimuli; the lateral geniculate nucleus may also have a role to play. Seasonal affective disorder (SAD) generally consists of recurrent depressive episodes in autumn and winter that alternate with euthmia or hypomania in spring and summer. The seasonal rhythms of mood, sleep and weight change seen in SAD patients resemble hibernation seen in animals. This led to the hypothesis that extension of the photoperiod in winter could counteract the depressive symptoms. Exposure to bright light had indeed been shown to be efficacious. Clinical studies show that carbohydrate craving, a common feature of

SAD, is possibly linked to a decreased serotonin turnover. Such a hypothesis is supported by the fact that the serotonin releasing agent D-fenfluramine is effective in treating SAD. Chronobiology is clearly an important area of research for the psychopharmacologist which needs more attention.

Theories of the mechanisms of action of antidepressants: is there a common mechanism of action?

Why is there a delay in the onset of the antidepressant response?

In an attempt to explain the reason for the delay in the onset of the therapeutic effect of antidepressants, which is clearly unrelated to the acute actions of these drugs on monoamine reuptake transporters or intracellular metabolizing enzymes, emphasis has moved away from the presynaptic mechanism governing the release of the monoamine transmitters to the adaptive changes that occur in pre- and postsynaptic receptors that govern the physiological expression of neurotransmitter function.

Antidepressant therapy is usually associated with a gradual onset of action over 2 to 3 weeks before the optimal beneficial effect is obtained. Much of the improvement seen early in the treatment with antidepressants is probably associated with a reduction in anxiety that often occurs in the depressed patient and improvement in sleep caused by the sedative action of many of these drugs. The delay in the onset of the therapeutic response cannot be easily explained by the pharmacokinetic profile of the drugs as peak plasma (and presumably brain) concentrations are usually reached in 7 to 10 days. Furthermore, the 2–3 weeks delay is also seen in many, though not all, patients given electroconvulsive therapy (ECT). Table 7.4 summarizes some of the changes in neurotransmitter receptors that occur in the cortex of rat brain following ECT or the chronic administration of antidepressants. From the results of such studies, it is apparent that adaptational changes occur in adrenoceptors, serotonin, dopamine and

Table 7.4. Changes in cholinergic and aminergic receptors in depression and following antidepressant treatment

---

1. Evidence that central muscarinic receptors are supersensitive in depressed patients and that chronic antidepressant treatments normalize the supersensitivity of these receptors. This effect does not depend on any intrinsic anticholinergic activity of the antidepressant (i.e. it is an indirect, adaptive effect).

2. Following chronic administration to rats, there is evidence that most antidepressants cause adaptive changes in $5-HT_{1A}$, $5-HT_{2A}$ alpha-1, alpha-2 and beta adrenoceptors, GABA-B receptors and possibly the NMDA-glutamate receptors.

GABA-B receptors. There is evidence that GABA-B receptors play a role in enhancing noradrenaline release in the cortex and in this respect differ fundamentally from the inhibitory GABA-A receptors which facilitate central GABAergic transmission. A decrease in the activity of GABA-B receptors may therefore contribute to the reduced central noradrenergic tone reported to occur in depression.

Changes in cholinergic function

In addition to these changes, recent evidence has shown that a decrease in cortical muscarinic receptors occurs in the bulbectomized rat model of depression that, like most of the changes in biogenic amine receptors, returns to control values following treatment with either typical (e.g. tricyclic antidepressants) or atypical (e.g. mianserin) antidepressants. Such findings are of particular interest as the anticholinergic activity of the tricyclic antidepressants is usually associated with their unacceptable peripheral side effects and most second generation antidepressants have gained in therapeutic popularity because they lack such side effects. Nevertheless, support for the cholinergic hypothesis of depression is provided by the finding that the short-acting reversible cholinesterase inhibitor pyridostigmine, when administered to drug-free depressed patients, causes an enhanced activation of the anterior pituitary gland as shown by the release of growth hormone secretion. This suggests that the muscarinic receptors are supersensitive in the depressed patient. However, the mechanism whereby the receptors are normalized by chronic (but not acute) antidepressant treatment vary and in most cases are unlikely to be due to a direct anticholinergic action. It has been postulated that depression arises as the result of an imbalance between the central noradrenergic and cholinergic systems; in depression the activity of the former system is decreased and, conversely, in mania it is increased. As most antidepressants, irrespective of the presumed specificity of their action on the noradrenergic and serotonergic systems, have been shown to enhance noradrenergic function, it is hypothesized that the functional reduction in cholinergic activity arises as a consequence of the increase in central noradrenergic activity.

In SUMMARY, irrespective of the specificity of the antidepressants following their acute administration, it can be speculated that a common feature of all these drugs is to correct the abnormality in neurotransmitter receptor function. Such an effect of chronic antidepressant treatment may parallel the time of onset of the therapeutic response and contribute to the receptor sensitivity hypothesis of depression and the common mode of action of antidepressants.

The link between the serotonergic and noradrenergic systems

Considerable attention has recently been focused on the interaction between serotonergic and beta-adrenergic receptors, which may be of particular relevance to our understanding of the therapeutic effect of antidepressants. Thus the chronic administration of antidepressants enhances the inhibitory response of forebrain neurons to micro-iontophoretically applied 5-HT. This enhanced response is blocked by lesions of the noradrenergic projections to the cortex. This dual effect could help to explain enhanced serotonergic function that arises after chronic administration of antidepressants or ECT. Conversely, impairment of serotonergic function by means of a selective neurotoxin (e.g. 5,7-dihydroxytryptamine) or 5-HT synthesis inhibitor (e.g. parachlorophenylalanine) largely prevents the decrease in functional activity of cortical beta-adrenoceptors that usually arises following chronic antidepressant treatment. 5-HT_{1B} receptors are located on serotonergic nerve terminals that act as autoreceptors, and, on stimulation by serotonin, decrease the further release of this amine. It has been hypothesized that the chronic administration of selective serotonin reuptake inhibitor antidepressants (such as fluoxetine, paroxetine, sertraline, citalopram and fluvoxamine) slowly desensitize the inhibitory 5-HT_{1B} receptors and thereby enhance serotonin release.

In addition to the importance of the 5-HT_{1B} autoreceptors in the regulation of serotonergic function, there is experimental and clinical evidence that the 5-HT_{1A} receptors play a fundamental role in both anxiety and depression. In brief, the 5-HT_{1A} somatodendritic receptors inhibit the release of serotonin and it is postulated that the enhanced release of the transmitter following the chronic administration of the selective serotonin reuptake inhibitors is a consequence of the adaptive down-regulation of the inhibitory 5-HT_{1A} receptors. The validity of this hypothesis is supported by the pharmacological effect of 5-HT_{1A} antagonists. Thus the beta-adrenoceptors antagonist and 5-HT_{1A} antagonist pindolol, in combination with fluoxetine or paroxetine, enhance the therapeutic efficacy of the SSRI and, in some studies, reduce the time of onset of the peak therapeutic effect. However, several investigators have not been able to replicate such findings.

Both clinical and experimental studies have provided evidence that 5-HT can also regulate dopamine turnover. Thus several investigators have shown that a positive correlation exists in depressed patients between the homovanillic acid (HVA), a major metabolite of dopamine, and 5-HIAA concentrations in the CSF. In experimental studies, stimulation of the 5-HT cell bodies in the median raphé causes reduced firing of the substantia nigra where dopamine is the main neurotransmitter. There is thus convincing evidence that 5-HT plays an important role in modulating dopaminergic

Table 7.5. Mechanism of action of antidepressants: changes in serotonergic function

---

1. There is experimental evidence that the chronic administration of antidepressants or ECT enhances the inhibitory effect of micro-iontophoretically applied 5-HT. This effect is blocked by lesions of the noradrenergic projections to the frontal cortex.

2. SSRIs after chronic administration down-regulate the inhibitory 5-HT$_{1A}$ receptors on the serotonergic cell body, thereby leading to an enhanced release of the transmitter from the nerve terminal.

3. 5-HT can also decrease dopamine release from the substantia nigra (an important dopaminergic nucleus). This may account for the observation that some SSRIs may cause dystonias and precipitate the symptoms of parkinsonism if given to such patients who are responding to L-dopa. Sertraline appears to differ from other SSRIs in this respect and may slightly enhance dopaminergic function by reducing the reuptake of this transmitter.

---

function in many regions of the brain, including the mesolimbic system. Such findings imply that the effects of some antidepressants that show an apparent selectivity for the serotonergic system could be equally ascribed to a change in dopaminergic function in mesolimbic and mesocortical regions of the brain. It has been postulated that the hedonic effect of antidepressants may be ascribed to the enhanced dopaminergic function in the mesocortex (Table 7.5).

The role of the glutamatergic system in the action of antidepressants

Whereas much emphasis has been placed on the monoamine neurotransmitters with respect to the mechanism of action of antidepressants, little attention has been paid to the changes in the glutamate system, the primary excitatory neurotransmitter pathway in the brain. Experimental evidence shows that tricyclic antidepressants inhibit the binding of dizolcipine to the ion channel of the main glutamate receptor, the N-methyl-D-aspartate receptor in the brain. The initial studies have more recently been extended to show that both typical and atypical antidepressants have a qualitatively similar effect by reducing the binding of dizolcipine to the NMDA receptors. Whether this is due to direct action of the antidepressants on the ion channel receptor sites, or an indirect effect possibly involving the modulation of the glycine receptor site, is uncertain, but there is evidence that glycine and drugs modulating the glycine site have antidepressant-like activity in animal models of depression. These results suggest that antidepressants act as functional NMDA receptor antagonists.

Intracellular changes that occur following chronic antidepressant treatment

The recent advances in molecular neurobiology have demonstrated how information is passed from the neurotransmitter receptors on the outer side of the neuronal membrane to the secondary messenger system on the inside. The coupling of this receptor to the secondary messenger is brought about by a member of the G protein family. Beta-adrenoceptors are linked to adenylate cyclase, and, depending on the subtype of receptors, 5-HT is linked to either adenylate cyclase (5-HT$_{1A}$, 5-HT$_{1B}$) or phospholipase (5-HT$_{2A}$, 5-HT$_{2C}$). Activation of phospholipase results in an intracellular increase in the secondary messengers diacylglycerol and inositol triphosphate (IP$_3$), the IP$_3$ then mobilizing intraneuronal calcium.

The net result of the activation of the secondary messenger systems is to increase the activity of the various protein kinases that phosphorylate membrane-bound proteins to produce a physiological response. Some researchers have investigated the effect of chronic antidepressant treatment on the phosphorylation of proteins associated with the cytoskeletal structure of the nerve cell. Their studies suggest that antidepressants could affect the function of the cytoskeleton by changing the component of the associated protein phosphorylation system. In support of their hypothesis, these researchers showed that both typical (e.g. desipramine) and atypical (e.g. (+) oxaprotiline, a specific noradrenaline reuptake inhibitor, and fluoxetine, a selective 5-HT uptake inhibitor) antidepressants increased the synthesis of a microtubule fraction possibly by affecting the regulatory subunit of protein kinase type II. These changes in cytoskeletal protein synthesis occurred only after chronic antidepressant treatments and suggest that antidepressants, besides their well-established effects on pre- and postsynaptic receptors and amine uptake systems, might change neuronal signal transduction processes distal to the receptor (Table 7.6).

Glucocorticoid receptors: adaptive changes following antidepressant treatment

Interest in the possible association of glucocorticoid receptors with central neurotransmitter function arose from the observation that such receptors have been identified in the nuclei of catecholamine and 5-HT-containing cell bodies in the brain. Experimental studies have shown that glucocorticoid receptors activate as DNA binding proteins which can modify the transcription of genes. The link to antidepressant treatments is indicated by the chronic administration of imipramine which increases glucocorticoid receptor immunoreactivity in rat brain, the changes being particularly pronounced in the noradrenergic and serotonergic cell body regions.

Table 7.6. Possible role of excitatory amino acids and intracellular second messengers in the action of antidepressants

1. In experimental studies, chronic antidepressant treatments have been shown to reduce the behavioural effects of the NMDA-glutamate receptor antagonist dizolcipine. This suggests that antidepressants may act as functional NMDA receptor antagonists and thereby reduce excitatory glutamate transmission which is mediated by NMDA receptors.

2. Intracellular protein phosphorylation is enhanced by chronic antidepressant treatment. This leads to the increased synthesis of microtubules that form an important feature of the cellular cytoskeleton. Thus antidepressants might change signal transduction with the neurone.

3. Enhanced synthesis and transport of neurotransmitter synthesizing enzymes (e.g. tyrosine and tryptophan hydroxylase).

Preliminary clinical studies have shown that lymphocyte glucocorticoid receptors are subsensitive in depressed patients. The failure of the negative feedback mechanism that regulates the secretion of adrenal glucocorticoids further suggests that the central glucocorticoid receptors are subsensitive. This leads to the hypersecretion of cortisol, a characteristic feature of many patients with major depression. Such findings lend support to the hypothesis that the changes in central neurotransmission occurring in depression are a reflection of the effects of chronic glucocorticoids on the transcription of proteins that play a crucial role in neuronal structure and function.

If the pituitary–adrenal axis plays such an important role in central neurotransmission, it may be speculated that glucocorticoid synthesis inhibitors (e.g. metyrapone) could reduce the abnormality in neurotransmitter function by decreasing the cortisol concentration.

Recent *in vitro* hybridization studies in the rat have demonstrated that typical antidepressants increase the density of glucocorticoid receptors. Such an effect could increase the negative feedback mechanism and thereby reduce the synthesis and release of cortisol. In support of this hypothesis, there is preliminary clinical evidence that metyrapone (and the steroid synthesis inhibitor ketoconazole) may have antidepressant effects. Recently several lipophilic antagonists of corticotrophin releasing factor (CRF) type 1 receptor, which appears to be hyperactive in the brain of depressed patients, have been shown to be active in animal models of depression. Clearly this is a potentially important area for antidepressant development.

Glucocorticoid receptors are present in a high density in the amygdala and neuroimaging studies have shown that the amygdala is the only structure in which the regional blood flow and glucose metabolism consistently correlate positively with the severity of depression. This

Table 7.7.   Role of glucocorticoids in modulating brain amines in depression

1. Glucocorticoid receptors occur on catecholamine and 5-HT cell bodies in the brain.
2. There is evidence that the glucocorticoid receptors are hyposensitive in the depressed patients.
3. Chronic antidepressant treatment sensitizes these receptors, thereby normalizing the noradrenergic and serotonergic function that is reduced by the hypercortisolaemia which occurs in major depression.

hypermetabolism appears to reflect an underlying pathological process as it also occurs in asymptomatic patients and in the close relatives of the patients (Table 7.7).

The effects of antidepressants on endocrine-immune functions

Stress is frequently a trigger factor for depression in vulnerable patients. There is clinical evidence to show that CRF is elevated in the cerebrospinal fluid of untreated depressed patients, which presumably leads to the hypercortisolaemia that usually accompanies the condition. One of the consequences of elevated plasma glucocorticoids is a suppression of some aspects of cellular immunity. It is now established that many cellular (for example, natural killer cell activity, T-cell replication) and non-cellular (for example, raised acute phase proteins) aspects are abnormal in the untreated depressed patient. Such observations could help to explain the susceptibility of depressed patients to physical ill health.

A link between CRF, the cytokines which orchestrate many aspects of cellular immunity, and the prostaglandins of the E series has been the subject of considerable research in recent years. There is clinical evidence to show that prostaglandin E_2 (PGE_2) concentrations are raised in the plasma of untreated depressed patients and are normalized following effective treatment with tricyclic antidepressants. Raised PGE_2 concentrations in the brain and periphery reflect increased proinflammatory cytokines (particularly tumour necrosis factor, interleukins 1 and 6) which occur as a consequence of increased macrophage activity in the blood and brain. In the brain the microglia functions as macrophages and produces such cytokines locally. Thus the increased synthesis of PGE_2 may contribute to the reduction in amine release in the brain that appears to underlie the pathology of depression. It has recently been postulated that several types of antidepressants (e.g. tricyclics, monoamine oxidase inhibitors) normalize central neurotransmission by reducing brain concentrations of both the cytokines and PGE_2 by inhibiting central and peripheral macrophage activity together with cyclooxygenase type 2 activity in the brain. Cyclooxygenase is the key enzyme in the synthesis of the prostaglandins. It is not without interest that the usefulness of tricyclic antidepressants in

Table 7.8. The possible role of prostaglandins and cytokines in depression

1. There is evidence that both cellular and non-cellular immunity are abnormal in the depressed patient.
2. The proinflammatory cytokines (interleukins 1 and 6 and tumour necrosis factor alpha) from macrophages are raised in depression. This leads to increased PGE_2 synthesis and release which may lead to a reduction in central monoamine release.
3. Chronic antidepressant treatments reduce both the proinflammatory cytokines and PGE_2.

severe rheumatoid arthritis can now be explained by the inhibitory action of such drugs on cyclooxygenase activity in both the periphery and brain. Such changes, together with those in glucocorticoid receptor function, may therefore incrementally bring about the normalization of defective central neurotransmission as a consequence of antidepressant treatment. Whether the inhibition of cyclooxygenase is a common feature of all classes of antidepressants is presently unknown (Table 7.8).

Antidepressants and changes in neuronal structure

Another possible mechanism whereby antidepressants may change the physical relationship between neurons in the brain is by inhibiting neurite outgrowth from nerve cells. In support of this view, it has been shown that the tricyclic antidepressant amitriptyline, at therapeutically relevant concentrations, inhibited neurite outgrowth from chick embryonic cerebral explants *in vivo*. While the relevance of such findings to the therapeutic effects of amitriptyline in man is unclear, they do suggest that a common mode of action of all antidepressants could be to modify the actual structure of nerve cells and possibly eliminate inappropriate synaptic contacts that are responsible for behavioural and psychological changes associated with depression.

There are several mechanisms whereby antidepressants can modify intracellular events that occur proximal to the postsynaptic receptor sites. Most attention has been paid to the actions of antidepressants on those pathways that are controlled by receptor-coupled second messengers (such as cyclic AMP, inositol triphosphate, nitric oxide and calcium binding). However, it is also possible that chronic antidepressant treatment may affect those pathways that involve receptor interactions with protein tyrosine kinases, by increasing specific growth factor synthesis or by regulating the activity of proinflammatory cytokines. These pathways are particularly important because they control many aspects of neuronal function that ultimately underlie the ability of the brain to adapt and respond to pharmacological and environmental stimuli. One mechanism whereby antidepressants could increase the synthesis of trophic factors is

Table 7.9. Changes in neuronal structure in depression

1. There is evidence that inadequately treated, or untreated, major depression is associated with a decrease in the hippocampal volume. This could be a consequence of the increase in proinflammatory cytokines and hypercortisol-aemia.
2. Experimental evidence suggests that chronic antidepressant treatments increase the formation of transcription factors within the brain which increases neuronal plasticity and leads to recovery.

by the activation of cyclic AMP-dependent protein kinase which indirectly increases the formation of the transcription factors. There is experimental evidence to show that the infusion of one of these transcription factors (brain derived neutrophic factor) into the midbrain of rats results in antidepressant-like activity, an action associated with an increase in the synthesis of tryptophan hydroxylase, the rate-limiting enzyme in the synthesis of serotonin (Table 7.9).

Summary of the pharmacological properties of antidepressants in general use in Europe

Tricyclic antidepressants (TCAs)

This group of drugs was introduced during the early 1960s following the chance discovery of the antidepressant effects of imipramine. The therapeutic efficacy of the TCAs has been ascribed to their ability to inhibit the reuptake of noradrenaline and serotonin into the neuron following the release of these transmitters into the synaptic cleft. In addition, these drugs inhibit the muscarinic receptors (causing dry mouth, impaired vision, tachycardia, difficulty in micturition), histamine type-1 receptors (causing sedation) and alpha-1 adrenoceptor antagonism (causing postural hypotension). Such side effects often lead to non-compliance (estimated to be at least 40% in general practice situations) and are more frequent in the elderly.

The excellent clinical efficacy of the TCAs has been well documented and the pharmacokinetic profiles are favourable. The most serious disadvantage of the TCAs lies in their cardiotoxicity. Thus, with the exception of lofepramine, all the tricyclic antidepressants, including maprotiline, block the fast sodium channels in the heart which can lead to heart block and death. Approximately 15% of all patients with major depression die by suicide and a high proportion of these (up to 25%) do so by taking an overdose of TCAs. Such a dose can be as low as 5–10 times the recommended daily dose.

Lofepramine differs from the other TCAs in that its structure seems to preclude it from causing the anticholinergic, antihistaminergic and antiadrenergic effects evident with the other TCAs. In addition, it does not appear to be any more cardiotoxic than most of the second-generation antidepressants. The reason for this is an enigma, as the main metabolite of lofepramine is desipramine, a typical cardiotoxic TCA. There is a suggestion that, due to its high lipophilicity, it impedes the access of desipramine to the sodium fast channels in the heart without interfering with their normal function. Thus lofepramine would appear to fulfil many of the requirements of a safe and effective TCA; it has been widely used, particularly in elderly depressed patients, in the past in both the UK and Ireland.

Irreversible inhibitors of monoamine oxidase (MAOIs)

Iproniazid, an MAOI no longer available because of its hepatotoxicity, was the first effective antidepressant to be discovered; it was introduced shortly before the discovery of imipramine. All MAOIs are presumed to have a similar mode of action, namely to inhibit the intra- and interneuronal metabolism of the biogenic amine neurotransmitters (noradrenaline, dopamine and serotonin). These amines are primarily metabolized by MAO-A (noradrenaline and serotonin) or MAO-B (dopamine). The irreversible MAOIs are inhibitors of MAO-A while selegiline (deprenyl), used as an adjunctive treatment for Parkinson's disease, is a selective, irreversible inhibitor of MAO-B.

The main limitation to the clinical use of the MAOIs is due to their interaction with amine-containing foods such as cheeses, red wine, beers (including non-alcoholic beers), fermented and processed meat products, yeast products, soya and some vegetables. Some proprietary medicines such as cold cures contain phenylpropanolamine, ephedrine, etc. and will also interact with MAOIs. Such an interaction (termed the "cheese effect"), is attributed to the dramatic rise in blood pressure due to the sudden release of noradrenaline from peripheral sympathetic terminals, an event due to the displacement of noradrenaline from its intraneuronal vesicles by the primary amine (usually tyramine). Under normal circumstances, any dietary amines would be metabolized by MAO in the wall of the gastrointestinal tract, in the liver, platelets, etc. The occurrence of hypertensive crises, and occasionally strokes, therefore limited the use of the MAOIs, despite their proven clinical efficacy, to the treatment of atypical depression and occasionally panic disorder.

The side effects of the MAOIs include, somewhat surprisingly, orthostatic hypotension. This is thought to be due to the accumulation of dopamine in the sympathetic cervical ganglia where it acts as an inhibitory transmitter, thereby reducing peripheral vascular tone. Other side effects include psychomotor restlessness and sleep disorder. The MAOIs are cardiotoxic but probably less so than the TCAs. Potentially fatal interactions can however occur when MAOIs are combined with SSRIs or any type of drug which enhances serotonergic function. The interaction can give rise to hyperexcitability, increased muscular tone, myoclonus and loss of consciousness. The analgesic pethidine is particularly dangerous in this respect (Figure 7.1).

Reversible inhibitors of monoamine oxidase (RIMAs)

Antidepressants of this class, such as moclobemide, have a high selectivity and affinity for MAO-A. However, unlike the MAOIs, the RIMAs are reversible inhibitors of the enzyme and can easily be displaced from the enzyme surface by any primary amine which may be present in the diet. This means that the dietary amines are metabolized by MAO in the wall of the gastrointestinal tract while the enzyme in the brain and elsewhere remains inhibited. Thus the RIMAs have brought the MAOIs back into use as antidepressants in general practice. It is now evident that the RIMAs are not as potent as most currently available antidepressants.

Selective serotonin reuptake inhibitors

Zimelidine was the first SSRI antidepressant to be launched in Europe and, despite its therapeutic success, was withdrawn in the late 1980s due to severe abdominal toxicity. Zimelidine was soon replaced by fluvoxamine which only slowly received acceptance in Europe because of the high incidence of nausea and vomiting; the recommended starting dose was initially too high. Fluoxetine was the third SSRI to be launched in Europe with the advantage of a fixed daily dose (20 mg) and relatively few side effects. Sertraline, paroxetine and citalopram followed so that by the end of the 1980s, the five SSRIs were well established throughout Europe and most of the world (Figure 7.2).

As the name implies, these drugs have a high affinity for the serotonin transporter both on neuronal and also platelet membranes. There is abundant evidence that the SSRIs inhibit the reuptake of 3H-5-HT into platelets, brain slices and synaptosomal fractions, as illustrated in Table 7.10, but it is clear that there is no direct relationship between the potency of the drug to inhibit 5-HT reuptake *in vitro* and the dose necessary to relieve depression in the clinic. In experimental studies, it is clear that the increased release of 5-HT from the frontal cortex only occurs following the chronic (2 weeks or longer) administration of any of the SSRIs. Thus the inhibition of 5-HT reuptake may be a necessary condition for the antidepressant activity, but it is not sufficient in itself.

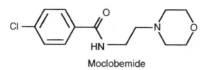

Moclobemide

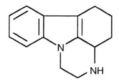

Pirlindole

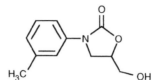

Toloxatone

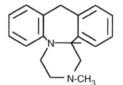

S-Mirtazapine

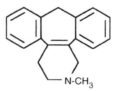

Setiptiline (teciptiline)

Figure 7.1. Structural formulae of some monoamine oxidase inhibitors (moclobemide, pirlindole and toloxatone) and alpha$_2$ adrenoceptor antagonists [S-mirtazapine and setiptiline (teciptiline)].

Despite their common ability to enhance serotonergic function *in vivo*, the SSRIs differ both in terms of their pharmacological profiles and their pharmacokinetics. Thus in addition to their direct inhibitory action on the serotonin transporter, they also affect other neurotransmitter systems which may have some clinical relevance. Citalopram has a modest antihistamine action which might account for its slightly sedative action. Sertraline has a

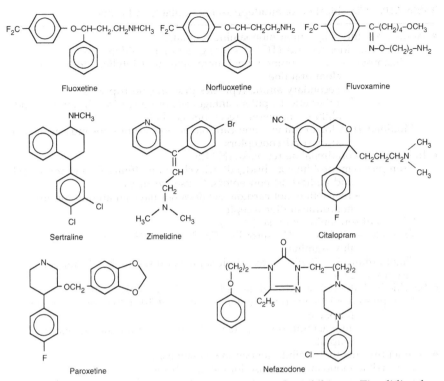

Figure 7.2. Chemical structure of some 5-HT uptake inhibitors. Zimelidine has been withdrawn due to serious adverse side effects. Norfluoxetine is an active metabolite of fluoxetine.

slight dopaminomimetic effect which may contribute to its alerting effect, while paroxetine is a muscarinic receptor antagonist. Both fluvoxamine and sertraline have affinity for sigma 1 receptors, the precise importance of which is uncertain but could contribute to the motor side effects which all the SSRIs are reputed to have, albeit very rarely. Fluoxetine, by activating 5-HT 2C receptors, may cause anxiety at least in some patients. Thus differences between the SSRIs are due not only to their different potencies as 5-HT reuptake inhibitors, but also because of their actions on other receptor systems. A comparison of the pharmacokinetic differences between the SSRIs is summarized in Table 7.10. These differences may be of clinical importance in terms of the special populations to whom the drugs should be administered (for example, the elderly may benefit particularly from citalopram because of its slightly sedative profile, and its lack of inhibition of cytochrome P450 enzymes in the liver, see p. 89). Sertraline could also be considered for this group and while drug interactions could be more problematic it does have a slightly alerting

Table 7.10. Classification of antidepressants available in Europe

---

- Antidepressants that inhibit monoamine reuptake
    Tricyclic antidepressants (TCAs) – first-generation antidepressants
        Examples – tertiary amine type: imipramine, amitriptyline, dothiepin,
            clomipramine
            – secondary amine type: desipramine, nortriptyline
            – other effects: potent antagonists of muscarinic, histaminic and
                alpha-1 adrenergic receptors; cardiotoxic
    Modified TCA-lofepramine – non-cardiotoxic; low affinity for muscarinic and
        alpha-1 adrenoceptors
- Inhibitors of noradrenaline reuptake (NARIs)
    Examples – maprotiline: a "bridged" tricyclic with affinity for histamine, H1,
        and alpha-1 adrenoceptors. Causes seizures
        – reboxetine: not cardiotoxic; does not have an affinity for any
            neurotransmitter receptors
- Inhibitors of serotonin reuptake (SSRIs)
    Examples – citalopram (1), sertraline (2), fluoxetine (3), paroxetine (4),
        fluvoxamine
    Slight affinity for (1) histamine, (2) dopamine, (3) serotonin, (4) muscarinic
    receptors (see text)
- Specific inhibitors of noradrenaline and serotonin reuptake (SNRIs)
    Examples – venlafaxine (more potent inhibitor of 5-HT than noradrenaline
        reuptake)
        – milnacipran (more potent inhibitor of noradrenaline than 5-HT
            reuptake)
- Antidepressants that inhibit monoamine metabolism
    Irreversible monoamine oxidase inhibitors (MAOIs)
    Examples – phenelzine, pargyline, tranylcypromine, isocarboxazid. All
        interact with dietary monoamine to cause the "cheese effect"
        (see text)
- Reversible inhibitors of monoamine oxidase A (RIMAs)
    Examples – moclobemide, pirlindole. At therapeutic doses unlikely to interact
        with dietary amines (see text)
- Tetracyclic antidepressants
    Examples – mianserin (1), mirtazepine (6-aza-mianserin) (2)
        (1) The first second-generation antidepressant; an alpha-2 adrenoceptor
            antagonist with some affinity for $5-HT_{1A}$, $5-HT_{2A}$ and $5-HT_3$, alpha-1
            adrenoceptors and H1 receptors
        (2) Known as a noradrenaline and specific serotonin antidepressant (NaSSA).
            More potent affinity for alpha-2 adrenoceptors and 5-HT receptors than
            mianserin; H1 antagonist
- Other antidepressants (sometimes called "atypical")
    Examples – trazodone, nefazodone: $5-HT_{1A}$ and $5-HT_2$ antagonists, weak SSRI
        activity; alpha-1 and H1 antagonism

---

profile which could be beneficial. Fluvoxamine has also been extensively
studied in the elderly, but nausea could be a problem while fluoxetine, with
its very long half-life (with its active metabolite norfluoxetine, amounting to
12 days in the elderly patient) could be beneficial for the non-compliant

patient. In the elderly, fluoxetine could cause some anorexia and weight loss however. Paroxetine should be administered with more care in the elderly because of its anticholinergic action.

In addition to their proven efficacy in the treatment of all types of depression, the SSRIs have been shown to be the drugs of choice in the treatment of panic disorder, obsessive–compulsive disorder, bulimia nervosa, and as an adjunct to the treatment of alcohol withdrawal and relapse prevention, premenstrual dysphoric disorder and post-traumatic stress disorder. The usefulness of these drugs in treating such a diverse group of disorders reflects the primary role of serotonin in the regulation of sleep, mood, impulsivity and food intake.

All the SSRIs have qualitatively similar side effects that largely arise from the increase in serotonergic function and the resulting activation of the different 5-HT receptor types in the brain and periphery. There are differences in the frequency of these effects however which would not be anticipated if all the SSRIs were essentially the same! These effects include nausea, vomiting, diarrhoea or constipation, insomnia, tremor, initial anxiety, dizziness, sexual dysfunction and headache. Loss in body weight may occur but this is rare. The behavioural toxicity of the SSRIs as indicated by their effects on psychomotor function, memory and learning, is low, particularly when compared to the TCAs and some of the sedative second-generation antidepressants such as mianserin, mirtazepine and trazodone. The SSRIs are not cardiotoxic and safety in overdose has been indicated for all these drugs. In general, the severity of the adverse effects is slight and seldom leads to non-compliance.

In addition to the five SSRIs currently available, many more compounds are in development which will no doubt be marketed in the near future. Of the new arrivals, escitalopram, the S-enantiomer of citalopram, has already become available in many European countries. A brief discussion of the properties of this drug has been presented on p. 98.

Noradrenaline reuptake inhibitors (NRIs)

Reboxetine is the only selective and reasonably potent noradrenaline reuptake inhibitor available clinically at the present time. Reboxetine has a chemical structure not dissimilar from viloxazine, an antidepressant which was of only limited clinical interest in the 1970s because of its weak efficacy and unacceptable side effects (nausea, vomiting and occasionally seizures). Unlike the secondary amine TCA antidepressants, such as maprotiline, desipramine, nortriptyline and protriptyline, reboxetine does not affect any other transporter or receptor system and therefore is largely devoid of TCA and SSRI-like side effects. In clinical trials, reboxetine has been shown to be as effective as the SSRIs in the treatment of depression but, unlike the SSRIs, reboxetine does not inhibit any of the cytochrome P450 enzymes in the liver.

In contrast to the widespread interest in 5-HT in depression research and in the development of antidepressants, there would appear to be little interest in developing antidepressants that selectively modulate the noradrenergic system. At the present time, there do not appear to be any drugs of this type in development.

For completeness, buproprion should be mentioned even though it is not widely registered as an antidepressant in Europe, partly because of its propensity to cause seizures in some patients. Buproprion, quite widely used in the USA as an antidepressant, appears to inhibit the reuptake of both dopamine and noradrenaline and therefore tends to have a slightly alerting action. In many European countries it has recently been introduced, at a lower than antidepressant dose, in the treatment of nicotine withdrawal in smoking cessation programmes.

Lastly, nomifensine was an interesting antidepressant that also had noradrenaline, dopamine and, due to its 4-hydroxy metabolite, serotonin reuptake properties. It was withdrawn some years ago because of the occurrence of haemolytic anaemia in a small number of patients. It was a particularly effective drug in the treatment of depression in patients with epilepsy as, unlike many antidepressants available at that time, it did not affect the seizure threshold.

Selective serotonin and noradrenaline reuptake inhibitors (SNRIs)

In an attempt to combine the clinical efficacy of the TCAs with the tolerability and safety of the SSRIs and NRIs, drugs showing selectivity in inhibiting the reuptake of both noradrenaline and serotonin were developed. Being structurally unrelated to the TCAs however, they lacked their side effects including their cardiotoxicity.

To date, venlafaxine is the most widely available of the SNRIs. Although it is known to enhance both serotonergic and noradrenergic function, at the lower clinical dose range it primarily enhances serotonergic function and therefore has the characteristic side effects of an SSRI. At higher therapeutic doses, venlafaxine also inhibits noradrenaline reuptake and therefore resembles a TCA antidepressant. While there is no evidence that venlafaxine is as cardiotoxic as the TCAs, recent studies have indicated that it is at least threefold more likely than the SSRIs to result in death if taken in overdose. Hypertension may occur in some patients when given a high therapeutic dose of venlafaxine.

A more potent, but qualitatively similar antidepressant to venlafaxine, duloxetine, is currently in advanced clinical development.

Milnacipran is also a dual-action antidepressant which, like venlafaxine, has been shown to be more effective than the SSRIs in the treatment of severe, hospitalized and suicidally depressed patients. At lower therapeutic doses, milnacipran blocks the noradrenaline transporters and therefore resembles the NRI antidepressants. Higher doses result in the serotonergic component becoming apparent (i.e. an SSRI-like action). The main problem with milnacipram appears to be its lack of linear kinetics with some evidence that it has a U-shaped dose–response curve (Figure 7.3).

Tetracyclic antidepressants

Mianserin was the first of the second-generation antidepressants to be developed. It lacked the amine reuptake inhibitory and MAOI actions of the first-generation drugs and also lacked the cardiotoxicity and anticholinergic activity of the TCAs. However, it was sedative (antihistaminic), caused postural hypotension (alpha-1 blockade) and also caused blood dyscrasias and agranulocytosis in a small number of patients. This has limited the use of mianserin in recent years.

Mirtazepine (called a Noradrenaline and Selective Serotonin Anti-depressant; NaSSA) is the 6-aza derivative of mianserin and shares several important pharmacological properties with its predecessor, namely its antihistaminic and alpha-1 adrenoceptor antagonistic actions. Like mianserin, mirtazepine also causes weight gain. Nevertheless, mirtazepine is better tolerated and there is no evidence of blood dyscrasias associated with its clinical use.

Regarding the mode of action of these tetracyclic compounds, both are potent alpha-2 adrenoceptor antagonists which cause an enhanced release of noradrenaline. The action of mirtazepine on serotonin receptors ($5\text{-}HT_{1A}$, $5\text{-}HT_{2A}$, $5\text{-}HT_3$) is both direct ($5\text{-}HT_{2A}$ and $5\text{-}HT_3$) and indirect ($5\text{-}HT_{1A}$). The complexity of the interaction of the drug with both adrenoceptors and serotonin receptors helps to emphasize the importance of the "cross talk" between these two neurotransmitter systems. Thus the antidepressant effects of both mirtazepine and mianserin are related to the enhancement of noradrenaline release (alpha-2 blockade) and $5\text{-}HT_{2A}$ receptor antagonism. In addition, mirtazepine (and to a lesser extent mianserin) blocks $5\text{-}HT_3$ receptors therefore reducing the anxiety and nausea normally associated with drugs that enhance serotonergic function. The anti-anxiety effect of mirtazepine is ascribed to its indirect activation of the $5\text{-}HT_{1A}$ receptors, an effect also seen following the administration of an SSRI. The probable sites of action of mirtazepine are shown in Figure 7.4.

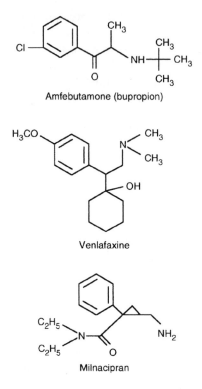

Amfebutamone (bupropion)

Venlafaxine

Milnacipran

Figure 7.3. Structural formulae of the noradrenaline (norepinephrine)/dopamine reuptake inhibitor amfebutamone (bupropion) and some nonselective noradrenaline and serotonin (5-hydroxytryptamine; 5-HT) reuptake inhibitors (venlafaxine, and milnacipran).

Other, or atypical, antidepressants

These include trazodone and a derivative of its metabolite nefazodone, both of which are strongly sedative, an effect which has been attributed to their potent alpha-1 receptor antagonism rather than to any antihistaminic effects. A main advantage of these drugs in the treatment of depression is that they appear to improve the sleep profile of the depressed patient. Their antidepressant activity is associated with their weak 5-HT reuptake inhibition and also a weak alpha-2 antagonism. However, unlike most of the second-generation antidepressants, neither drug is effective in the treatment of severely depressed patients. Furthermore, there is some evidence that trazodone can cause arrythmias, and priapism, in elderly patients.

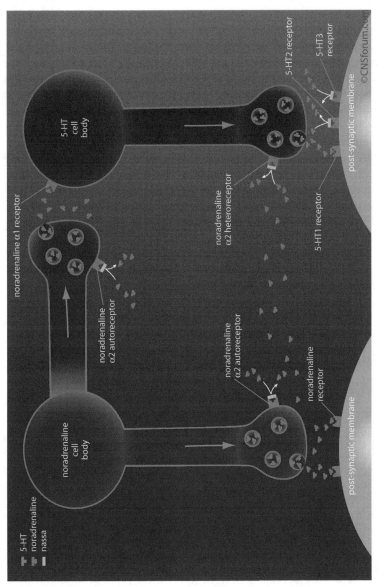

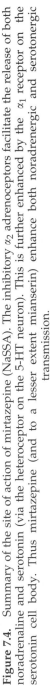

Figure 7.4. Summary of the site of action of mirtazepine (NaSSA). The inhibitory α_2 adrenoceptors facilitate the release of both noradrenaline and serotonin (via the heteroceptor on the 5-HT neuron). This is further enhanced by the α_1 receptor on the serotonin cell body. Thus mirtazepine (and to a lesser extent mianserin) enhance both noradrenergic and serotonergic transmission.

Herbal antidepressants – St John's Wort (Hypericum officinalis)

St John's Wort in recent years has become widely used in Europe and North America for the treatment of mild depression. Unlike all other antidepressants mentioned above, St John's Wort is obtained through herbalists and health food shops in such countries, the exception being Ireland where it can only be obtained on prescription like any other antidepressant. There are at least 12 placebo-controlled studies proving the efficacy of St John's Wort against standard antidepressants; all these studies show that the mixture of compounds present in St John's Wort is effective in mild to moderate, but not severe, depression. Of the main active ingredients of the plant, it would appear that hyperfolin is largely responsible for the antidepressant activity. This compound is an inhibitor of the reuptake of noradrenaline, dopamine and serotonin. In addition, it appears to have some NMDA-glutamate receptor antagonist activity, a property which it shares with many other antidepressants.

A diagram summarizing the sites of action of most classes of antidepressants is illustrated in Figure 7.5.

Physical pain and depression

Major depression is a triad of psychological, somatic and physical symptoms. Over 75% of depressed patients report painful physical symptoms involving the neck, back, head, stomach and the skeleto-muscular system. Not only can chronic pain lead to depression, but also vice versa.

Fibromyalgia, accounting for 2–4% of the general population, is a common cause of chronic pain. It has been estimated that 20–40% of such patients have co-morbid depression with a lifetime prevalence of about 70%. This raises the question whether there is a common mechanism linking pain and depression.

Neuroanatomically both the locus coeruleus and the raphé nuclei project to the spinal cord where they gate sensory pathways from the skeletomuscular areas. As there is evidence that both noradrenaline and 5-HT are dysfunctional in depression, it is perhaps not surprising to find that the pain threshold is often reduced in patients with depression. Conversely, different types of antidepressants have been shown to have an antinociceptive effect in both rodent models of neuropathic pain, and clinically in fibromyalgia, chronic fatigue syndrome, postherpetic neuralgia and diabetic neuropathy. In general, it would appear that the dual action antidepressants (such as the TCAs and SNRIs) are more effective than the SSRIs.

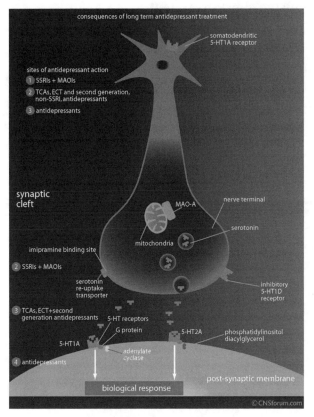

Figure 7.5. Summary of the sites of action of antidepressants and ECT on the serotonergic neuron.

Treatment decisions for unipolar depression

- Treatment of choice – second-generation antidepressants such as a SSRI, venlafaxine, mirtazepine, reboxetine, moclobemide.
- Switching – alternative second-generation antidepressant, usually from another group.
- Augmentation of antidepressant response – add lithium, thyroid hormone, an atypical antipsychotic (e.g. risperidone, olanzepine), pindolol, buspirone.
- Other options – ECT, St John's Wort.

Note: In a survey of 13 studies, switching from an SSRI to either another SSRI or to imipramine, venlafaxine, mirtazepine or buproprion resulted in a response rate of 30–90%.

Electroconvulsive shock treatment

One of the pioneers in the application of electroconvulsive shock treatment (ECT) was the Italian clinician Cerletti who stated that the ". . . electricity itself is of little importance . . . the important and fundamental factor is the epileptic-like seizure no matter how it is obtained". ECT is undoubtedly an effective treatment for a range of psychiatric diseases varying from severe depression and mania to some forms of schizophrenia. Despite the considerable use of ECT over the last 50 years, it still arouses intense emotional and scientific debate. While the opposition to the use of ECT has been more evident in some Continental European countries and the United States than in Britain or Ireland, it was a British study of the use of ECT which, following a survey of over 100 centres, found that many units were badly equipped and had poor facilities and staff training. This report resulted in a considerable improvement in the application of ECT, with the establishment of guidelines governing the management and use of the technique; somewhat similar guidelines were instituted by the American Psychiatric Association.

It is now generally agreed that ECT is singularly effective and useful. There has been controversy over the relative merits in using unilateral or bilateral ECT. In general, it would appear that unilateral ECT is effective in the treatment of most depressed patients, whereas manic patients appear to respond best to bilateral ECT. Following a course of treatment, twice weekly for several weeks, the success rate in treating depression is about 80%. This is more successful than using antidepressants (up to 70% for a single course of treatment). Seizure monitoring is essential to ensure an adequate response. The principal side effect of ECT is a temporary cognitive deficit, specifically memory loss. There is evidence that such impairment is reduced if unilateral ECT is applied to the non-dominant hemisphere. Brief pulse-current ECT machines are now favoured in Britain and the United States to ensure optimal efficacy and minimal side effects. As Cerletti hypothesized in 1938, chemically induced seizures are equally effective as ECT and at one time pentamethylenetetrazole or flurothyl were used to produce seizures. However, the safety and ease of application of ECT means that such methods have been largely replaced.

How does ECT work?

While there are various psychological, neurophysiological and neuroendocrine theories that have been developed to explain the beneficial effects of ECT, most attention has been given to the manner in which ECT causes changes in those neurotransmitters that have been implicated in psychiatric illness. It is known that the rise in the seizure threshold during the course of treatment, and the corresponding alteration in cerebral blood flow, may reflect profound changes in cerebral metabolism that could be of crucial importance regarding the action of ECT. Changes in the hypothalamo–pituitary–adrenal axis have also been reported, but most studies suggest that such changes are secondary to the clinical response. The major emphasis of research has therefore been in the functional changes in brain neurotransmission, but it must be emphasized that most detailed studies have been conducted in rodents and therefore their precise relevance to changes in the human brain are a matter of conjecture.

Experimental studies in rodents have largely centred on the changes in biogenic amine neurotransmitters following chronic ECT treatments. Under these conditions, noradrenaline and 5-HT have been shown to be increased; the number of presynaptic $alpha_2$ receptors and their functional activity has been shown to be decreased, as has the functional activity of the dopamine autoreceptors. Such changes have also been found following the chronic administration of antidepressant drugs. The most consistent changes reported have been those found in postsynaptic receptor function. The functional activity of the postsynaptic beta adrenoceptors is decreased, a change which is also found with antidepressants. The postsynaptic 5-HT$_2$ receptor sensitivity is enhanced by chronic ECT and antidepressant treatment. Thus there appears to be a consistency between the chronic effects of both ECT and antidepressants in enhancing 5-HT responsiveness and diminishing that of noradrenaline. Regarding the dopaminergic system, while there is speculation that changes in the activity of this system may be important in the action of novel antidepressants such as bupropion, the only consistent changes found following chronic application of ECT and antidepressants is a functional decrease in the dopamine autoreceptor activity. This would lead to a reduction in the release of this transmitter.

In contrast to the plethora of animal studies, few clinical studies have shown consistent changes in the biogenic amines. There is evidence that the urinary and CSF concentrations of the noradrenaline metabolites normetanephrine and MHPG are decreased, suggesting that the turnover of noradrenaline is decreased, the opposite to that found in animals. Neuroendocrine challenge tests that have been used as probes to assess central noradrenergic function (e.g. with clonidine) show no consistent changes in patients following chronic ECT. Consistent changes have been reported in serotonergic function, however, with enhanced prolactin release occurring in response to a thyroid-stimulating hormone challenge. This is in agreement with the view that chronic ECT sensitizes postsynaptic 5-HT$_2$ receptors. Furthermore, platelet imipramine binding, which according to the results of some studies is increased in the untreated depressed patient, is attenuated by both antidepressant and ECT treatments, although it must be emphasized that not all investigators can replicate these findings. The transport of $[^3H]$5-HT into the platelets of depressed patients is also normalized following ECT and chronic antidepressant treatments. There is no evidence of any change in the dopaminergic system in depressed patients following ECT.

The central cholinergic system has been implicated in the pathogenesis of affective disorder and in memory function, which is frequently found to be malfunctioning in depressed patients. The memory deficit elicited by chronic ECT in both patients and animals may be related to the decreased density and function of central muscarinic receptors, but it should be emphasized that the changes reported in cholinergic function are small and their relevance to the clinical situation remains to be established.

Brain GABA is closely associated with the induction of seizures. In animals, chronic ECT decreases GABA synthesis in the limbic regions. While consistent changes in GABA-A receptor activity have not been reported, it would appear that GABA-B receptor density increases in the limbic regions following chronic ECT. This is qualitatively similar to the changes that have been reported following antidepressant treatment. The recent interest in the involvement of GABA in the aetiology of depression and in the mode of action of antidepressants is based on the hypothesis that GABA plays a key role not only in the induction of seizures but also in modulating the changes in the serotonergic system that are induced by both antidepressants and ECT.

Due to the ubiquitous distribution of peptides as cotransmitters and neuromodulators in the brain, it is not surprising to find that ECT produces changes in their concentrations and in their possible functional activity. Increased metenkephalin concentrations have been reported following chronic ECT. Such changes may be due to increased opioid receptor binding sites. Opioid-mediated behavioural changes such as catalepsy and reduced pain responses are increased following ECT in animals. Whether such changes are relevant to the effects of ECT and antidepressants in depressed patients is still unknown.

Other possibilities that have been suggested as a cause of the antidepressant action of ECT include an enhanced adenosine₁ receptor density in the cortex; agonists at these receptor sites are known to have anticonvulsant properties, while antagonists such as caffeine can cause convulsions, at least in high doses. Thyroid-stimulating hormone activity has also been shown to be enhanced. This peptide may exert antidepressant effects in its own right, but may also act by modulating both serotonergic and dopaminergic activity.

In SUMMARY, it would appear that ECT produces a number of changes in central neurotransmission that are common to antidepressants. These include a decrease in the functional activity of beta adrenoceptors and an enhanced activity of 5-HT$_2$ and possibly GABA-B receptors. The functional defect in central muscarinic receptors may be associated with the memory deficits caused by ECT treatment. It must be emphasized that the changes reported have largely been derived from animal experiments and their precise relevance to the mode of action of ECT in man is still a matter of conjecture.

Adverse effects of drug treatment for depression

TCAs

Significant side effects have been estimated to occur in about 5% of patients on TCAs, most of these effects being attributed to their antimuscarinic properties, for example, blurred vision, dry mouth, tachycardia and disturbed gastrointestinal and urinary tract function. Orthostatic hypotension due to the block of alpha$_1$ adrenoceptors and sedation resulting from antihistaminic activity frequently occur at therapeutic doses, particularly in the elderly. Excessive sweating is also a fairly common phenomenon, but its precise mechanism is uncertain. In the elderly patient, the precipitation of prostatic hypertrophy and glaucoma by the TCAs is also a frequent cause of concern.

Adverse effects of the TCAs on the brain include confusion, impaired memory and cognition and occasionally delirium; some of these effects have been reported to occur in up to 30% of patients over the age of 50. These effects may occasionally be confused with a recurrence of the symptoms of depression and are probably due to the central antimuscarinic activity of these drugs. Tremor also occurs frequently, particularly in the elderly, and may be controlled by the concurrent administration of propranolol. Neuroleptics are normally not recommended to be used in combination with TCAs as they are liable to accentuate the side effects of the latter drugs. The risk of seizures, and the switch from depression to mania in bipolar patients, has also been reported following TCA administration.

Weight gain is a frequent side effect and is of considerable concern, particularly in the female patient, an effect probably associated with increased appetite. Other less common side effects include jaundice (particularly with imipramine), agranulocytosis and skin rashes.

Acute poisoning

This occurs all too frequently with the TCAs and can be life threatening. Death has been reported with doses of 2000 mg of imipramine, or the equivalent quantity of other TCAs, which approximates to 10 daily doses or less! Severe intoxication has been reported at doses of 1000 mg. Because of

Table 7.11.   Relative toxicity of antidepressants in overdose (UK data for period 1985–1990)

Drug	Deaths per million prescriptions
Tricyclics	
Amitriptyline	46.5
Dothiepin	50.0
Nortriptyline	39.2
Doxepin	31.3
Imipramine	28.4
Clomipramine	11.1
Maprotiline	37.6
Lofepramine	0.0*
Non-tricyclics	
Nomifensine	2.5
Trazodone	13.6
Mianserin	5.6
Viloxazine	9.4
Fluoxetine	0.0
Fluvoxamine	6.4
MAOIs	
Tranylcypromine	58.1
Phenelzine	22.8
Isocarboxazid	12.9

Mortality data obtained from Office of Population and Statistics of England and Wales and Registrar-General of Scotland. Data for single drug or single drug+alcohol.
*Since above data were reported, six cases of mortality following overdose have been identified in which lofepramine may be the causative agent.

the toxicity of these drugs and the nature of the illness, in which suicidal thoughts are a common feature, it is generally recommended that no more than a 1 week's supply should be given at any one time to an acutely depressed patient.

The symptoms of overdose are to some extent predictable from the antimuscarinic and adrenolytic activity of these drugs. Excitement and restlessness, sometimes associated with seizures, and rapidly followed by coma, depressed respiration, hypoxia, hypotension and hypothermia are clear signs of TCA overdose. Tachycardia and arrhythmias lead to diminished cardiac function and thus to reduced cerebral perfusion, which exacerbates the central toxic effects. It is generally accepted that dialysis and forced diuresis are useless in counteracting the toxicity, but activated charcoal may reduce the absorption of any unabsorbed drug. The risk of cardiac arrhythmias may extend for several days after the patient has recovered from a TCA overdose.

It is partly due to the toxicity of the TCAs that the newer non-tricyclic drugs have been developed. All the evidence suggests that the non-tricyclics are much safer in overdose. Table 7.11 gives a survey of the relative toxicity of the older and newer antidepressants in overdose.

Drug interactions

Another area of concern regarding the use of the TCAs is their interaction with other drugs which may be given concurrently. Such interactions may arise due to the drugs competing for the plasma protein binding sites (e.g. phenytoin, aspirin and the phenothiazines) or for the liver microsomal enzyme system responsible for the common metabolism of the drugs (e.g. steroids, including the oral contraceptives, sedatives, apart from the benzodiazepines, and the neuroleptics). All of the TCAs potentiate the sedative effects of alcohol and any other psychotropic drug with sedative properties given concurrently. Smoking potentiates the metabolism of the TCAs. There is a well-established interaction between the TCAs and the adrenergic neuron blocking antihypertensives (e.g. bethanidine and guanethidine) which results from the TCA impeding the uptake of the neuron blocker into the sympathetic nerve terminal, thereby preventing it from exerting its pharmacological effects.

There is also a rare, but occasionally fatal, interaction between TCAs and MAOIs in which hyperpyrexia, convulsions and coma can occur. The precise mechanism by which this is brought about is unclear, but it may be associated with a sudden release of 5-HT.

Following prolonged TCA administration, abrupt withdrawal of the drug can lead to generalized somatic or gastrointestinal distress, which may be associated with anxiety, agitation, sleep disturbance, movement disorders and even mania. Such symptoms may be associated with central and peripheral cholinergic hyperactivity that is a consequence of the prolonged muscarinic receptor blockade caused by the TCAs.

MAOIs

The toxic effects of these drugs may arise shortly after an overdose, the effects including agitation, hallucinations, hyperreflexia and convulsions. Somewhat surprisingly, both hypo- and hypertension may occur, the former symptoms arising due to the accumulation of the inhibitory transmitter dopamine in the sympathetic ganglia leading to a marked reduction in ganglionic transmission, while hypertension can result from a dramatic release of noradrenaline from both central and peripheral sources. Such toxic effects are liable to be prolonged, particularly when the older irreversible inhibitors such as phenelzine and tranylcypromine are used. Treatment of such adverse effects should be aimed at controlling the temperature, respiration and blood pressure.

The toxic effects of the MAOIs are more varied and potentially more serious than those of the other classes of antidepressants in common use. Hepatotoxicity has been reported to occur with the older hydrazine type of MAOIs and led to the early demise of iproniazid; the hepatotoxicity does not appear to be related to the dose or duration of the drug administered.

Excessive central stimulation, usually exhibited as tremors, insomnia and hyperhidrosis, can occur following therapeutic doses of the MAOIs, as can agitation and hypomanic episodes. Peripheral neuropathy, which is largely restricted to the hydrazine type of MAOI, is rare and has been attributed to a drug-induced pyridoxine deficiency. Such side effects as dizziness and vertigo (presumably associated with hypotension), headache, inhibition of ejaculation (which is often also a problem with the TCAs), fatigue, dry mouth and constipation have also been reported. These side effects appear to be more frequently associated with phenelzine use. They are not associated with any antimuscarinic properties of the drug but presumably arise from the enhanced peripheral sympathetic activity which the MAOIs cause.

Drug interactions

Predictable interactions occur between the MAOIs and any amine precursors, or directly or indirectly acting sympathomimetic amines (e.g. the amphetamines, phenylephrine and tyramine). Such interactions can cause pronounced hypertension and, in extreme cases, stroke.

MAOIs interfere with the metabolism of many different classes of drugs that may be given concurrently. They potentiate the actions of general anaesthetics, sedatives, including alcohol, antihistamines, centrally acting analgesics (particularly pethidine due to an enhanced release of 5-HT) and anticholinergic drugs. They also potentiate the actions of TCAs, which may provide an explanation for the use of such a combination in the treatment of therapy-resistant depression.

The *"cheese effect"* is a well-established phenomenon whereby an amine-rich food is consumed while the patient is being treated with an irreversible MAOI. Foods which cause such an effect include cheeses, pickled fish, yeast products (red wines and beers, including non-alcoholic varieties), chocolate and pulses such as broad beans (which contain dopa). It appears that foods containing more than 10 mg of tyramine must be consumed in order to produce a significant rise in blood pressure. Furthermore, it is now apparent that there is considerable variation in the tyramine content of many of these foods even when they are produced by the same manufacturer. Therefore it is essential that all patients on MAOIs should be provided with a list of foods and drinks that should be avoided.

Changing a patient from one MAOI to another, or to a TCA, requires a "wash-out" period of at least 2 weeks to avoid the possibility of a drug interaction. There is evidence to suggest that a combination of an MAOI with clomipramine is more likely to produce serious adverse effects than occurs with other TCAs. Regarding the newer non-tricyclic antidepressants, it is recommended that a "wash-out" period of at least 5 weeks be given before a patient on fluoxetine is given an MAOI; this is due to the very long half-life of the main fluoxetine metabolite norfluoxetine.

Although it is widely acknowledged that the older MAOIs have the potential to produce serious adverse effects, the actual reported incidence is surprisingly low. Tranylcypromine was one of the most widely used drugs, involving several million patients by the mid 1970s, and yet only 50 patients were reported to have severe cerebrovascular accidents and, of these, only 15 deaths occurred. Nevertheless, it is generally recommended that this drug should not be given to elderly patients or to other patients with hypertension or cardiovascular disease.

Second-generation antidepressants

With the possible exception of maprotiline, which is chemically a modified TCA with all the side effects attributable to such a molecule, all of the newer non-tricyclic drugs have fewer anticholinergic effects and are less cardiotoxic than the older tricyclics. *Lofepramine* is an example of a modified tricyclic that, due to the absence of a free NH_2 group in the side chain, is relatively devoid of anticholinergic side effects. Thus by slightly modifying the structure of the side chain it is possible to retain the efficacy while reducing the cardiotoxicity.

Of the plethora of new *5-HT uptake inhibitor antidepressants* (e.g. zimelidine, indalpine, fluoxetine, fluvoxamine, citalopram, sertraline and paroxetine), the most frequently mentioned side effects following therapeutic administration are mild gastrointestinal discomfort, which can lead to nausea and vomiting, occasional diarrhoea and headache. This appears to be more frequent with fluvoxamine than the other SSRI antidepressants. Such changes are attributable to increased peripheral serotonergic function. Some severe idiosyncratic and hypersensitivity reactions such as the Gullain–Barré syndrome and blood dyscrasias have led to the early withdrawal of zimelidine and indalpine. For the well-established antidepressants such as fluoxetine, the side effects appear to be mild and well-tolerated, although akathisia and agitation have been reported and may be more pronounced in elderly patients.

Nomifensine and bupropion are examples of non-tricyclic antidepressants that facilitate *catecholaminergic function*. These drugs have the advantage over the TCAs of being non-sedative in therapeutic doses. The rare, although fatal, occurrence of haemolytic anaemia and pyrexia following therapeutic administration of nomifensine led to its withdrawal from the market a few years ago. Bupropion was also temporarily withdrawn from clinical use following evidence of seizure induction, but it has now returned to the market in the United States. Idiosyncratic reactions have been reported to occur with the tetracyclic antidepressant *mianserin*, several cases of agranulocytosis have been reported in different countries. Elderly patients would appear to be most at risk from such adverse effects. Whether such side effects are a peculiarity of the mianserin structure or will also be found with the 6-aza derivative, mirtazepine, is uncertain but preliminary evidence from post-marketing surveys suggests that this is unlikely. Other frequent side effects associated with therapeutic doses of mianserin are sedation and orthostatic hypotension; sedation and weight gain are also problems with mirtazepine.

Clearly the major advantage of all the recently introduced antidepressants lies in their relative safety in overdosage and reduced side effects. These factors are particularly important when considering the need for optimal patient compliance and in the treatment of the elderly depressed patient who is more likely to experience severe side effects from antidepressants.

Treatment-resistant depression

It has been estimated that at least 30% of patients with major depression fail to respond to a 6-week course of a TCA antidepressant. A major problem arises however in the definition of "treatment resistance". To date, there appears to be no internationally acceptable definition of the condition. A practical definition which many clinicians find useful is that treatment resistance occurs when the patient fails to respond to:

1. An antidepressant given at maximum dose for 6–8 weeks.
2. An antidepressant from another group administered for 6–8 weeks.
3. A full course of ECT.

The following possibilities may then be considered should the patient fail to respond:

1. Add lithium to a standard antidepressant (e.g. an SSRI) maintaining the plasma lithium concentration at 0.4–0.6 mmol/l. This is a well-established method with approximately 50% of the patients responding. However, the plasma lithium concentration must be monitored.
2. Administer a high therapeutic dose of a "dual action" antidepressant such as venlafaxine or possibly mirtazepine. A discontinuation syndrome may occur if venlafaxine is abruptly withdrawn. The

symptoms of the discontinuation reaction, which also occur occasionally when some of the SSRIs are abruptly withdrawn, include dizziness, "electroshock" sensations, anxiety and agitation, insomnia, flu-like symptoms, diarrhoea and abdominal pain, parathesis, nausea.

3. Add tri-iodothyronine to a standard antidepressant. This combination is usually well tolerated but monitoring the plasma T_3 concentration is important.

4. Add tryptophan to a standard antidepressant (usually an SSRI). There is a danger that the serotonin syndrome may occur however and occasionally the eosinophilia myalgia syndrome. The symptoms that occur with increasing severity are restlessness, diaphoresis, tremor, shivering, myoclonus, confusion, convulsions, death.

5. Add pindolol (a $5-HT_{1D}$ antagonist as well as a beta adrenoceptor antagonist), which is well researched but there are contradictory findings in the literature with regard to its efficacy. So far, the clinical data suggest that the response to a standard antidepressant is accelerated.

6. Add dexamethasone to a standard antidepressant. This combination is well tolerated for a short course of treatment but so far there is only limited evidence of efficacy from the literature.

7. Add lamotrigine to a standard antidepressant. Again, the support for this approach is largely anecdotal.

8. Add buspirone to a standard antidepressant (usually an SSRI). The evidence in favour of this combination is largely anecdotal.

9. Add an atypical antipsychotic (e.g. olanzapine or risperidone). There is some "open trial" evidence in favour of such combinations.

10. Add mirtazepine to a standard antidepressant (usually an SSRI). Again, the evidence is largely anecdotal.

There are a number of other methods mentioned in the literature, some of which (such as the combination of a TCA with an MAOI) are potentially cardiotoxic and not to be recommended. More recently, a combination of an SSRI with a TCA has become popular but is not to be recommended because of the probability of metabolic interactions involving the cytochrome P450 system that can increase the tissue concentration of even a modest dose of a TCA to a cardiotoxic level.

In CONCLUSION it appears that the chemically and pharmacologically diverse drugs that act as antidepressants have two properties in common. Firstly, they demonstrate approximately equal clinical efficacy and require several weeks' administration to produce an optimal therapeutic effect. Secondly, they all modulate a number of different types of mainly postsynaptic neurotransmitter receptors in animals and in depressed patients. Such effects occur irrespective of their specific effects on a particular neurotransmitter system that may arise after their short-term administration. Thus, the amine hypothesis of depression, in which it was postulated that depression arises from a deficiency in one or more of the biogenic amine neurotransmitters, which is corrected following effective antidepressant treatment, has now evolved into the "receptor sensitivity hypothesis". This hypothesis explains the delay in the therapeutic effects of antidepressant treatments as being due to time-dependent adaptational changes in neurotransmitter receptors. Thus, depression may be related to an underlying abnormality in neurotransmitter receptor function. Whether this is sufficient to cause the abnormal affect state is still a matter of debate. It is possible, for example, that the changes in receptor function that ultimately produce the behavioural changes associated with depression are a consequence of changes in gene expression, nerve growth factor synthesis and central glucocorticoid receptor activity that reflect the response of the patient to prolonged hypercortisolaemia.

Clearly, more research is needed to elucidate the precise mechanisms of action of antidepressants and the psychopathology of the condition. Only then may it be possible to develop antidepressants that show a clear therapeutic superiority over those available today.

8 Drug Treatment of Mania

Introduction

The term "bipolar disorder" originally referred to manic-depressive illnesses characterized by both manic and depressive episodes. In recent years, the concept of bipolar disorder has been broadened to include subtypes with similar clinical courses, phenomenology, family histories and treatment responses. These subtypes are thought to form a continuum of disorders that, while differing in severity, are related. Readers are referred to the *Diagnostic and Statisticial Manual of Mental Disorders* of the American Psychiatric Association (DSM–IV) for details of this classification.

The diagnosis of mania is made on the basis of clinical history plus a mental state examination. Key features of mania include elevated, expansive or irritable mood accompanied by hyperactivity, pressure of speech, flight of ideas, grandiosity, hyposomnia and distractibility. Such episodes may alternate with severe depression, hence the term "bipolar illness", which is clinically similar to that seen in patients with "unipolar depression". In such cases, the mood can range from sadness to profound melancholia with feelings of guilt, anxiety, apprehension and suicidal ideation accompanied by anhedonia (lack of interest in work, food, sex, etc.).

Mania, manic-depression and depression, which comprise the affective disorders, are relatively common; it has been estimated that there is an incidence of at least 2% in most societies throughout the world. There is good evidence to suggest that *genetic factors* play a considerable role in predisposing a patient to an affective disorder. In a seminal Danish twin register study, in which the incidence of affective disorders was determined in all twins of the same sex born in Denmark between 1870 and 1920, a total of 110 pairs of twins were identified in which one or both had manic-depression. The concordance rates, that is the rate of coexistence of the disorder in twin pairs, for all types of affective disorder were found to be

Fundamentals of Psychopharmacology. Third Edition. By Brian E. Leonard
© 2003 John Wiley & Sons, Ltd. ISBN 0 471 52178 7

47% for the mono- and 20% for the dizygotic twins. Further analysis showed that the discrepancy in concordance rates for manic-depression was even greater between the mono- and the dizygotic pairs, being 79% for the former and 25% for the latter. There was no difference in the concordance rate for bipolar and unipolar affective disorders in the dizygotic twins, the values being 24% and 19%, respectively. Such findings strongly suggest that affective disorders are inherited. Nevertheless, despite the apparent differences in the genetic loading for monopolar and bipolar affective illness, there is increasing evidence that both types of illness can be associated with the same genetic make-up. Thus a substantial portion of unipolar patients have the same genetic and biological vulnerability as bipolar patients. What causes some patients to display mania or hypomania whereas others do not is unknown.

More recently attempts have been made to define the mode of genetic transmission of affective disorders. A study of single autosomal locus markers in such patients has concluded that there is a lack of evidence to indicate single locus transmission, and that a polygenic model is more consistent with the available data. Linkage markers (e.g. the link between the X chromosome and colour blindness), autosomal markers such as those associated with human leucocyte antigen (HLA), and restriction fragment length polymorphism (RFLP) have also been studied in populations of patients with affective disorders. There was much excitement generated by the discovery that the RFLP analysis of the manic patients in the unique Amish population in Pennsylvania showed a link between the disorder and the insulin-*ras*-1 oncogene on chromosome 11. Unfortunately, a more detailed analysis of the data has failed to confirm these initial findings. At present it must be concluded that, while the heritability of manic-depression is evident from clinical studies, the mode of transmission and the identity of the transmitted defect have not been demonstrated. Nevertheless, with the spectacular developments in molecular genetics now taking place, one may expect considerable advances in the identification of the locus of inheritance to be made in the coming decade. Figure 8.1 illustrates the location of some of the genes implicated in bipolar disorder.

Biochemical changes associated with mania

The various hypotheses that have been advanced regarding the biochemical cause of mania mainly centre on the idea that it is due to a relative excess of noradrenaline, and possibly dopamine, with deficits also arising in the availability of 5-hydroxytryptamine (5-HT) and acetylcholine. This simplistic view forms the basis of the *amine theory of affective disorders*

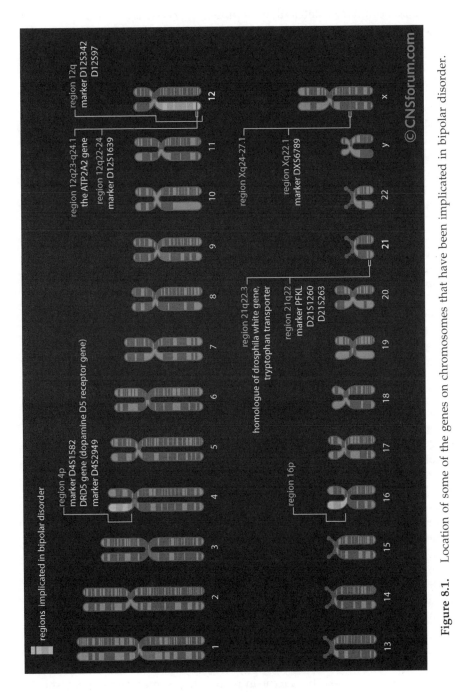

Figure 8.1. Location of some of the genes on chromosomes that have been implicated in bipolar disorder.

which, in summary, states that depression arises as a consequence of biogenic amine deficit, while mania is due to an excess of these amines in central synapses. In mania, evidence in support of this hypothesis comes from the limited studies that have been undertaken on patients before and after effective treatment. An alternative approach has been to study drugs such as lithium that have been used to treat the condition.

Most studies of the changes in the urine concentration of the main central metabolite of noradrenaline, 3-methoxy-4-hydroxyphenylglycol (MHPG), have shown abnormalities in manic patients. However, there is a discrepancy in the literature regarding the duration and extent of the change. Urinary noradrenaline concentrations have, however, been found to be increased during the active phase of the illness and to return to normal following effective treatment; the increase is said to reflect a rise in the concentration of MHPG in the cerebrospinal fluid (CSF). The concentration of the main dopamine metabolite, homovanillic acid (HVA), is also reported to rise in mania, but whether such changes are causally related to the core symptoms of the illness is debatable as it would be anticipated that an increase in the sympathetic drive would be necessarily associated with the illness.

While there have been a number of studies of changes in the sympathetic system in mania, few studies have attempted to assess changes in the serotonergic system. Hypomania has been reported to occur in depressed patients being treated with 5-hydroxytryptophan, the precursor amino acid of 5-HT, in combination with the peripheral decarboxylase inhibitor carbidopa. Mania has also been reported to occur in depressed patients following treatment with tryptophan in combination with clomipramine, a 5-HT uptake inhibitor. Nevertheless, there are no reports of a 5-HT agonist exacerbating the symptoms of mania in patients who are hypomanic! This suggests that a serotonergic stimulus may trigger a manic episode but alone is not a sufficient cause. Regarding the changes in serotonergic function in mania, only one study to date has investigated [^{3}H]5-HT transport into the platelets of patients before and after effective treatment. Unlike depression, where the [^{3}H]5-HT uptake is reduced, in mania the uptake is enhanced before treatment and normalized on recovery.

Regarding the dopaminergic system, there is experimental evidence to show that dopaminomimetic agents such as amphetamine, piribedil, bromocriptine and L-dopa can initiate mania in predisposed patients during remission. Indeed, the behavioural excitation and hypomania following D-amphetamine withdrawal has been proposed as a model of mania. Other evidence implicating a change in the dopaminergic system has been derived from the efficacy of neuroleptics (dopamine antagonists), which effectively attenuate the symptoms of the illness.

Unlike the biogenic amines, the cholinergic system has received relatively little attention as a possible factor in mania. Experimental evidence shows

that cholinomimetic drugs and anticholinesterases have antimanic properties, although their effects appear to be short-lived. Furthermore, their
effects appear to be associated with a reduction in the affective core
symptoms and locomotor components of the illness, but not in the
grandiose thinking and expansiveness.

Which, if any, of these different types of neurotransmitters is causally
involved in the illness is still a matter for conjecture.

In SUMMARY, it would appear that the noradrenergic, serotonergic and
dopaminergic systems are all overactive in acute mania while the inhibitory
GABAergic system is underactive. This view would concur with the actions
of drugs used to treat mania which primarily enhance inhibitory
neurotransmission (which also explains their use as antiepileptics) and/or
decrease excitatory neurotransmission. The changes thought to occur in
mania with respect to these neurotransmitter pathways are illustrated in
Figures 8.2, 8.3, 8.4 and 8.5.

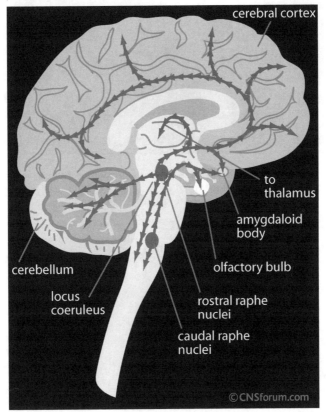

Figure 8.2. Diagrammatic representation of noradrenergic system in mania. All
main noradrenergic pathways thought to be overactive in mania.

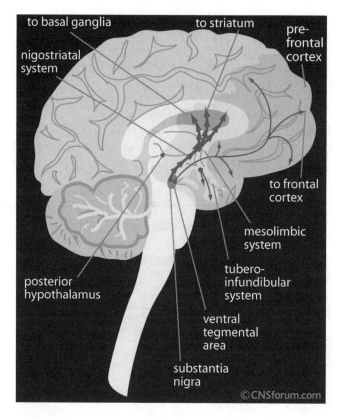

Figure 8.3. Diagrammatic representation of dopaminergic system in mania. Dopaminergic tracts to basal ganglia thought to be overactive thereby causing hyperactivity. Other dopaminergic tracts are probably unaffected.

Pharmacological treatment of mania

Lithium salts

Of the various types of psychotropic drugs which have been used to treat mania, lithium salts are universally acclaimed to be the most important and effective treatment of mania and manic-depression.

It can be argued that the introduction of lithium salts into the practice of psychiatry in 1949 heralded the beginning of psychopharmacology, as it predated the discovery of chlorpromazine, imipramine, monoamine oxidase inhibitors and resperine. Lithium came into clinical use serendipitously, the Australian psychiatrist Cade having by chance given it to a small group of manic patients and found that it had beneficial effects,

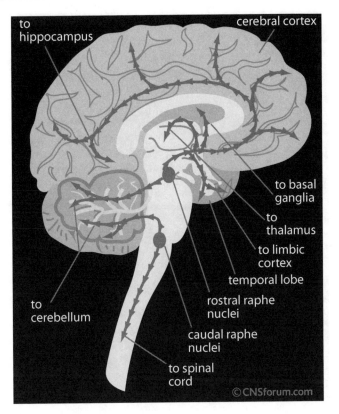

Figure 8.4. Diagrammatic representation of serotonergic system in mania. All serotonergic tracts may be overactive in mania.

whereas it appeared to lack activity when given to schizophrenics and depressives. However, lithium salts did not come into regular use in most industrialized countries until the early 1970s, partly because of the toxicity of the drug and partly because of the lack of commercial interest in a drug that could be dug out of the soil!

Lithium salts, generally in the form of the carbonate or bicarbonate, are rapidly absorbed from the gastrointestinal tract and reach a peak plasma concentration after 2–4 hours. Extreme fluctuations in blood lithium levels, which are associated with side effects such as nausea, diarrhoea and abdominal cramp, are reduced by using sustained release preparations. Lithium is not protein bound and therefore is widely distributed throughout the body water, which accounts for the adverse effects it has on most organ systems should it reach toxic levels. To avoid toxicity, and ensure optimal

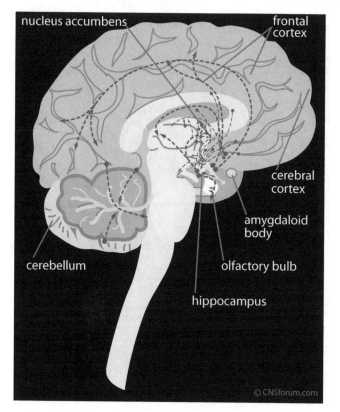

Figure 8.5. Diagrammatic representation of GABAergic system in mania. Some evidence that the main GABAergic tracts are hypoactive in mania.

efficacy, it is essential to monitor the plasma levels at regular intervals to ensure that they lie between 0.6 and 1.2 mEq/litre; there is evidence that lower levels (0.4–0.6 mEq/litre) may be sufficient when lithium salts are used to prevent relapse in the case of patients with unipolar depression.

As lithium is an alkaline earth metal which readily exchanges with sodium and potassium, it is actively transported across cell membranes. The penetration of kidney cells is particularly rapid, while that of bone, liver and brain tissue is much slower. The plasma : CSF ratio in man has been calculated to be between 2:1 and 3:1, which is similar to that found for the plasma : red blood cell (RBC) ratio. This suggests that the plasma : RBC ratio might be a useful index of the brain concentration and may be predictive of the onset of side effects, as these appear to correlate well with the intracellular concentration of the drug.

Most of the lithium is eliminated in the urine, the first phase of the elimination being 6–8 hours after administration, followed by a slower phase which may last for 2 weeks. Sodium-depleting diuretics such as frusemide, ethacrynic acid and the thiazides increase lithium retention and therefore toxicity, while osmotic diuretics as exemplified by mannitol and urea enhance lithium excretion. The principal side effects of lithium are summarized in Table 8.1.

Table 8.1.   Main side effects of lithium

Gastrointestinal tract
Anorexia
Nausea
Vomiting
Diarrhoea
Thirst
Incontinence

Neuromuscular changes
General muscle weakness
Ataxia
Tremor
Fasciculation and twitching
Choreoathetoid movements
Hyperactive tendon reflexes*

Central nervous system
Slurred speech*
Blurring of vision
Dizziness
Vertigo
Epileptiform seizures
Somnolence
Confusion*
Restlessness*
Stupor*
Coma*

Cardiovascular system
Hypotension
Pulse irregularities
ECG changes
Circulatory collapse

Other effects
Polyuria
Glycosuria
General fatigue* and lethargy*
Dehydration

*Side effects usually associated with the toxic effects of lithium.

The *mode of action* of lithium is still the subject of debate! Because of its similarity to sodium it was initially believed that it acted by competing with sodium in the brain and other tissues. However, it is now known that lithium interacts equally well with potassium, calcium and magnesium ions, all of which are widely distributed and essential for the functioning of most biological processes. It seems likely that lithium displaces sodium and potassium from their intracellular compartments and thereby substitutes for them; calcium, magnesium and phosphate concentrations are also altered. These effects of lithium on the electrolyte balance were once considered to be related to an action of the drug on sodium/potassium dependent adenosine triphosphatase (Na^+K^+-ATPase), an enzyme primarily involved in the repolarization of excitable membranes. Lithium appears to compete with a common binding site on the carrier, the site having a greater affinity for the lithium than the sodium ion. This could account for the ability of the drug to slow the speed of repolarization of nervous tissue. Other effects on brain function may be associated with an increase in the permeability of the blood–brain barrier resulting from an interaction of lithium with membrane phospholipids. The increased concentration of amino acids in the CSF may be a reflection of this.

It has long been apparent that the uptake, storage, release and metabolism (i.e. the turnover) of biogenic amines can be affected by both mono- and divalent cations. The effect on dopamine receptor sensitivity may be a particularly important action of lithium. It has been speculated that dopamine receptor hypersensitivity is closely associated with the onset of mania. Both acutely and chronically administered lithium can reduce the supersensitivity of both pre- and postsynaptic dopamine receptors, an effect which may help to explain its mood-stabilizing action but not its somewhat controversial ability to initiate tardive dyskinesia. Regarding the effects of lithium on noradrenergic function, it has long been known that it increases the reuptake of noradrenaline into neurons, increases the turnover of this amine in the brain without markedly affecting its turnover in the periphery, decreases its release and enhances its metabolism. The net effect of lithium is therefore to lead to a reduction in noradrenergic function which presumably is reflected in its antimanic properties.

At the postsynaptic level, lithium has been shown to reduce the function of beta adrenoceptors, presumably by affecting the coupling between the receptor and the secondary messenger system. This effect only becomes apparent following chronic treatment, which may help to explain the delay of several days, or even weeks, before an optimal beneficial effect is observed. All antidepressants are known to reduce the functional activity of postsynaptic beta receptors, which may explain why lithium has both an antimanic and an antidepressant effect in patients with manic-depression.

Relationship between the mode of action of lithium and its side effects

Many of the adverse effects of lithium can be ascribed to the action of lithium on adenylate cyclase, the key enzyme that links many hormones and neurotransmitters with their intracellular actions. Thus antidiuretic hormone and thyroid-stimulating-hormone-sensitive adenylate cyclases are inhibited by therapeutic concentrations of the drug, which frequently leads to enhanced diuresis, hypothyroidism and even goitre. Aldosterone synthesis is increased following chronic lithium treatment and is probably a secondary consequence of the enhanced diuresis caused by the inhibition of antidiuretic-hormone-sensitive adenylate cyclase in the kidney. There is also evidence that chronic lithium treatment causes an increase in serum parathyroid hormone levels and, with this, a rise in calcium and magnesium concentrations. A decrease in plasma phosphate and in bone mineralization can also be attributed to the effects of the drug on parathyroid activity. Whether these changes are of any clinical consequence is unclear.

Prolactin secretion, at least in experimental animals, is increased following chronic lithium treatment, probably as a consequence of the enhanced sensitivity of postsynaptic 5-HT receptors and the decreased sensitivity of dopamine receptors. In patients on therapeutic doses of the drug, however, the plasma prolactin levels would not appear to be markedly altered. There is little evidence that circulating gonadotrophin concentrations are affected by therapeutic doses of lithium.

One major side effect of lithium that causes great concern to patients is weight gain; this has been estimated to occur in up to 60% of patients according to some investigators. In addition to increased food intake, lithium also has an effect on the intermediary metabolism of carbohydrates. During the acute phase of lithium administration, insulin release is decreased leading to a raised plasma glucose; the insulin concentration then rises and increased fat synthesis could then occur. This appears to be due to an inhibition of several enzymes at the beginning of the glycolytic pathway, which could lead to enhanced lipid synthesis.

Recently research has focused on the action of lithium on serotonergic function. Lithium has been shown to facilitate the uptake and synthesis of 5-HT, to enhance its release and to increase the transport of tryptophan into the nerve terminal, an effect which probably contributes to the increased 5-HT synthesis. The net effect of these changes is to produce postsynaptic receptor events, which might explain why lithium, in combination with tryptophan and a monoamine oxidase inhibitor or a 5-HT uptake inhibitor, is often effective in therapy-resistant depression.

Drugs which enhance the activity of the central cholinergic system have been shown to have antimanic effects. Experimental studies have shown that lithium increases acetylcholine synthesis in the cortex, which is probably associated with an increase in the high affinity transport of choline into the neuron; the release of this transmitter is also increased. Whether these effects on the cholinergic system are relevant to its therapeutic action in manic patients remains to be proven.

So far attention has concentrated on the effects of lithium on excitatory transmitters. There is evidence that the drug can also facilitate inhibitory transmission, an effect that has been attributed to a desensitization of the presynaptic gamma-aminobutyric acid (GABA) receptors, which results in an increase in the release of this inhibitory transmitter. The increased conversion of glutamate to GABA may also contribute to this process. Thus it would appear that lithium has a varied and complex action on central neurotransmission, the net result being a diminution in the activity of excitatory transmitters and an increase in GABAergic function.

When receptors are directly linked to ion channels, fast excitatory or inhibitory postsynaptic potentials occur. However, it is well established that slow potential changes also occur and that such changes are due to the receptor being linked to the ion channel indirectly via a secondary messenger system. For example, the stimulation of beta adrenoceptors by noradrenaline results in the activation of adenylate cyclase. The antimanic and antidepressant effects of lithium are linked to a reduction in the functional activity of postsynaptic beta adrenoceptor-linked cyclase, combined with a reduction in the activity of the presynaptic noradrenergic neuron. The adverse effects of the drug on renal and thyroid function are due to the inhibition of the hormone-linked cyclases in these organs. Undoubtedly, transmitter receptor changes (e.g. serotonergic, noradrenergic, dopaminergic and GABAergic) play a major role in the therapeutic effects of lithium. Such changes may be related to the ability of the drug to re-synchronize disrupted circadian rhythms, which appear to be an essential feature of the affective disorders.

Other drug treatments for mania

The long-term toxic effects of lithium, such as nephrogenic diabetes insipidus, which has been calculated to occur in up to 5% of patients, and the rare possibility of lithium combined with neuroleptics being neurotoxic, has stimulated the research for other drug treatments. However, apart from the neuroleptics, these drugs have not been studied as extensively in the treatment of acute mania, but are worthy of consideration because of their reduced side effects.

Neuroleptics

Most psychotic and non-compliant patients are difficult to treat with lithium alone and need to be treated with neuroleptics. Haloperidol has been widely used alone to control the more florid symptoms of mania, but doubts have arisen concerning its toxic interactions with lithium. Such considerations are based on a report that such a combination caused neurotoxicity in a small group of manic patients, but it should be emphasized that a variety of other neuroleptics have also been rarely found to cause these effects. The symptoms of neurotoxicity include ataxia, confusion, hyperactive reflexes, chorea, slurred speech and even coma. It seems likely that some of these patients suffered from the malignant neuroleptic syndrome rather than enhanced lithium toxicity, but problems such as dehydration and over-sedation may have enhanced the drug interaction. More recently, atypical antipsychotics such as olanzapine and risperidone have been shown to be effective in the treatment of acute mania. These drugs have advantages over haloperidol, and the first-generation neuroleptics, due to the improved side-effect profiles and better patient compliance.

Tardive dyskinesia can occur in manic patients on neuroleptics alone, the frequency may be greater than in schizophrenics who are more likely to be on continuous medication. One possible explanation for this lies in the fact that neuroleptics are often administered to manic patients for short periods only, sufficient to abort the active episode, and then abruptly stopped. Thus high doses of neuroleptics are separated by drug-free periods, leading to a situation most likely to precipitate tardive dyskinesia. The recent increase in prescribing high potency neuroleptics such as haloperidol instead of low potency drugs such as chlorpromazine or thioridazine has undoubtedly increased the frequency of tardive dyskinesia. Clearly, use of the atypical antipsychotics with the very low frequency of EPS makes them the treatments of choice.

Valproate

Valproic acid (dipropylacetic acid) is a single branched chain carboxylic acid that is structurally unlike any of the other drugs used in the treatment of bipolar disorder or epilepsy. The amide derivative, valproamide, is available in Europe as a more potent form of valproate. Valproate was first developed in France as an antiepileptic agent in 1963. As an antiepileptic agent, it was shown to be active against a variety of epilepsies without causing marked sedation.

The mechanism of action of valproate is complex and still the subject of uncertainty. The drug appears to act by enhancing GABAergic function. Thus it increases GABA release, inhibits catabolism and increases the density of GABA-B receptors in the brain. There is also evidence that it increases the sensitivity of GABA receptors to the action of the inhibitory transmitter. Other actions that may contribute to its therapeutic effects include a decrease in dopamine turnover, a decrease in the activity of the NMDA-glutamate receptors and also a decrease in the concentration of somatostatin in the CSF. Unlike carbamazepine, valproate does not bind to peripheral benzodiazepine receptors (see p. 230).

Numerous open studies, and seven controlled studies, have shown that valproate is effective in the treatment of acute mania. It has also been claimed to have an antidepressant action. Recent studies have shown that valproate is effective in the long-term treatment of bipolar disorder.

Valproate is generally well tolerated and less likely to cause cognitive impairment than other antiepileptic drugs such as carbamazepine. It does frequently cause gastrointestinal upset and a benign elevation of liver transaminases however. Because valproate is highly plasma protein bound, and is partially metabolized by the cytochrome P450 system, it can interact with many other drugs. For example, aspirin can enhance the efficacy and toxicity of valproate by displacing it from the plasma proteins while microsomal enzyme-inducing drugs such as carbamazepine can decrease its plasma and tissue concentrations. The general properties of valproate are further discussed in Chapter 12.

Carbamazepine

This is a tricyclic compound somewhat similar to imipramine that is an anticonvulsant widely used in the treatment of temporal lobe epilepsy. Following its widespread use as an antiepileptic, it soon became evident that it had psychotropic effects. These included an improvement in mood, reduced aggressiveness and improved cognitive function. *Kindling* refers to the development of seizures after repeated delivery of a series of subthreshold stimuli to any region of the brain. This phenomenon can most readily be induced in limbic structures and, whereas conventional anticonvulsants such as phenytoin and phenobarbitone have little effect in attenuating kindled seizures, carbamazepine and the benzodiazepine anticonvulsants prevent such seizure development. It is now well established that carbamazepine is relatively selective in attenuating seizure activity in the hippocampus and amygdala, which suggests that it acts preferentially at limbic sites in the brain.

The mechanism of action of carbamazepine is complex, and is complicated by the fact that it has a long half-life metabolite, carbamazepine epoxide, which also has pronounced psychotropic properties.

The anticonvulsant properties of the drug would appear to be due to its ability to inhibit fast sodium channels, which may be unrelated to its psychotropic effects. Like lithium, it has been shown to decrease the release of noradrenaline and reduce noradrenaline-induced adenylate cyclase activity; unlike lithium, it seems to have little effect on tryptophan or 5-HT levels in patients at therapeutically relevant concentrations. It also reduces dopamine turnover in manic patients and increases acetylcholine synthesis in the cortex, an effect also seen with lithium. The effect of carbamazepine on GABAergic function appears to be related to its interaction with GABA-B type receptors, which may be relevant to its usefulness in the treatment of trigeminal neuralgia. There is no evidence that it changes GABA levels in the CSF of patients. Furthermore, while it would appear that the drug has no effect on central benzodiazepine receptors, there is evidence that it has a high affinity for the peripheral type of benzodiazepine receptor. These receptors are found in the mammalian brain but differ from the central receptors in that they are not linked to GABA receptors and therefore do not affect chloride ion flux. The main function of the peripheral type of benzodiazepine receptor would seem to be to control calcium channels. This may help to explain some of the psychotropic effects of carbamazepine, particularly as calcium channel antagonists such as *verapamil* have antimanic effects.

Changes in the activity of adenosine receptors have been implicated in the stimulant effects of drugs like caffeine. Carbamazepine exhibits a partial agonist effect on adenosine receptors, and experimental evidence suggests that the reduced reuptake and release of noradrenaline caused by the drug are due to its interaction with these receptors. The precise relevance of these findings to its anticonvulsant and psychotropic effects is presently unclear.

Of the various peptides (e.g. the opioids, vasopressin, substance P and somatostatin) thought to be involved in the actions of carbamazepine, there is evidence that the reduction in the CSF concentration of somatostatin might be important in explaining its effects on cognition and also on the hypothalamo–pituitary–adrenal axis; somatostatin is a major inhibitory modulator of this axis and hypercortisolism frequently occurs in patients following carbamazepine administration.

There is still controversy regarding the general usefulness of carbama- zepine as an alternative to lithium. It is apparent that the nature of the illness alters throughout the lifetime of the patient, so that pharmacological interventions may differ according to the stage of the illness. Preliminary clinical studies suggest that lithium may be particularly beneficial during the early and intermediate stages of the illness, whereas carbamazepine and related anticonvulsants may be more useful, either alone or in combination with lithium, at later stages, particularly, when the patient shows rapid, continuous cycling between mania and depression.

Other drugs

Other drugs that are reported to have beneficial effects but which have not undergone such extensive evaluation as the neuroleptics or carbamazepine include the *calcium channel antagonists* such as verapamil. A small open study has suggested that the alpha$_2$ adrenoceptor agonist *clonidine* may have some activity. More substantial studies have been conducted on the benzodiazepines *lorazepam* and *clonazepam*, and the anticonvulsant *sodium valproate*. All these drugs facilitate GABAergic function in some way, the first two by acting as agonists at benzodiazepine receptor sites and the latter by desensitizing the GABA autoreceptor and thereby enhancing the release of this inhibitory transmitter. Lastly, electroconvulsive shock treatment (ECT) has been claimed to be effective in attenuating the symptoms of an acute manic attack, but there is evidence that patients treated with ECT should not receive lithium concomitantly to reduce the possibility of neurotoxic side effects.

In addition to these drugs, many of the newer antiepileptic drugs such as lamotrigine have found a place in the therapeutic management of mania. These are extensively covered in Chapter 12.

Maintenance treatments for bipolar disorder

The pharmacological management of bipolar disorder involves treatment of both the acute and the longer-term maintenance phase of the illness. Long-term maintenance is necessary to reduce or prevent the recurrence of the symptoms, and to minimize the risk of suicide.

For many years, lithium salts have been used for maintenance treatment. However, naturalistic studies have reported a relatively high failure rate in patients on lithium and therefore other therapeutic approaches have been considered.

With regard to the use of lithium in maintenance therapy, the studies which were published in the 1970s clearly demonstrated the efficacy of lithium in preventing relapse into mania or depression in patients with bipolar disorder. However, subsequent longer-term naturalistic studies raised doubts over the validity of these findings. In particular, these studies have shown that up to 50% of patients respond poorly to lithium. Some of the reasons for the re-evaluation of the early reports on the efficacy of lithium as a maintenance treatment are due to the methodological limitations of the placebo-controlled studies which include a lack of diagnostic criteria and a limited consideration of those patients withdrawing from the clinical trial prematurely.

In contrast to the large number of studies that have investigated lithium as a maintenance treatment for bipolar disorder, relatively few studies have been made of divalproex sodium, despite its widespread use in the acute treatment of mania. There is evidence from one placebo-controlled study in which lithium was compared with divalproex sodium that the latter drug was better tolerated but that the prevention of relapse did not differ between the drugs. It would therefore appear that a switch to divalproex sodium may be particularly useful in bipolar patients who are experiencing cognitive deficits, loss of creativity and functional impairments consequent on lithium use.

Again there are relatively few studies that have investigated the use of carbamazepine in maintenance therapy. The results of the studies published suggest that carbamazepine is not as effective as lithium or divalproex. In the controlled studies of carbamazepine, the majority of patients required adjunctive treatment to prevent a breakthrough for the manic or depressive symptoms.

Despite the widespread use of neuroleptics in maintenance treatment of bipolar disorder, there have not been any systematic studies of their suitability for this role. Through clinical experience it has been widely accepted that neuroleptics are useful adjunctive treatments to lithium and related drugs. Treatment refractory patients frequently respond to atypical antipsychotics such as clozapine or risperidone. Such adverse effects as EPS, cognitive dysfunction and weight gain frequently limit the long-term use of classical neuroleptics. For this reason, the atypical neuroleptics such as olanzapine and risperidone should now be considered as alternatives for maintenance treatment.

Treatment decisions for bipolar disorder

- Treatment of choice – mood stabilizer with or without an antidepressant (e.g. lithium, valproate, carbamazepine, lamotrigine). Antidepressants include an SSRI, venlafaxine, mirtazepine as possibilities but few controlled trials to substantiate choice.
- Switching – alternative mood stabilizer plus alternative second-generation antidepressant.
- Augmentation of the response – combine two mood stabilizers; add thyroid hormone to mood stabilizer.
- Other options – ECT; possibly calcium channel blockers such as verapamil or nimodipine.

In CONCLUSION, lithium is universally accepted as a mood-stabilizing drug and an effective antimanic agent whose value is limited by its poor therapeutic index (i.e. its therapeutic to toxicity ratio). Neuroleptics are effective in attenuating the symptoms of acute mania but they too have serious adverse side effects. High potency typical neuroleptics appear to increase the likelihood of tardive dyskinesia. Of the less well-established treatments, carbamazepine would appear to have a role, particularly in the more advanced stages of the illness when lithium is less effective.

9 Anxiolytics and the Treatment of Anxiety Disorders

Introduction

Until the late 1960s, the symptoms of anxiety and insomnia were mainly treated with barbiturates. The barbiturates are known to cause dependence, and severe withdrawal effects were sometimes reported following the abrupt termination of their administration. Furthermore, their efficacy in the treatment of anxiety disorders was limited. The discovery of the benzodiazepine anxiolytic chlordiazepoxide some 30 years ago, and the subsequent development of numerous analogues with an essentially similar pharmacological profile, rapidly led to the replacement of the barbiturates with a group of drugs that have been widely used for the treatment of anxiety disorders, insomnia, muscle spasm and epilepsy and as a preoperative medication. The benzodiazepines have also been shown to have fewer side effects than the barbiturates, to be relatively safe in overdose and to be less liable to produce dependence than the barbiturates. They have now become the most widely used of all psychotropic drugs; during the last 25 years it has been estimated that over 500 million people worldwide have taken a course of benzodiazepine treatment.

In recent years there has been growing concern among members of the public and the medical profession regarding the problem of dependence and possible abuse of the benzodiazepines, and the recent decrease in the number of prescriptions of these drugs for the treatment of anxiety reflects this concern. And yet, despite the decline in the short-term use of benzodiazepine drugs to treat anxiety, their use as hypnotic sedatives is largely unchanged. Furthermore, their long-term use for the treatment of anxiety and/or insomnia continues. Thus in the UK approximately 1.5% of the adult population have taken benzodiazepines continuously for 1 year or more, while nearly half of these have taken the drugs for at least 7 years. It has been variously estimated that approximately 0.25 million people have

Fundamentals of Psychopharmacology. Third Edition. By Brian E. Leonard
© 2003 John Wiley & Sons, Ltd. ISBN 0 471 52178 7

Table 9.1. Benzodiazepines on the "selected list" for the NHS

	Half-life (range in hours)	Accumulation
Drugs used for anxiety		
Chlordiazepoxide*	20–90	+++
Diazepam*	20–90	+++
Oxazepam	6–28	+
Lorazepam	8–24	±
Alprazolam	6–16	+
Drugs used for insomnia		
Nitrazepam	16–40	+++
Temazepam	6–10	+
Lormetazepam	8–12	+
Loprazolam	6–12	+
Triazolam	4–10	–

*Includes active metabolites.
+++=marked accumulation; +=some accumulation; ±=?some accumulation; –=no accumulation.

taken benzodiazepines continuously for several years in the UK. The benzodiazepines commonly available are shown in Table 9.1.

The pharmacological properties of all these drugs are essentially similar, despite the fact that they may be prescribed for the treatment of anxiety or for insomnia. There is little objective evidence to suggest that the drugs listed are more specific for the treatment of anxiety or of insomnia; an anxiolytic benzodiazepine given at night is likely to be an effective hypnotic, while a low dose of a hypnotic benzodiazepine given in the morning may be an effective anxiolytic. The reason for the similarity in the pharmacological profile of these drugs lies in the similarity of their mechanism of action and also in their metabolite inter-relationship (see Figure 9.1).

In essence, all of the older benzodiazepines that are structurally related to chlordiazepoxide and diazepam are termed 1,4-benzodiazepines. The chemical structure of some commonly used benzodiazepines is shown in Figure 9.2. They enhance the actions of the inhibitory neurotransmitter gamma-aminobutyric acid (GABA) in the brain. As a consequence, they affect the activities of the cerebellum (concerned with balance and coordination), the limbic areas of the brain and the cerebral cortex (thought and decision making, fine movement control).

The half-life of a benzodiazepine is not predictive either of its onset of action or of the therapeutic response of the patient. However, the rate of absorption and distribution within the body are important parameters in determining the pharmacodynamic response. The period for maximal response to treatment may be as long as 6 weeks, and there is no evidence

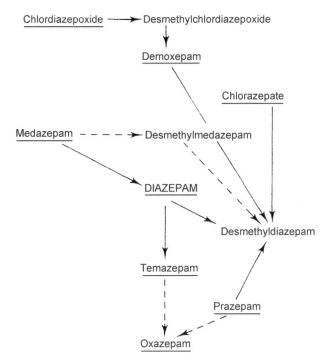

Figure 9.1. The metabolic pathways for the principal 1,4-benzodiazepines. The major pathway is shown with solid arrows and the minor pathway with broken arrows. Commercially available drugs are underlined.

that prolongation of the treatment, or increasing the dose of the drug, will lead to additional improvement in the response.

Chemical pathogenesis of anxiety

Although different authors have ascribed different meanings to the term "anxiety", and have often used the terms "fear" and "anxiety" interchangeably, it is generally accepted that anxiety is an unpleasant state accompanied by apprehension, worry, fear, nervousness and some-times conflict. Arousal is usually heightened. An increase in the autonomic sympathetic nervous system is often associated with these psychological changes and may be manifest as an increase in blood pressure and heart rate, an erratic respiratory rate, decreased salivary flow leading to dryness in the mouth and throat, and gastrointestinal disturbances (Figure 9.3). Whilst "physiological" anxiety is usually short-lived, often with a rapid onset and abrupt cessation once the aversive event has terminated, "pathological" anxiety occurs when the response of the individual to an

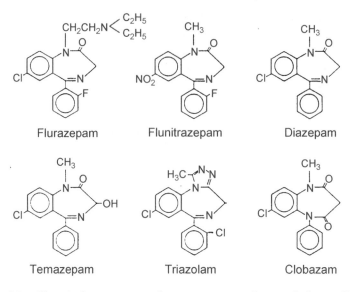

Figure 9.2. Chemical structure of some commonly used benzodiazepines. Clobazam differs from the other benzodiazepines shown, being a 1,5- rather than a 1,4-benzodiazepine.

anxiety-provoking event becomes excessive and affects the ability of the individual to lead a normal life. It has been estimated that 2–4% of the population suffer from pathological anxiety and frequently no causative factor can be identified. The benzodiazepines, and non-benzodiazepine anxiolytics such as buspirone, may be useful in alleviating the symptoms of pathological anxiety. The three neurotransmitters that appear to be most directly involved in different aspects of anxiety are noradrenaline, 5-hydroxytryptamine (5-HT) and GABA (Figure 9.4).

Noradrenaline is the neurotransmitter most closely associated with the peripheral and central stress response (Figure 9.5). There is experimental evidence to show that drugs such as yohimbine that block the noradrenergic autoreceptors (e.g. on cell bodies and nerve terminals) and thereby enhance noradrenaline release cause fear and anxiety in both man and animals. Conversely, drugs that stimulate these autoreceptors (as exemplified by clonidine) diminish the anxiety state because they reduce the release of noradrenaline. Benzodiazepines have been shown to inhibit the fear-motivated increase in the functional activity of noradrenaline in experimental animals, but it is now widely believed that the action of the benzodiazepines on the central noradrenergic system is only short term and may contribute to the sedative effects which most conventional benzo-diazepines produce, at least initially. Nevertheless, altered noradrenergic

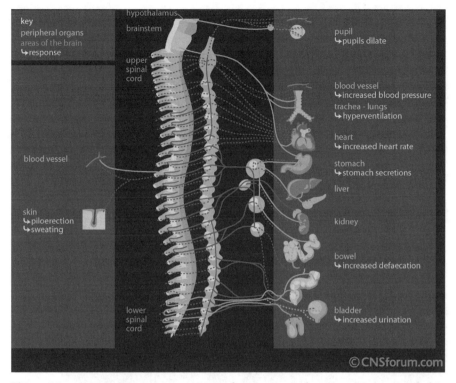

Figure 9.3. Autonomic nervouse system showing typical panic responses in phobia and reflecting increased sympathetic nervous system activity.

function may underlie certain forms of severe anxiety such as that seen in patients with panic attacks or anxiety states associated with major depression. Such forms of anxiety generally respond to treatment with antidepressants or benzodiazepines that also have some mild antidepressant properties (e.g. alprazolam).

Several experimental studies have suggested that a reduction in the activity of 5-HT in the brain results in anxiolysis, and therefore the anxiolytic effects of the benzodiazepines may be at least partly mediated by a reduction in central serotonergic neurotransmission. Other studies have shown that benzodiazepines inhibit the firing of serotonergic neurons in the midbrain raphé region, an area that contains serotonergic cell bodies which send projections to the limbic and cortical regions of the brain (Figure 9.8).

The link between the serotonergic pathways and the control of anxiety has been further strengthened by the introduction of non-benzodiazepine anxiolytics such as buspirone, ipsapirone and gepirone, which decrease central serotonergic function by stimulating a subclass of 5-HT receptors (5-

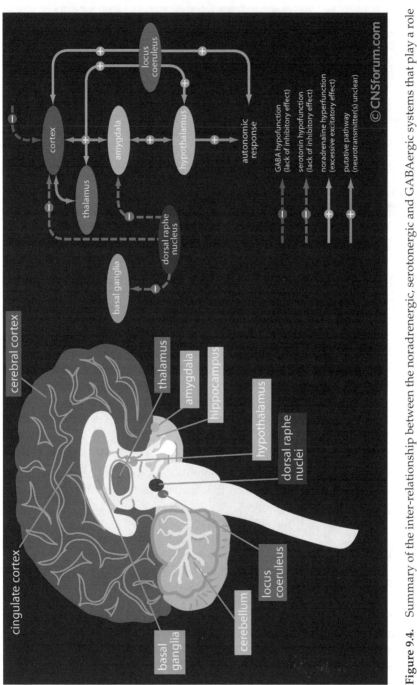

Figure 9.4. Summary of the inter-relationship between the noradrenergic, serotonergic and GABAergic systems that play a role in generalized anxiety disorder.

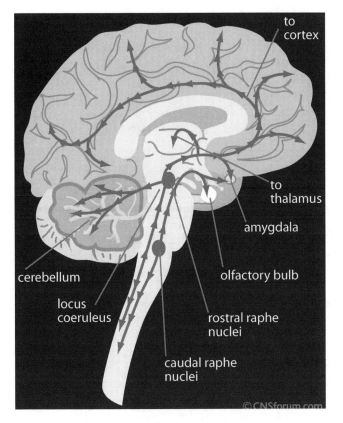

Figure 9.5. Diagram of the main noradrenergic tracts that are thought to be hyperactive in generalized anxiety disorder.

HT_{1A}), leading to a decrease in serotonergic release. Despite the connection between the decreased functional activity of the serotonergic system and the anxiolytic effects of the benzodiazepines, it would appear that their effect on serotonergic transmission is indirect and probably mediated via a facilitation of the principal inhibitory neurotransmitter, GABA.

Unlike the biogenic amines, noradrenaline and 5-HT, GABA is one of the most widely distributed neurotransmitters in the mammalian brain, occupying some 40% of all synapses. Whereas noradrenaline and 5-HT are primarily excitatory in their actions, GABA is an inhibitory transmitter and therefore reduces the firing rate of excitatory neurons with which it is in contact. In various animal models of anxiety, the facilitation of GABAergic activity is associated with a reduction in anxiety. Conversely, drugs such as bicuculline, which specifically block GABA receptors, precipitate the symptoms of anxiety. There is also experimental evidence to show that the anti-anxiety effects of the benzodiazepines may be inhibited by GABA receptor antagonists or by drugs that reduce the synthesis of GABA. From such studies it may be concluded that the primary action of "classical" benzodiazepines such as diazepam is to facilitate central GABAergic transmission but, due to the modulatory effects of GABAergic neurons on other neurotransmitter systems in the brain, secondary changes occur in noradrenergic and serotonergic pathways which may contribute to their anxiolytic effects.

Role of peptide neurotransmitters in anxiety

Several neuropeptides have been shown to play a role in anxiety but so far none has been developed as a drug largely because of their poor pharmacokinetic properties and difficulty in penetrating the blood–brain barrier. This situation may change in the future when drugs are developed that, though they may not be peptides, have a high affinity for the peptide receptors.

Angiotensin peptides – the angiotensin converting enzyme inhibitor (ACE), captopril, has anxiolytic activity in both experimental and clinical studies. It has recently been shown that the angiotensin 1 receptor antagonist, losartin, has anxiolytic properties whereas the angiotensin 2 antagonists are inactive.

Cholecytokinin ligands – agonists of the central CCK receptors cause anxiety and precipitate panic attacks in predisposed individuals. Two types of CCK receptors have been identified, CCK-A and -B (from the alimentary tract and brain respectively), both of which occur in the mammalian brain. CCK-B agonists initiate anxiety while the antagonists are anxiolytic in both experimental and clinical situations. So far the poor bioavailability and side effects have limited their clinical development.

Neurokinin receptor ligands – there are two types of NK receptors in the brain. NK2 agonists have been found to be anxiogenic while the antagonists are anxiolytic at least in animal studies. Some NK1 antagonists have also been shown to be anxiolytic in experimental studies.

Corticotrophin releasing factor ligands – alpha helical CRF has been shown to block the anxiogenic effects of alcohol withdrawal in rats. It is possible that CRF interacts with neuropeptide Y receptors; NPY 1 receptor agonists to have anticonflict effects in animal studies.

NMDA-glutamate ligands – the glycine antagonist, HA-966, has anxiolytic effects in animal studies.

Adenosine receptor ligands – the adenosine receptor antagonist, caffeine, induces anxiety in both animals and man while agonists have anxiolytic effects.

Pathophysiological basis of panic disorder and obsessive–compulsive disorder: pharmacological treatment

A number of models of anxiety disorder have been proposed which help to explain differences in human behaviour in terms of their possible genetic and biological determinants. Of these models the one developed by Gray is particularly appealing to the neuroscientist in that it seeks to link three interdependent systems in the brain to specific behavioural functions. Thus one system is concerned with behavioural variations in response to signals of reward and non-punishment, a system concerned with impulsiveness. The second is located in the septohippocampal area and is concerned with behavioural inhibition; this is particularly relevant to the genesis of anxiety. The third system controls the escape and defensive–aggressive behaviour (the fight–flight response) and involves the amygdala–hypothalamus–midbrain regions. Thus the model of Gray regards anxiety disorders as arising from variations in the activities of several interdependent regions of the limbic system (Figure 9.6).

An integrated theory of anxiety

In 1987, Jeffrey Gray proposed that the septohippocampal system acted as a "comparator" in that it compared anticipated anxiety with threatening stimuli. He postulated that when the anticipated anxiety did not match with the threatening stimulus then an inhibitory system operating through the septohippocampal circuit was activated which blocked the defensive behaviour, increased the vigilance and suppressed reward behaviour. The noradrenergic and serotonergic systems were thought to play a complementary role in these events.

An additional "defence" system mediates the fight–flight response. This involves the amygdala, hypothalamus and central grey matter of the midbrain (PAG). The fight–flight response occurs when the PAG is activated by the input from the amygdala. Figure 9.7 summarizes the inter-relationship between the septohippocampal system, the PAG and the hypothalamus. The original theory of Gray has been modified more recently by Deakin and Graeff to include the role of the serotonergic system.

Biology of panic disorder

In recent years there has been considerable interest in the neurobiological basis of the anxiety disorders. It is generally accepted that the noradrenergic and serotonergic systems are causally involved in the pathogenesis of these disorders. Both the locus coeruleus and the dorsal raphé project to the

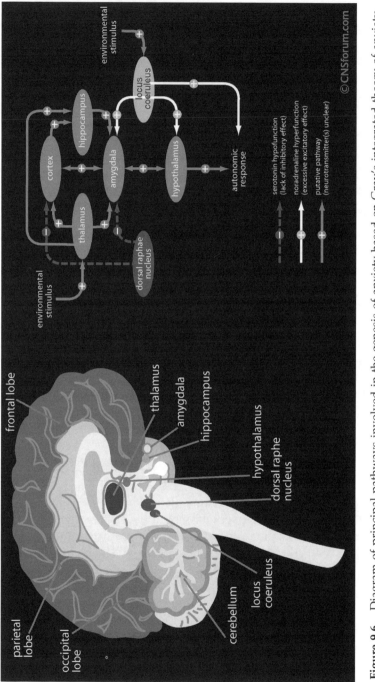

Figure 9.6. Diagram of principal pathways involved in the genesis of anxiety based on Gray's integrated theory of anxiety.

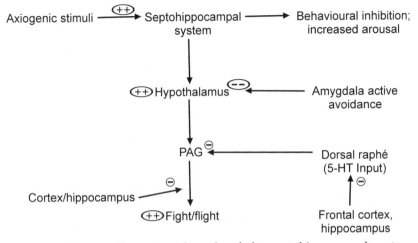

Figure 9.7. Diagram illustrating the role of the septohippocampal system in anxiety.

septohippocampal circuit which, in turn, projects to the other regions of the limbic system that mediate anxiety. The hippocampus and the amygdala are of particular importance in that they are interconnected and also project to both subcortical and cortical nuclei. Their main neurophysiological function appears to involve the integration of external and internal sensory perception. It is well established that infusion of lactate in patients who are vulnerable to panic attack can initiate the full symptoms of the attack. Positron emission tomography (PET) imaging studies on such patients show that there is an abnormal hemispheric asymmetry in the para-hippocampal gyrus blood flow and oxygen consumption together with an increase in glucose utilization in this area of the brain. Such studies help to locate the sites of the anxiety disorders in subcortical regions of the brain and also to provide a rational basis for defining the sites of action of the drugs that are used to treat them. They also suggest which of the numerous neurotransmitter systems found in these areas may be causally connected with the disorders.

Panic disorder is one of the most prevalent psychiatric disorders in industrialized countries. It is often associated with agoraphobia and has an estimated prevalence of between 1% and 6%. The use of imipramine in the treatment of anxiety by Klein and Fink, and the discovery by William Sargant that monoamine oxidase inhibitors (MAOIs) were effective in the treatment of "atypical depression" over 30 years ago led to the investigation of the efficacy of such treatments in patients with panic disorder. Since that time, such drugs have been shown to attenuate the symptoms of panic in addition to those of phobic avoidance and anticipatory anxiety. As both the

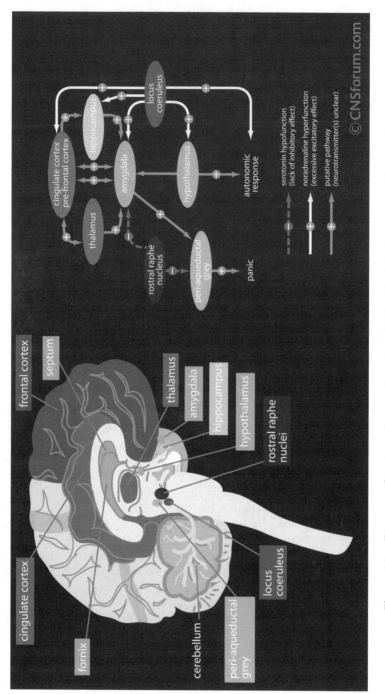

Figure 9.8. Diagram of main pathways thought to be involved in the genesis of panic disorder.

tricyclic antidepressants (TCAs) and the non-specific MAOIs such as phenelzine affect both the noradrenergic and serotonergic systems it was unclear which of these neurotransmitters was causally related to the beneficial effects of antidepressant treatment. However, by determining the plasma concentrations of imipramine (which inhibits the reuptake of both noradrenaline and serotonin) and its major metabolite desipramine (which is selective in inhibiting noradrenaline reuptake) it has been shown that the antipanic action of imipramine is largely attributable to its effect on serotonergic function. This view has been strengthened in recent years by the widespread use of clomipramine, the most specific inhibitor of 5-HT reuptake of the conventional TCAs, in the treatment of panic disorder. However, there is convincing clinical evidence that other TCAs such as the "second generation" tricyclic lofepramine which inhibits both noradrenaline and 5-HT uptake, is equi-effective with clomipramine and has an advantage of fewer adverse effects.

Undoubtedly one of the major advances in the treatment of panic disorder in the last two decades has resulted from the introduction of the selective 5-HT reuptake inhibitors (the SSRIs). Detailed double-blind placebo-controlled studies have shown that these drugs are effective in reducing the frequency of panic attacks, anxiety and the associated symptoms of the disorder. The importance of the serotonergic system in the therapeutic response to the SSRIs is indicated by studies in which fluvoxamine was compared with the selective noradrenaline reuptake inhibitor maprotiline. Whereas the number of panic attacks and the severity of anxiety significantly decreased following fluvoxamine, no such beneficial effects were seen following maprotiline treatment. Thus the SSRIs would appear to exhibit specific antipanic properties which are related to their chronic modulatory effects on serotonergic transmission. Generally all the SSRIs show a latency of several weeks before the optimal antipanic effect is established. This suggests that major changes in 5-HT receptor function must occur before the full clinical effect is manifest, a situation which is similar to that occurring when these drugs are used in the treatment of depression. In support of this hypothesis it has been found that a transient increase in anxiety frequently occurs when patients start treatment on an SSRI; this generally disappears as treatment proceeds and has been explained by an initial hypersensitivity of $5-HT_{1A}$ receptor subtypes which normalize following chronic drug treatment.

Despite the clear evidence that the serotonergic system is involved in the therapeutic efficacy of the antidepressants, it should be noted that the antipanic effect of the triazolobenzodiazepine alprazolam does not appear to be directly mediated by changes in the serotonergic system. This further emphasizes the complexity of the inter-relationships between the various biogenic amine and peptide (for example, cholecystokinin which has been implicated in the aetiology of panic disorder) neurotransmitters and also accounts for the diverse range of drugs that have been used in the treatment of the disorder.

Biology of obsessive–compulsive disorder

According to the DSM-IV classification, anxiety as a disorder can be divided into panic disorder with or without agoraphobia, generalized anxiety disorder, obsessive–compulsive disorder (OCD) and social phobia. Patients with generalized anxiety disorder appear to respond best to anxiolytic benzodiazepines; the properties and adverse effects of these drugs have been discussed in detail elsewhere. In recent years there have been a number of "open" and "placebo-controlled" studies showing that the SSRIs and the reversible MAOI moclobemide are effective in the treatment of social phobia. However considerable attention has been paid recently to the pharmacological treatment of OCD, a condition which, until it was discovered that clomipramine could effectively attenuate some of the symptoms, was largely unaffected by drug treatment including anti-depressants that enhance noradrenergic function.

By using imaging methods it has been shown that blood flow rates were greater in parts of the cortex in OCD patients than in matched control subjects. Similarly PET imaging studies in which the uptake of fluorodeoxyglucose was used to determine the activity of different brain regions, showed that the activity of the inferior prefrontal cortex was significantly greater in untreated OCD patients (Figure 9.9). There is evidence that these

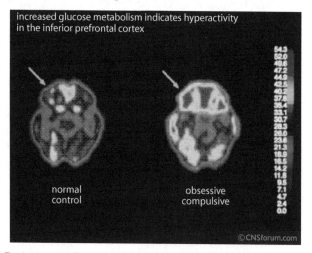

Figure 9.9. Brain image (by positron emission tomography) of glucose utilization of patient with OCD compared to a normal control.

abnormalities are reversed following effective treatment with clomipramine or an SSRI.

Despite the convincing evidence that the SSRIs are effective in the treatment of OCD, whereas antidepressants that lack an inhibitory effect on 5-HT reuptake (such as desipramine and nortriptyline) are largely ineffective, direct evidence implicating an abnormality in serotonergic function is limited. Thus there is evidence that the non-specific $5-HT_1$ receptor agonist m-chlorophenyl piperazine (mCPP) (a metabolite of trazodone and the related antidepressant nefazodone) can enhance the anxiety and obsessional state of some OCD patients but these changes are not associated with an increase in plasma cortisol and prolactin which would be indicative of $5-HT_1$ receptor hypersensitivity. Other clinical studies have shown that in patients responding to fluoxetine, there is no correlation between changes in $5-HT_{1A}$ receptor function and the reduction in the OCD symptoms. Thus it would appear that while the serotonergic system may be abnormal in OCD, and that drugs which selectively enhance serotonergic function are therapeutically effective in treating the condition, the nature of the abnormality in serotonergic function remains obscure. There is evidence, for example, that the dopaminergic system in the basal ganglia is hyperactive in OCD which may contribute to the main symptoms of the disorder (Figure 9.10). Nevertheless, there is now abundant clinical evidence that clomipramine and the SSRIs have made a major contribution to the pharmacological treatment of this disorder. In addition to drug treatments for OCD, it is sometimes necessary to consider psychosurgery when drug treatment fails. Cingulotomy (a lesion of the cingulate gyrus) has been shown to be effective.

In CONCLUSION, the recognition of the high frequency of such anxiety states as panic disorder in the general population in recent years has led to the widespread interest in the aetiology and treatment of the condition. The introduction of the SSRIs has been important not only because of their proven efficacy in the treatment of panic disorder and OCD but also because of the light they have thrown on the possible abnormality in the serotonergic system which may underlie the cause of such anxiety disorders.

Pathophysiological basis of social phobia and post traumatic stress disorder

Social phobia is a disorder marked by the intense fear and/or avoidance of situations in which the individual feels that he/she may be scrutinized by others. Social phobia may thus be considered to be an extreme form of shyness.

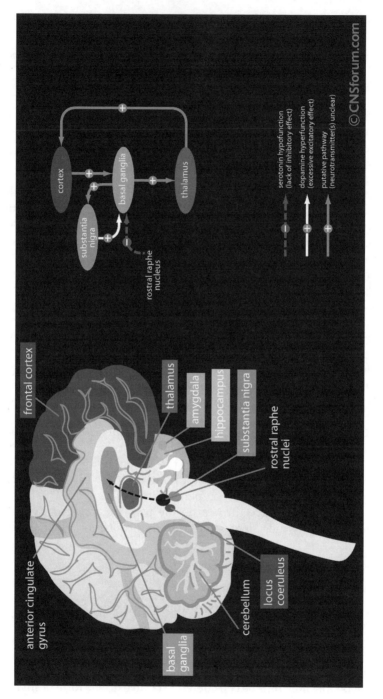

Figure 9.10. Main brain regions and neurotransmitter pathways thought to be involved in OCD.

It is uncertain whether, unlike generalized anxiety disorder, panic disorder and obsessive–compulsive disorder, social phobia has a genetic basis.

The biological basis of social phobia appears to reflect a hyperactivity of the central and peripheral sympathetic systems. Patients with the condition complain of tachycardia, tremor and blushing when placed in difficult social situations. Both the hypothalamic–pituitary–thyroid and adrenal axes appear to be normal, although there is evidence that the cortisol response to fenfluramine (a 5-HT releasing agent) is enhanced. It has also been suggested that the 5-HT$_{2C}$ receptors are hyperactive in these patients. In addition, SPECT studies have indicated that the density of the dopamine transporters in the basal ganglia are reduced.

Thus it would appear that the neurobiology of social phobia remains obscure. Nevertheless, the use of SSRI and MAOI antidepressants suggests that the primary disorder is related to a disorder of the serotonergic system.

Post traumatic stress disorder (PTSD) is the only psychiatric condition whose definition demands a particular stressor to precede its appearance. Unlike the other anxiety disorders, it is only in the past decade that the biology of PTSD has come under scrutiny. Furthermore, although PTSD can occur following various traumatic events (for example, sexual abuse, accidents and torture), most emphasis has been placed on combat-related disorders.

With regard to the neurobiology of PTSD, there is only limited evidence that the sympathetic system is hyperfunctional. A disrupted sleep pattern is a common feature of the disorder, particularly involving REM sleep dysregulation (flashbacks during the day and anxiety dreams during the night). Unlike other stress-related and anxiety disorders, patients with PTSD have reduced plasma cortisol and 24-hour cortisol excretion. Combat veterans have also shown a greater suppression of cortisol with low doses of dexamethasone (0.5 mg) than control subjects. This suggests that there is an increased glucocorticoid receptor sensitivity in these patients.

Imaging studies (MRI) have shown that combat veterans have a reduced hippocampal volume which may relate to their short-term memory deficits. However, the possibility that alcohol abuse, a common co-morbid condition, is also responsible has not been ruled out.

A major problem in interpreting the biological factors that are causally related to PTSD arises from the difficulty in differentiating the changes due to depression and drug abuse, which are common co-morbid conditions, and the limitation of most studies to combat victims.

Treatment of PTSD has largely been dependent on antidepressants (TCAs, MAOs and more recently the SSRIs) but other approaches have been to use anti-adrenergic drugs (such as propranolol and clonidine), carbamazepine (to reduce anger and aggressive outbursts) and lithium. However, the evidence for the efficacy of such drugs is largely based on "open" trials or anecdotal case reports. Benzodiazepines will reduce many of the symptoms but can also increase the frequency of anger and aggression due to cortical dysinhibition.

In SUMMARY, it is apparent that the biological basis of PTSD remains obscure although there is evidence that the hypothalamic–pituitary–adrenal axis is hypofunctional. So far there is no convincing evidence that any of the classical neurotransmitter pathways are directly involved although there is limited evidence that the opioid system could be hyperactive which might contribute to the suppression of memory recall which is often exhibited by victims of torture and sexual abuse.

Summary of the treatment decisions for the anxiety disorders

Treatment decisions for panic disorder

- Treatment of choice – SSRI.
- Switching – alternative SSRI; a second-generation antidepressant; a high potency benzodiazepine such as alprazolam.
- Augmentation – add a high potency benzodiazepine.
- Other options – a non-specific MAOI (e.g. phenelzine), RIMA (e.g. moclobemide), clomipramine.

Treatment decisions for social anxiety

- Treatment of choice – an SSRI (plus cognitive behavioural therapy).
- Switching – an alternative SSRI; MAOI; moclobemide.
- Augmentation – SSRI plus buspirone (? efficacy).

Treatment decisions for post traumatic stress disorder

- Treatment of choice – an SSRI.
- Switching – a second-generation antidepressant.
- Augmentation – a mood stabilizer; an atypical antipsychotic.
- Other options – nefazodone, venlafaxine.

Treatment decisions for obsessive–compulsive disorder

- Treatment of choice – an SSRI.
- Switching – an alternative SSRI; clomipramine.
- Augmentation – an atypical antipsychotic; clonazepam.
- Other options – venlafaxine, MAOI.

The benzodiazepine receptor and GABA function

Schmidt and colleagues in 1967 were the first to show that diazepam could potentiate the inhibitory effect of GABA on the cat spinal cord. Later it was shown that the effect of diazepam could be abolished if the endogenous GABA content was depleted, thus establishing that diazepam, and related benzodiazepines, did not act directly on GABA receptors but in some way modulated inhibitory transmission via GABA. It was subsequently demonstrated that the benzodiazepines bind with high affinity and specificity to neuronal elements in the mammalian brain and that there is an excellent correlation between their affinity for these specific binding sites and their pharmacological potencies in alleviating anxiety in both man and animals. The binding of a benzodiazepine to this receptor site is enhanced in the presence of GABA or a GABA agonist, thereby suggesting that a functional, but independent, relationship exists between the GABA receptor and the benzodiazepine receptor.

The *barbiturates*, and to some extent *alcohol*, also seem to produce their anxiolytic and sedative effects by facilitating GABAergic transmission. This action of chemically unrelated compounds can be explained by their ability to stimulate specific sites on the GABA receptor complex, the most marked effect being due to the benzodiazepines when they activate their specific receptor site. Thus benzodiazepines bind with high affinity to the benzodiazepine receptor and, as a result, change the structural conformation of the GABA receptor so that the action of GABA on its receptor is enhanced. This enables GABA to produce a stronger inhibition of the postsynaptic neuron than would occur in the absence of the benzodiazepine, the anxiolytic effect being produced by an allosteric enhancement of the action of GABA. The relationship between the various components of the GABA receptor and the GABA nerve terminal is shown in Figure 2.11 (see p. 56).

The inhibitory effect of GABA is mediated by chloride ion channels. When the GABA receptor is occupied by GABA, or by a drug acting as an agonist such as muscimol, the chloride channels open and chloride ions diffuse into the cell (see p. 56 for details). The chloride ion channel contains at least two binding sites. One of these sites is activated by barbiturates that have weak anxiolytic and hypnotic properties (e.g. pentobarbitone and phenobarbitone). Such drugs facilitate inhibitory transmission by increasing the duration of opening of the chloride ion channel. Another class of experimental anxiolytic agents that are not structurally related to the benzodiazepines (the pyrazolopyridines, of which etazolate is a clinically active example) also act at a specific site within the chloride ion channel and enhance GABAergic function by increasing the frequency of channel opening. The structure of the various sub-units that comprise the GABA-A receptor are shown in Figure 9.11.

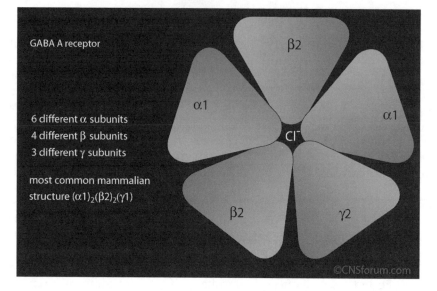

Figure 9.11. Structure of the sub-units that comprise the GABA-A receptor.

Thus it may be concluded that the "classical" benzodiazepines such as diazepam, and structurally related drugs, act as anxiolytics by activating a specific benzodiazepine receptor which facilitates inhibitory GABAergic transmission. Other drugs with anxiolytic properties, such as some of the barbiturates and alcohol, also facilitate GABAergic transmission by acting on sites associated more directly with the chloride ion channel.

Types of benzodiazepine receptors

Two types of receptor have been identified, termed Bz1 and Bz2. These receptors occupy different sub-units of the GABA-A receptor and therefore have different affinities for the benzodiazepine ligands. For example, the potent hypnotic zolpidem binds to the Bz1 receptor that is linked to the alpha-1 site on the GABA-A receptor while the hypnotic zopiclone binds to the Bz2 receptor which occupies both the alpha-2 and 3 sites on the GABA receptor. This selectivity for the Bz1 receptor may account for the fewer side effects of zolpiden in comparison to other hypnotic benzodiazepines.

The third type of benzodiazepine receptor is the so-called peripheral benzodiazepine receptor (pBz). This was first discovered in the rat adrenal gland, hence the term "peripheral". However, it is now known to occur on the platelet membrane, on immune cells and also in the mammalian brain.

The pBz receptor is distinct from the Bz1 and 2 receptors and does not activate GABA-A receptors. It is occupied by the isoquinoline PK 11195 and the benzodiazepine Ro 4864, neither of which has affinity for the brain Bz1 or 2 receptors. In the brain the pBz receptor is associated with the outer membrane of the mitochondria and with the glia cells.

The primary function of the pBz receptor is in the regulation of cholesterol uptake and the synthesis of neurosteroids. The latter compounds have an affinity for the GABA-A receptors which provide an indirect coupling between the pBz and the GABA receptors in the brain.

Most of the benzodiazepines that are currently available are full agonists occupying the Bz1 and 2 receptors. However, several drugs have been developed which act as partial agonists (for example, bretazenil which is a non-sedative anxiolytic) and partial inverse agonists such as sarmazenil. The beta carboline abercarnil is in development as a partial agonist. The properties of agonists and inverse agonists will be discussed further.

Diversity of drugs acting on the benzodiazepine receptor

Until about 1980, it was widely accepted that the benzodiazepine structure was a prerequisite for the anxiolytic profile and for the recognition of and binding to the benzodiazepine receptor. More recently, however, a chemically unrelated drug, the *cyclopyrrolone* zopiclone, has been shown to be a useful sedative hypnotic with a benzodiazepine-like profile. Other chemical classes of drugs that are also structurally dissimilar to the benzodiazepines (e.g. triazolopyridazines) have also been developed and shown to have anxiolytic activity in man; these non-benzodiazepines also act via the benzodiazepine receptor. Thus the term *"benzodiazepine receptor ligand"* has been introduced to describe all drugs, irrespective of their chemical structure, that act on benzodiazepine receptors and thereby modulate inhibitory transmission in the brain.

Over the last decade there has been an increase in our knowledge of the relationship between the structure of benzodiazepine receptor ligands and their pharmacological properties. This has led to the development of potent receptor *agonists* that stimulate the receptor and produce pharmacological effects qualitatively similar to diazepam and related "classical" benzodiazepines, *antagonists*, which block the effects of the agonists without having any effects themselves, and a group of drugs that have a mixture of agonist and antagonist properties (so-called *partial agonists*). In addition, an intriguing group of compounds have been developed that have the opposite effect on the benzodiazepine receptor to the pure agonists. These are known as *inverse agonists*. The pharmacological properties of these different types of benzodiazepine receptor ligands are summarized in Figure 9.12.

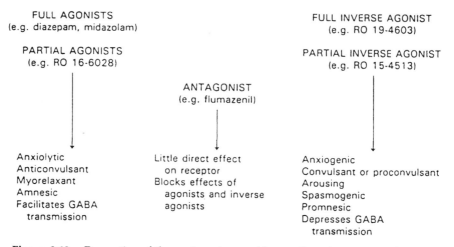

Figure 9.12.   Properties of the various types of benzodiazepine receptor ligands.

At the molecular level, the differences between the agonist and antagonist benzodiazepines are ascribed to the ability of the drug to induce a conformational change in the fine structure of the receptor molecule that produces functional consequences in terms of cellular changes. The partial agonists have intrinsic activity that lies between the full agonists and the antagonists. When administered they have qualitatively similar effects to full agonists, but may not be quite as potent; when given with full agonists they reduce the potency of the full agonist. Some 12 years ago, the Danish investigators Braestup and Nielsen found that a group of non-benzodiazepine compounds, the beta-carbolines, not only antagonized the actions of the full agonists but also had intrinsic activity themselves. Such compounds were clearly not pure antagonists, which lack intrinsic activity, but were found to be inverse agonists because they had the exact opposite biological effects to the pure agonists, i.e. they caused anxiety, convulsions and facilitated memory function. Thus the benzodiazepine receptor is so far unique in that it has a bidirectional function. This discovery could be of major importance in designing drugs in which the adverse effects of the "classical" benzodiazepines could be reduced but their beneficial effects maintained. The development of partial agonists may be particularly important in the production of anxiolytics that lack the sedative and amnestic properties of full agonists such as diazepam.

Are there natural ligands for the benzodiazepine receptor in the brain?

The presence of benzodiazepine receptors in the brain would suggest that there are natural ligands present which modulate these receptors. To date, a

Table 9.2. Putative endogenous ligands for the benzodiazepine receptor in the mammalian brain

Nicotinamide
Inosine and hypoxanthine
Ethyl-beta-carboline-3 carboxylate
Tribulin
Nephentin
Diazepam-displacing activity in human cerebrospinal fluid
Diazepam-binding inhibitor (DBI)

specific compound has not been unequivocally identified, but a number of candidates have been isolated that show agonist or inverse agonist activity. Some of these candidates are listed in Table 9.2.

Of the putative ligands for the benzodiazepine receptors that are listed in Table 9.2, diazepam-binding inhibitor (DBI), nephentin and tribulin appear to be particularly interesting. *DBI* is a polypeptide that has been isolated, and its structure elucidated, from mammalian and human brain. It is called "diazepam-binding inhibitor" because it can inhibit the binding of tritiated diazepam to the benzodiazepine receptor; recently it has also been shown to inhibit the binding of antagonists and inverse agonists to this receptor. Pharmacological studies show that DBI has anxiogenic properties and its concentration in the brain appears to be sufficiently high to block benzodiazepine receptors under appropriate conditions. It is only present in trace amounts in tissues other than the brain.

Tribulin is a relatively low molecular weight compound with acidic or neutral properties that has been isolated from human urine by Sandler and colleagues in the UK. The presence of this compound increases following stress and it has been found to inhibit the binding of benzodiazepines to their receptor site. In 1983 Sandler suggested that tribulin might be related to the endogenous anxiogenic factor and structurally related to the beta-carbolines. More recently it has been shown that tribulin is a mixture of at least three low molecular weight compounds.

Nephentin is also a large polypeptide that has been shown to have a relatively high affinity for the benzodiazepine receptor and does not have any effect upon other neurotransmitter receptors. Unlike DBI, however, the concentration of nephentin is much higher in non-nervous peripheral tissues such as the bile duct than it is in the brain. Furthermore, the distribution of nephentin in the brain does not coincide with that of the benzodiazepine receptors. It is possible, nevertheless, that nephentin is a precursor of a lower molecular weight peptide that can block the benzodiazepine receptor.

Less progress has been made in the detection of natural compounds that may act as agonists on the benzodiazepine receptor. Three non-peptides (nicotinamide, inosine and hypoxanthine) have been shown to have low affinities for the benzodiazepine receptor and there is some experimental evidence suggesting that they have mixed agonist–antagonist properties. Nevertheless, the consensus of opinion would appear to suggest that these substances are not the endogenous ligands for the benzodiazepine receptor. It is possible that purinergic mechanisms are activated by inosine and hypoxanthine and that the modulation of benzodiazepine receptor function is a secondary consequence of this.

There is some evidence to suggest that the benzodiazepines exist not only in plants such as the potato but also in the mammalian brain, including the brains of individuals who have never taken benzodiazepine anxiolytics or hypnotics. While such findings are still controversial, they do point to the possibility that the benzodiazepines are endogenous modulators of the GABA receptor and that a defect in their synthesis may have a role to play in the aetiology of anxiety disorders.

It may be concluded that there is some evidence to suggest that anxiety arises as a consequence either of a deficiency of an endogenous agonist or the presence of an endogenous inverse agonist acting on the benzodiazepine–GABA receptor complex. Thus one possible approach to drug design in the future may be the development of drugs that either facilitate the synthesis of endogenous agonists or reduce the synthesis of inverse agonists at the benzodiazepine receptor sites.

Changes in benzodiazepine receptor function following chronic administration of benzodiazepines

It is a well-established biological phenomenon that receptors adapt to the prolonged presence or absence of an agonist by changing their sensitivity, thereby attempting to return their function to normal levels. Thus prolonged blockade of dopamine receptors in the basal ganglia by neuroleptics such as chlorpromazine or haloperidol causes a *super-sensitivity* of these receptors. Conversely, conditions in which the receptor is chronically stimulated by its endogenous neurotransmitter, or by an agonist drug, result in a decrease in the functioning of the postsynaptic receptors; this phenomenon is known as *subsensitivity*, an event which may be accompanied by a decrease in the number of receptors. Such changes, sometimes termed "up"- or "down"-regulation, may develop slowly or rapidly, the former being due to changes in the synthesis of the receptor while the latter probably reflects the movement of receptors into, or out of, the neuronal membrane.

Experimental studies in rodents have clearly demonstrated that high doses of "classical" benzodiazepines such as diazepam, lorazepam and flurazepam cause a decrease in benzodiazepine receptors in the cortex of the brain but the number of receptors rapidly returns to normal (after approximately 5 days) following the abrupt cessation of drug treatment. There is also electro-physiological evidence to show that the functional activity of the GABA receptors that are linked to the benzodiazepine receptors is also decreased following prolonged treatment with chlordiazepoxide, even though the actual number of GABA receptors is increased. *In vitro* evidence suggests that chronic benzodiazepine treatment results in an uncoupling of the benzodiazepine receptor from the GABA receptor complex.

Functional tolerance following chronic treatment with the benzodiazepines is well documented in animals and man and represents a pharmacody-namic rather than pharmacokinetic phenomenon. Tolerance appears to occur more rapidly with the sedative and anticonvulsant rather than the anxiolytic properties of the "classical" benzodiazepines. However, since clinically relevant tolerance develops with therapeutic doses, but changes in receptor tolerance only occur with very high doses of the drugs that are usually far in excess of those used clinically, little experimental evidence exists at present whereby the functional tolerance to benzodiazepines can be explained on the basis of benzodiazepine receptor desensitization. However, one must be cautious in extrapolating the results of animal experiments to the patient with an anxiety disorder who is being treated with a benzodiazepine. The benzodiazepine receptor complex shows marked plasticity in the animal brain, but relatively few changes have been noted in this receptor system in samples obtained from post-mortem human brain, even when the patients suffered from epilepsy at the time of death. This suggests that the regulation or plasticity of the benzodiazepine receptor in the human brain differs considerably from that in the brain of the experimental animal, although the molecular properties of the benzodiazepine receptor appear to be remarkably similar.

Adverse effects of benzodiazepines

The short-term effects are mainly those of sedation but following longer-term use accumulation may occur, particularly in the case of drugs like diazepam and chlordiazepoxide that have long half-lives due to their active metabolites. After long-term administration (weeks to months) *tolerance* develops. While most patients rapidly become tolerant to the sedative side effects of these drugs, some patients, particularly the elderly, experience excessive sedation, poor memory and concentration, motor incoordination and muscle weakness. In extreme cases in the elderly, an acute confusional state may arise which simulates dementia. All sedatives, including the benzodiazepines, interact with alcohol and therefore these drugs should not be taken in combination.

In addition to the tolerance that occurs following the long-term treatment of a patient with a benzodiazepine, *dependence* also arises. Dependence is defined as a situation occurring as a consequence of the compensatory adaptive changes in the brain as a result of chronic drug administration. Evidence for *physical dependence* is obtained from the *withdrawal* effects that arise on discontinuation of the medication. *Rebound* effects are defined as an increase in the severity of the initial symptoms beyond that occurring in the patient before treatment started. Rebound insomnia following abrupt discontinuation of benzodiazepine hypnotics is well described, and rebound anxiety arises not uncommonly in those patients in whom an anxiolytic benzodiazepine has been suddenly terminated. Slowly tapering the dose of a benzodiazepine over a period of many days or weeks largely overcomes the problem of rebound effects.

Sudden withdrawal from a high chronic dose of benzodiazepine has long been known to provide a variety of side effects, including seizures and paranoid behaviour in extreme cases. Withdrawal symptoms include psychological changes such as anxiety, apprehension, irritability, insomnia and dysphoria, bodily symptoms such as palpitations, tremor, vertigo and sweating, and perceptual disturbances, including hypersensitivity to light, sound and pain, and depersonalization. The perceptual disturbances that occur on withdrawal are not generally seen in those patients exhibiting rebound effects and it therefore may be possible to distinguish between these two phenomena. It has been estimated that 15–30% of patients on benzodiazepines for longer than a year may encounter problems in trying to discontinue their medication.

Use of non-benzodiazepines in the treatment of anxiety disorders

The *barbiturates* and *meprobamate* have been entirely superseded by the benzodiazepines and because of their low benefit-to-risk ratio (dependence producing, lethality in overdose, potent sedative effects) they should never be used as anxiolytics. Despite their popularity as short-term sedatives, *antihistamines* are ineffective anxiolytics, while the use of *sedative antidepressants* such as amitriptyline should be limited to the treatment of patients with symptoms of both anxiety and depression due to their limited efficacy and the poor patient compliance associated with their adverse effects. However, patients with panic disorder do appear to show a beneficial response to antidepressants (see Chapter 6). A similar argument can be made regarding the use of low doses of *antipsychotics*, although drugs such as chlorpromazine may have some value in treating severely anxious patients who had previously been dependent on sedatives. *Beta adrenoceptor antagonists* such as propranolol may have a place in the treatment of anxious patients with pronounced autonomic symptoms (palpitations, tremor and gastrointestinal upset).

The azaspirodecanedione anxiolytics

A series of non-benzodiazepine anxiolytics have recently been introduced which, unlike the benzodiazepines, do not facilitate GABAergic function but appear to act as agonists at 5-HT$_{1A}$ receptors. *Buspirone* is an example of this novel class of anxiolytics, and is structurally similar to gepirone and ipsapirone. The latter compounds are reported to show both anxiolytic and antidepressant properties. The structure of these novel compounds is shown in Figure 9.13.

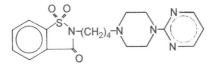

Buspirone

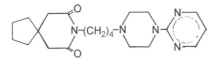

Gepirone

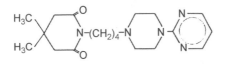

Ipsapirone

1-Pyrimidylpiperazine
(1-PP) metabolite of buspirone, gepirone
and ipsapirone

Figure 9.13.   Chemical structure of some azaspirodecanedione anxiolytics.

In vitro ligand binding studies have shown that buspirone binds with high affinity to 5-HT$_{1A}$ and D$_2$ receptor sites. However, it is known that *in vivo* the main metabolite of buspirone and ipsapirone is 1-pyrimidylpiperazine (1-PP), which also has a high affinity for alpha$_2$ adrenoceptors. Thus the pharmacological activity of buspirone and related compounds may be the result of a complex interaction between the parent compound and the pharmacologically active metabolite. It seems possible that the antagonist effect of the 1-PP metabolite on alpha$_2$ adrenoceptors might account for the presumed antidepressant action of such drugs, as it is known that some atypical antidepressants such as mianserin and idazoxan also show an antagonistic activity on such receptors. Another interesting aspect of the action of buspirone lies in its specificity of action of 5-HT$_{1A}$ receptors in the brain. Thus experimental studies have shown that it has a more marked effect in reducing the turnover of 5-HT in the hippocampus, and to a lesser extent the cortex, than it does in the striatum. From such studies of the effects of buspirone-like drugs on central neurotransmission, it may be concluded that their anxiolytic action is due to a reduction in 5-HT turnover in the limbic region of the brain, while the possible antidepressant effect could be attributed to a selective enhancement of noradrenaline turnover in this region. Such an explanation must be treated with caution, however, as it is well established that alpha$_2$ adrenoceptor antagonists such as yohimbine induce anxiety states in both man and animals. Whether buspirone-like drugs selectively enhance noradrenaline turnover only in the limbic region, and do not cause a hyperarousal state which could induce anxiety, is a matter of conjecture. The pharmacological consequences of the interaction of buspirone with D$_2$ receptor sites is uncertain; there is little evidence that buspirone has neuroleptic properties at those doses which are known to be anxiolytic. The slight abdominal discomfort occasionally associated with the initial administration of buspirone could be due to the stimulation of 5-HT receptors in the gastrointestinal tract.

Clinical trials of buspirone have shown the drug to be slower in onset of action compared with diazepam, but it produces significantly less sedation and fewer detrimental effects on psychomotor function than the benzodiazepines. The main advantage of buspirone would therefore appear to be in its lack of dependence, amnestic and sedative effects. However, its slower onset of action and its lower efficacy in alleviating the somatic symptoms of anxiety make it unlikely that it will replace the therapeutically effective and proven benzodiazepines, despite the greater frequency of their side effects. Whether ipsapirone and gepirone, which are still in clinical development, will be therapeutically superior to buspirone can only be assessed after they become more widely available for clinical use.

Clinical studies show that buspirone is an effective anxiolytic with an advantage over the benzodiazepines of lacking a sedative effect, not interacting with alcohol and not exhibiting any dependence effects following prolonged use. Its main clinical disadvantage lies in the delay in onset of its therapeutic effect (up to 2 weeks in some cases) and its limited efficacy in attenuating anxiety in those patients who had previously responded to benzodiazepines. Furthermore, unlike the benzodiazepines, it does not appear to have beneficial effects in patients with panic disorder.

The failure of buspirone to exhibit cross-tolerance with the benzodiazepines in both animal and man suggests that the drug alleviates anxiety by a different mechanism. Experimental studies have shown that buspirone, gepirone and ipsapirone act as full or partial agonists on 5-HT_{1A} receptor subtypes. Experimental studies show that potent 5-HT_{1A} agonists such as 8-hydroxy-2-(dipropylamino)tetralin (8OH-DPAT) are anxiolytic in some animal models of anxiety. This suggests that this novel class of anxiolytics modulate central serotonergic transmission, which probably accounts for the relative lack of those side effects that the benzodiazepines exhibit due to their facilitating action on GABA receptors (sedation, dependence, etc.). Modulation of 5-HT_{1A} receptor function may also account for the antidepressant properties which this series of drugs are claimed to show.

In CONCLUSION, evidence has been presented to show that the benzodiazepines produce their variety of pharmacological effects by activating specific receptors that form part of the main inhibitory neurotransmitter receptor system, the GABA receptor, in the mammalian brain. Different classes of benzodiazepine receptor ligands have been developed which can alleviate anxiety or produce anxiety according to the fine structural changes that occur when the drugs interact with the benzodiazepine receptor.

There is some evidence that natural substances occur in the human brain that can cause either an increase or a reduction in the anxiety state by acting on the benzodiazepine receptor. The unique nature of the benzodiazepine receptor, and the disparate properties of the drugs that act on this receptor, should allow plenty of scope for the development of novel compounds with selective anxiolytic and other properties in the future. Despite the evidence from animal studies that benzodiazepine receptor function changes in response to chronic drug treatment, there is little evidence from human brain studies that such changes are relevant to the phenomena of tolerance, dependence and withdrawal effects that have been the recent cause for public concern. Novel anxiolytics such as buspirone that are structurally unrelated to the benzodiazepines and which do not modulate GABAergic function have the advantage of lacking the sedative and dependence-producing effects of the benzodiazepines. Nevertheless, the relative lack of efficacy of such drugs, and the delay in their onset of therapeutic effect, make it unlikely that they will replace the benzodiazepines as the drugs of choice in the treatment of anxiety disorders.

10 Drug Treatment of Insomnia

Introduction

Apart from the benzodiazepines, the sedative hypnotics are a group of drugs that depress the brain in a relatively non-selective manner. This results in a progressive change from drowsiness (sedation), sleep (hypnosis) to loss of consciousness, surgical anaesthesia, coma and finally cardiovascular and respiratory collapse and death. The central nervous system (CNS) depressant drugs include general anaesthetics, barbiturates and alcohols, including ethanol. Before the advent of the benzodiazepines, barbiturates in low doses were widely used as anxiolytics. A *sedative* drug is one that decreases CNS activity, moderates excitement and generally calms the individual, whereas a *hypnotic* produces drowsiness and facilitates the onset and maintenance of sleep from which the individual may be easily aroused.

Historically the first sedative hypnotics to be introduced were the bromides in the mid 19th century, shortly followed by chloral hydrate, paraldehyde and urethane. It was not until the early years of this century that the first barbiturate, sodium barbitone, was developed and this was shortly followed by over 50 analogues, all with essentially similar pharmacological properties. The major breakthrough in the development of selective, relatively non-toxic sedative hypnotics followed the introduction of chlordiazepoxide in 1961. Most of the benzodiazepines in current use have been selected for their high anxiolytic potency relative to their central depressant effects. Because of their considerable safety, the benzodiazepines have now largely replaced the barbiturates and the alcohols, such as chloral hydrate and trichloroethanol, as the drugs of choice in the treatment of insomnia.

The hypnotics are some of the most widely used drugs, over 15 million prescriptions being given for this group of drugs in Britain in 1985; the number of prescriptions for hypnotics has remained fairly constant over the last decade despite the reduction in anxiolytic prescriptions by about 50% over this same period. This situation is hard to reconcile with the fact that

Fundamentals of Psychopharmacology. Third Edition. By Brian E. Leonard
© 2003 John Wiley & Sons, Ltd. ISBN 0 471 52178 7

all benzodiazepines in current use have hypnotic properties if given in slightly higher therapeutic doses. This implies that what determines their use as anxiolytics, for day-time administration, or hypnotics, for night-time use, is largely a question of dose and marketing. As discussed in considerable detail elsewhere (see p. 213), there is a metabolic inter-relationship between the commonly used 1,4-benzodiazepines and their mode of action is similar. It is of interest that the hypnotic benzodiazepines have received little media attention, in contrast to the anxiolytics of the same class, regarding their possible dependence-forming effects.

Physiology of sleep

Although there is no evidence for a specific sleep "centre" in the brain, it is generally accepted that the level of consciousness is located in the diffuse network of nerve cells that comprise the reticular formation. This region consists of tegmental parts of the medulla, pons and midbrain. Lesions of the reticular formation result in somnolence or coma, sensory stimuli failing to arouse the animal. Such observations led to the conclusion that the brain stem reticular activity system maintains alertness and wakefulness, while lack of sensory stimulation results in sleep. Arousal from sleep by sensory stimuli is attributed to collateral pathways that link the main sensory pathways to the reticular formation. Undoubtedly this is a gross simplification of the anatomical substrate for sleep and wakefulness. There is evidence, for example, that animals may recover consciousness following lesions of the reticular formation and that the forebrain is not completely dependent on inputs from the reticular formation to maintain consciousness. Nevertheless, it is generally accepted that the reticular formation plays an important, if not a key role, in sleep and wakefulness.

Physiological basis of sleep – circadian rhythmicity

It is a well-known fact that the circadian rhythm is entrained for diurnal cues to approximately 24 hours. However, a non-entrained rhythm, which operates in the absence of external cues, lasts between 25 and 27 hours. Thus the human sleep–wake cycle normally shows a 24-hour rhythm but not all physiological processes (for example, body temperature) follow the sleep–wake cycle.

It is now known that circadian rhythms are controlled by clock genes which are found in species as wide apart as insects and mammals. It would appear that the clock genes are activated by light falling on the retina. The activated retina neurons then stimulate the retinohypothalamic tract which projects to the suprachiasmatic nucleus and thence to the anterior pituitary. This pathway is responsible for coupling the circadian rhythm with the

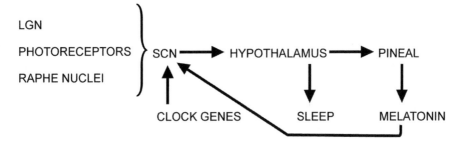

Figure 10.1.   Pathways involved in the entraining of the circadian rhythm.

light cycle. The lateral geniculate nucleus (LGN) activates the suprachiasmatic nucleus (SCN) in the case of the non-light-based stimuli such as motor activity. The raphé nuclei also impact on the SCN. Thus several pathways appear to be involved in the entraining process (see Figure 10.1).

Sleep and the EEG

In general, the sleep cycle is synchronized via the SCN. All sensory stimuli activate the ascending reticular activating system, thereby causing cortical arousal and preventing the cortex reverting to its basic slow-wave oscillating rhythm. The excitatory, arousing mechanisms are complemented by inhibitory inputs from the hypothalamus. At least four different types of neurotransmitters are involved in regulating the EEG pattern in the sleep–wake cycle. Thus acetylcholine causes a desynchronization of the cortical EEG while REM sleep is induced by cholinomimetic drugs (such as arecoline and physostigmine) but blocked by atropine.

The central histamine 1 receptors are active in the posterior hypothalamus during the waking phase but inactive during the slow-wave sleep and REM stages of the sleep–wake cycle. Antagonists of the H_1 histamine receptors cause sedation.

There is evidence that the histaminergic tract that passes from the posterior hypothalamus to the cortex via the thalamus is inhibited by a GABAergic pathway. It is now known that H_3 receptors act as autoreceptors on histaminergic neurons and that agonists of H_3 receptors augment slow-wave sleep. In addition, histamine can increase cortical arousal by enhancing excitatory cholinergic neurons from the basal forebrain and also inhibits the hypothalamic pre-optic area which normally promotes sleep. With respect to the control of the circadian rhythm, histamine has both excitatory (H_1) and inhibitory (H_2) effects on the SCN. Thus in addition to acetylcholine, noradrenaline and 5-HT, histamine would also appear to play a crucial role in regulating the sleep pattern.

Noradrenaline – the EEG is aroused by stimulants such as the amphetamines and methylphenidate whereas drugs such as reserpine which deplete brain noradrenaline have the opposite effect. Similar effects to the stimulants may be obtained by the electrical stimulation of the locus coeruleus which has been shown to decrease in activity during the REM sleep phase of the sleep cycle. The precise role that noradrenaline plays in sleep is uncertain. While it may be involved in sleep induction, noradrenaline also has many other physiological functions including control of the heart rate, blood pressure, autonomic activity, etc. which play a role in the entraining process.

Dopamine – low doses of the dopamine agonist apomorphine increase slow-wave sleep and, like other dopaminometics, cause somnolence in patients with Parkinson's disease. Conversely, dopamine autoreceptor antagonists, which enhance dopamine release, reduce both REM and non-REM sleep. Stimulants such as cocaine cause arousal by activating D_2 postsynaptic receptors, effects which are blocked by most neuroleptics.

Serotonin – the reduction in the release of 5-HT in the brain (for example, by blocking 5-HT synthesis with parachlorophenyl alanine) induces sleep while the electrical stimulation of the raphé nuclei causes excitation. It would appear that the activity of the raphé nuclei is decreased in slow-wave sleep. However, the role of specific 5-HT receptors in mediating the effects of 5-HT is unclear. This is due to the relative lack of specificity of the drugs available but also due to the fact that 5-HT modulates the activity of other neurotransmitter systems involved in the regulation of sleep. For example, 5-HT_{1A} receptor agonists increase the frequency of slow-wave sleep which may be due to its inhibitory effect on the release of acetylcholine from the nucleus basalis. It would appear however that the serotonergic system is active during the waking phase but reduced during the sleep phase of the sleep–wake cycle.

In animals, two main types of sleep pattern may be identified termed *non-rapid eye movement sleep* (non-REM or slow-wave sleep) and *rapid eye movement sleep* (REM sleep). Normal sleep is composed of several REM and non-REM cycles. *Non-REM sleep* is divided into light sleep (stages 1 and 2) and slow-wave or delta sleep (stages 3 and 4). *Stage 1* sleep is characterized by alpha rhythm on the EEG and forms the transition between wakefulness and sleep; it occupies approximately 5% of the time. Muscle tone is relatively weak and while a certain amount of mental activity persists, concentration and imagination fluctuate. As the sleep deepens, hypnagogic hallucinations may occur. *Stage 2* sleep represents over 50% of the total sleeping time and is marked by characteristic sleep spindles and K complexes in the EEG; delta waves are also present occasionally. Muscle tone is weak and there are no eye movements. *Stages 3 and 4*, slow-wave sleep, occupy approximately 20% of the sleep time. The EEG is characterized by more than 50% of the sleep pattern being in the form of delta waves. This stage of sleep is the recuperative phase which is associated with growth hormone secretion and tissue repair; the secretion of prolactin is not associated with any specific phase of sleep. Dreaming may occur but tends to be of brief duration and of a rational nature. Nocturnal terrors and sleep walking are associated with stage 4 sleep.

REM sleep occupies approximately 20% of the sleep time in the normal adult, up to 30% in the young child and less than 20% in the aged or mentally handicapped. The cortical EEG activity resembles that of wakefulness, but is accompanied by muscular weakness; 4 Hz "sawtooth" waves herald the onset of REM sleep. The precise physiological function of REM sleep is unknown but it is associated with dreaming sleep, the dreams being long, emotional and animated. The physiological changes accompanying REM sleep include hypertension, tachycardia alternating with bradycardia, pelvic congestion in the female and penile tumescence in the male. Cortisol secretion appears to peak during the latter part of the sleep cycle when REM sleep is most pronounced. This type of sleep is also characterized by bursts of eye movement and small sporadic muscular twitches of the face and extremities.

The typical sleep pattern of the young adult is composed of four to six cycles of non-REM sleep alternating with REM sleep at approximately 90 minute intervals. The subject first goes into non-REM sleep and then gradually descends from stage 1 through to stage 4 sleep, the frequency of the waves becoming slower and their amplitude greater. The depth of sleep then briefly (for a few minutes) returns to stage 2, after which the first episode of REM sleep appears. Bodily movements often occur at this stage. This may be illustrated by means of a hypnogram, as shown in Figure 10.2.

It should be noted that stages 3 and 4 are more pronounced during the early part of the sleep period, whereas REM sleep tends to increase during the sleep cycle. The actual period of sleep is to some extent genetically determined, some individuals requiring at least 8 hours while others need only 4 hours to function normally. The sleep pattern becomes more fragile with advancing age, so that in the elderly the number of nocturnal awakenings increases and REM sleep becomes more evenly distributed throughout the night.

The sleep architecture may be modified by disease and by certain drugs. In the healthy individual, the duration of the first phase of REM sleep is usually 3 minutes. In patients with depression or narcoplexy, the time of onset of the first REM phase is shorter than usual, while those with anxiety

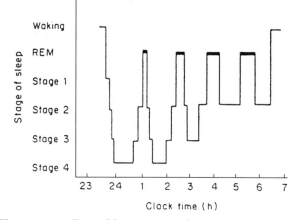

Figure 10.2. Typical hypnogram of a normal young adult.

disorders have a delayed time of onset of the first REM phase. The duration of the first REM phase is also increased in depressed patients.

All hypnotics in current clinical use alter the sleep architecture by reducing the quantity and quality of the REM sleep phase in particular. Thus a single dose of a hypnotic *benzodiazepine* suppresses REM during the period in which it is present, but for up to the two following nights the amount of REM sleep is generally increased (so-called REM rebound). When the hypnotic is given for a prolonged period, the REM sleep gradually returns to normal, but abrupt withdrawal can lead to prolonged rebound in REM sleep, which is often associated with intense and unpleasant dreams and anxiety on wakening. Most hypnotics also affect the quality of the non-REM sleep, particularly the slow-wave sleep pattern. Thus stage 3 and stage 4 sleep are suppressed and remain so during the period of drug administration. Following drug withdrawal, the slow-wave sleep gradually returns to normal, but this may take up to 15 days. However, no rebound effect appears to occur in slow-wave sleep. All hypnotics in current use also decrease stage 1 of non-REM sleep and prolong stage 2 sleep; this may be the reason why the nocturnal awakenings decrease, so that the individual feels that the quality of sleep under the influence of the hypnotic has improved! The effect of a hypnotic on the quality of the REM and slow-wave sleep is shown diagrammatically in Figure 10.3.

Disturbance in the sleep pattern commonly occurs in the alcoholic. The sleep pattern in this type of patient is characterized by frequent awakenings and decreased REM and slow-wave sleep. Concomitantly, stages 1 and 2 are increased but shallower than usual. After withdrawal from alcohol, the

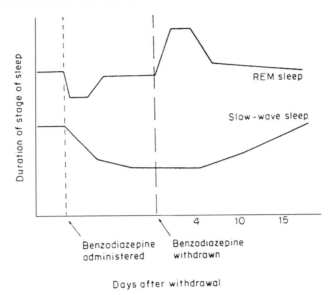

Figure 10.3. Illustration of the rebound effect following 15 days' continuous treatment with a benzodiazepine.

patient experiences insomnia and REM rebound occurs. The sleep profile of the alcoholic often remains abnormal for 1–2 years following withdrawal.

Most *antidepressants* decrease the quantity of REM sleep in the depressed patient, although it is difficult to say whether this is a reflection of the action of the drugs or due to the underlying pathology. Abrupt withdrawal of antidepressants, particularly the monoamine oxidase inhibitors, is often associated with REM rebound.

Use of hypnotics

Despite the fact that man spends approximately one-third of his life asleep, the purpose of sleep still remains a mystery. The clinical importance of sleep is reflected in the frequency and severity of complaints about insomnia, a condition that signifies unsatisfactory or insufficient sleep. Problems may involve difficulty in getting to sleep, disturbing dreams, early wakening, and day-time drowsiness due to poor sleep at night. In most cases, these symptoms are fairly transient and may be associated with a specific or identifiable event such as a family or work situation, a temporary financial problem, etc. Should the sleep disturbance persist for longer than 3 weeks, specific treatment may be indicated. The Association of Sleep Disorders Centres has classified sleep disorders into two broad classes – *disorders of initiating and maintaining sleep* (DIMS) and *disorders of excessive somnolence* (DOES); these definitions have now been appended to the DSM–IV.

The hypnogram of a patient with an underlying psychiatric illness may be characterized by a delay in sleep onset, the presence of residual muscular activity causing frequent awakenings, fragmented sleep, reduced REM and slow-wave sleep, and day-time drowsiness. Such disorders are generally not associated with a recent or transient event and the cause cannot usually be identified. Often such changes in the sleep architecture are associated with major psychiatric disorders such as depression, mania, psychosis or severe anxiety states.

For the purpose of considering the prescribing of hypnotics, insomnia may be classified into three major types:

1. *Transient insomnia.* This occurs in normal sleepers who experience an acute stress or stressful situation lasting for a few days, for example, air travel to a different time zone or hospitalization.
2. *Short-term insomnia.* This is usually associated with situational stress caused, for example, by bereavement or which may be related to conflict at work or in the family.
3. *Long-term insomnia.* Studies suggest that insomnia in up to 50% of patients in this category is related to an underlying psychiatric illness. Of the remainder of the patients in this category, chronic alcohol or drug abuse may be the cause of the sleep disruption.

Whenever the use of hypnotics is considered appropriate, it is universally agreed that patients should be given the smallest effective dose for the shortest period of time necessary. This recommendation applies particularly to elderly patients. For transient and short-term insomnia there is no clear consensus, although in practice the use of a medium or short half-life hypnotic for a few days is sometimes recommended when sleep disturbance is associated with shift work or "jet-lag". For chronic insomnia, careful investigation of the underlying cause of the condition is essential before hypnotics are routinely prescribed. Should the insomnia be associated with a psychiatric condition or drug abuse, specific treatment of the core illness will often obviate the need for hypnotics.

For all practical purposes, the benzodiazepines are the group of drugs most widely used to treat insomnia. These may be divided into three classes based on their pharmacokinetic characteristics:

1. *Short half-life drugs,* such as triazolam, midazolam and brotizolam, with elimination half-lives of about 6 hours.

Table 10.1.   Plasma elimination half-lives of hypnotic benzodiazepines and their active metabolites

Drug	Elimination half-life of parent compound (hours)	Active metabolite	Elimination half-life of metabolite (hours)
Short half-life			
Brotizolam	5.0 (3–5)	1-Methylhydroxy derivative	Short
Triazolam	2.3 (1.4–3.3)	1-Methylhydroxy derivative	Short
Midazolam	2.5 (1–3)	1-Methylhydroxy derivative	Short
Intermediate half-life			
Loprazolam	6.3 (4–8)	None	–
Lormetazepam	9.9 (7–12)	None	–
Temazepam	12.0 (8–21)	None	–
Long half-life			
Flunitrazepam	15.0 (9–25)	7-Amino derivative	23
Flurazepam	Very short	N-Desalkyl-flurazepam	87
Nitrazepam	18 (20–34)	None	–
Benzodiazepine ligands			
Zaleplon	1.0	None	–
Zolpidem	1.5–4.5	None	–

2. *Intermediate half-life drugs*, such as temazepam, lormetazepam and loprazolam, with half-lives of 6–12 hours.
3. *Long half-life drugs*, such as nitrazepam, flurazepam and flunitrazepam, with half-lives over 12 hours.

The elimination half-lives of a number of commonly used hypnotics are shown in Table 10.1. It should be noted that many of the drugs in current use have active metabolites which considerably prolong the duration of their pharmacological effect. This is particularly true for the elderly patient in whom the half-life of the hypnotic is prolonged due to decreased metabolism and renal clearance; such individuals are also more sensitive to the sedative effects of any psychotropic medication.

   In general, the efficacy of hypnotics for short-term use is well established and there is a close relationship between their pharmacokinetic and pharmacodynamic profiles. The most widely used hypnotic in the UK, for example, is temazepam, which is relatively slowly absorbed and therefore has only a marginal effect on the sleep latency but facilitates sleep duration.

The short elimination half-lives of drugs such as brotizolam ensure that residual sedative effects do not occur during the day. In contrast, fast elimination hypnotics such as midazolam and triazolam, which are effective in treating sleep onset insomnia, often give rise to rebound insomnia on withdrawal. It should be emphasized that the abrupt withdrawal of hypnotics, particularly when they have been given for several weeks or longer, is generally accompanied by REM rebound which results in an increased frequency of dreams and nightmares and can precipitate disturbed sleep and anxiety. Slow reduction in the night-time dose of the hypnotic over several days may reduce the risk of such a rebound.

Regarding the efficacy of hypnotics when used long-term, there is evidence that sleep latency shows more tolerance than sleep time. Furthermore, it is generally accepted that each hypnotic has a minimal effective dose and that increasing this does little to improve the duration of sleep but is more likely to increase the side effects.

Summary of the drugs used to treat insominia

1. Benzodiazepine receptor agonists
   Benzodiazepines (triazolam, temazepam, midazolam, lorazepam, estazolam).
   Non-benzodiazepines (imidazopyridines, e.g. zolpidem; pyrazopyrimidines, e.g. zaleplon; cyclopyrolones, e.g. zopiclone).
2. Pharmacological effects
   Benzodiazepines – shorter latency to sleep, longer duration of sleep, decreased REM sleep, increased slow-wave sleep.
   Zopiclone – similar to benzodiazepines.
   Zaleplon and zolpidem – stated to have little adverse effect on sleep profile. There is evidence that the therapeutic efficacy is maintained even after several months of treatment.
3. Main side effects
   Long half-life benzodiazepines cause day-time sedation.
   Dose-related anterograde amnesia.
   Impaired reaction time and vigilance.
   In elderly, cognitive impairment; falls causing fractures.
   Rebound insomnia can occur after withdrawal of short half-life drugs.
   Recurrence of original symptoms can occur when drug is stopped.
   Withdrawal effects on abrupt discontinuation of drug. These include: dizziness, confusion and dysphoria.
   Because of the frequency of side effects, benzodiazepine ligands are only recommended for the short-term (4 weeks) treatment of insomnia.

4. Other treatments include:
    Sedative antidepressants (venlafaxine, trazodone, nefazodone, TCAs, mianserin, mirtazepine).
    Antihistamines (diphenhydramine, doxylamine).
    Melatonin (may shorten sleep latency but little effect on sleep time).
    Valerian extract (evidence of efficacy in double-blind studies).
    It should be noted that all these alternative treatments for insomnia also have side effects, some of which (e.g. TCAs) are potentially more serious than those occurring with the benzodiazepine group.

Non-benzodiazepine hypnotics

These drugs comprise the barbiturates, alcohols and a new class of cyclopyrrolone hypnotics. Because of the severity of their side effects and their dependence potential, the barbiturates should not be used to treat insomnia.

The alcohol type of hypnotics include the chloral derivatives, of which *chloral hydrate* and *chlormethiazole* are still occasionally used in the elderly, and *ethchlorvynol*. Chloral hydrate is metabolized to another active sedative hypnotic *trichlorethanol*. These drugs all have a similar effect on the sleep profile. They are short half-life drugs (about 4–6 hours) that decrease the sleep latency and number of awakenings; slow-wave sleep is slightly depressed while the overall REM sleep time is largely unaffected, although the distribution of REM sleep may be disturbed. Chloral hydrate and its active metabolite have an unpleasant taste and cause epigastric distress and nausea. Undesirable effects of these drugs include lightheadedness, ataxia and nightmares, particularly in the elderly. Allergic skin reactions to chloral hydrate have been reported. Chronic use of these drugs can lead to tolerance and occasionally physical dependence. Like the barbiturates, overdosage can lead to respiratory and cardiovascular depression. Therapeutic use of these drugs has largely been superseded by the benzodiazepines.

Any new hypnotic should induce and maintain natural sleep without producing residual sedative effects during the day; it should not cause dependence or interact adversely with other sedatives, including alcohol. The *ideal hypnotic* should not cause respiratory depression or precipitate cardiovascular collapse when taken in overdose. *So far no drug fulfils all these criteria.*

Several new anxiolytic and sedative drugs act at the benzodiazepine receptor site, or one of the subsets that comprise this receptor site even though the chemical structure of these molecules differs substantially from the benzodiazepines. One of the first of these compounds to be developed was the cyclopyrrolone *zopiclone*. A structurally somewhat similar molecule

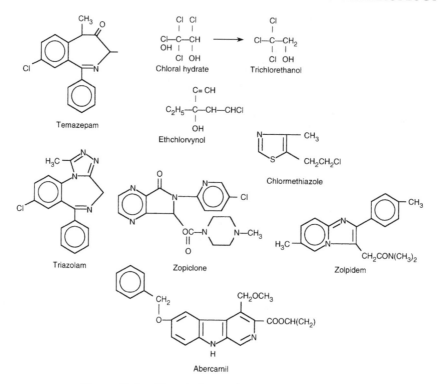

Figure 10.4. Chemical structure of some hypnotics.

zolpidem, an imidazopyridine, has also been marketed recently as has the beta-carboline *abercarnil*. Of the newer benzodiazepines, the tetracyclic 2,4 benzodiazepine *bretazenil* has also been introduced as a short-acting sedative–hypnotic. The chemical structure of these molecules is illustrated in Figure 10.4.

The therapeutic profile and adverse effects of the non-benzodiazepine sedative–hypnotics

Zopiclone was the first of the new sedative–hypnotics to be launched in the late 1970s and has been shown to be equi-effective with the standard sedative–hypnotic benzodiazepines such as flurazepam and temazepam. There is evidence that zopiclone may cause less "hang-over" effects than the conventional benzodiazepines but some studies have shown that this drug does produce performance decrement when this is tested shortly after treatment. A similar profile has been reported for zolpidem while abercarnil has been reported to cause a performance decrement for the first few days of treatment that then largely disappears. Bretazenil has been shown to cause dose-related disruptions in psychomotor performance, but these effects are not as prominent as occurs following an equivalent dose of diazepam or alprazolam. A somewhat unusual side effect has been described by patients taking zopiclone – a bitter, unpleasant taste and a dry mouth. The cause of these effects is presently unknown.

Regarding abuse liability, to date there have been only few studies in which newer sedative–hypnotics have been investigated. Nevertheless there is some evidence that those with a history of sedative abuse preferred high doses of triazolam and zopiclone to placebo. There is some evidence that bretazenil has a lower abuse potential than the benzodiazepines. Abuse liability of these novel sedative hypnotics has also been evaluated in primates. Abercarnil causes a lower incidence of withdrawal effects than conventional benzodiazepines. This may be due to the differences in the intrinsic efficacy rather than the bioavailability of these drugs for the brain. However, zopiclone and bretazenil did lower the seizure threshold to electroshock-induced seizures in mice whereas the seizure threshold was unaffected by zolpidem, tracozalate and C1 218,872. In baboons zolpidem may cause physiological dependence; similar studies in monkeys show that mild withdrawal effects occur after the abrupt withdrawal of zopiclone, whereas withdrawal from diazepam caused severe symptoms. It may be concluded that sedative–hypnotic drugs with a limited efficacy such as bretazenil and zolpidem are also limited in their ability to cause physiological dependence.

In human studies, there is some evidence that withdrawal signs such as nervousness, anxiety and vertigo occur following sub-chronic administration of zopiclone but the frequency and intensity of the withdrawal effects are greater after conventional 1,4-benzodiazepines. No rebound effects have been seen in patients with insomnia who received zolpidem daily for 7–180 days. By contrast, after 3 weeks of abercarnil treatment of patients with generalized anxiety disorder possible signs of withdrawal resulted, the incidence of these withdrawal effects being related to doses of abercarnil administered.

From the published clinical studies, it would appear that the partial agonists bretazenil and abercarnil are less likely to cause physiological dependence, have lower reinforcing effects and a lower incidence of subjective effects associated with abuse liability than the conventional 1,4-benzodiazepine sedative–hypnotics. It is presently unclear whether the full agonists for the GABA-A receptor, zolpidem and zopiclone, offer a real advance in the treatment of insomnia although their adverse effect profiles and abuse liability may be lower than that of the conventional benzodiazepines.

In CONCLUSION, hypnotics are a widely used group of drugs accounting for about 15% of all prescriptions over the last four decades. The condition for which these drugs are prescribed, insomnia, is ill-defined. Various types of insomnia exist, and there are many possible causes. Most short-term insomnia is associated with stress and can be alleviated by the short-term administration of a hypnotic. Most long-term insomnia is associated with psychiatric illness or drug or alcohol abuse and therefore careful investigation and evaluation of the patient is necessary before hypnotics should be considered. As with all psychotropic drugs, the elderly patient is most likely to experience unwanted side effects such as sedation and day-time drowsiness. Of the different classes of hypnotics available, the benzodiazepines, particularly those with medium or short elimination half-lives, are the most widely used. The rule which should always be applied in the prescribing of hypnotics is that the smallest effective dose should be prescribed for the shortest time necessary to treat the sleep disturbance.

11 Drug Treatment of Schizophrenia and the Psychoses

Introduction

Schizophrenia is a group of illnesses of unknown origin that occur in approximately 1% of the adult population in most countries in which surveys have been conducted. The economic and social cost is considerable, as approximately 40% of all hospitalized psychiatric patients in most industrialized countries suffer from schizophrenia and related disorders. At least 25 major family studies have been published in the last three decades that have consistently shown that the risk for the disease in the relatives of schizophrenics is substantially greater than that expected in the general population. While most of these studies have been criticized on methodological grounds, it is generally accepted that schizophrenia does have a genetic basis.

Schizophrenia usually begins during adolescence or young adulthood and is characterized by a spectrum of symptoms that typically include disordered thought, social withdrawal, hallucinations (both aural and visual), delusions of persecution (paranoia) and bizarre behaviour. These symptoms are sometimes categorized as "positive" (e.g. hallucinations) and "negative" (e.g. social withdrawal and apathy) (Figure 11.1). So far, there is no known cure and the disease is chronic and generally progressive. Nevertheless the introduction of the phenothiazine neuroleptic chlorpromazine by Delay and Denecker in France in 1952 initiated the era of pharmacotherapy in psychiatric medicine and has led to the marketing of many dozens of chemically diverse antipsychotic drugs that have played a major role in limiting the disintegration of the personality of the schizophrenic patient. Drugs used to treat psychotic disorders such as schizophrenia are called *neuroleptics, antipsychotics* or *major tranquillizers*.

Although the discovery that chlorpromazine and related phenothiazine neuroleptics were effective in the treatment of schizophrenia was

Fundamentals of Psychopharmacology. Third Edition. By Brian E. Leonard
2003 John Wiley & Sons, Ltd. ISBN 0 471 52178 7

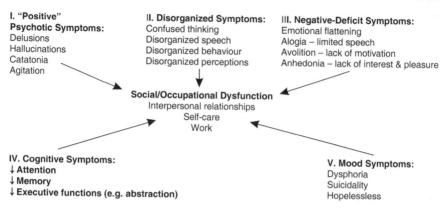

Figure 11.1. Schizophrenia's core symptom clusters.

serendipitous, investigators soon attempted to define the mechanism of action of this group of drugs that had begun to revolutionize psychiatric treatment. It was hoped that the elucidation of the mechanism of action of such neuroleptics would not only enable more selective and potent drugs to be discovered, but also give some insight into the pathology of schizophrenia.

A major advance came with the discovery that chlorpromazine, haloperidol and other related neuroleptics not only antagonized the stimulant action of L-dopa (levodopa) in animals but also enhanced the accumulation of the main metabolites of dopamine and noradrenaline in rat brain. These findings led to the suggestion that the neuroleptics must be blocking the postsynaptic receptors for dopamine, and to some extent noradrenaline, thereby leading to a stimulation of the presynaptic nerve terminal through a feedback mechanism. The seminal paper by Carlsson and Lindqvist in 1963 helped to lay the basis for the dopamine hypothesis for schizophrenia and the mode of action of neuroleptic drugs. Later studies in Canada and the United States of America showed that there is a good correlation between the average clinical dose of neuroleptic administered and the affinity of the drug for postsynaptic dopamine receptors. The dopamine hypothesis of schizophrenia has reasonably good support from pharmacological studies, but the supporting evidence from post-mortem material, and from studies on schizophrenic patients using techniques such as positron emission tomography (PET), are more controversial. Whatever the final outcome, however, the dopamine hypothesis has had a major impact on drug development and, even though dopamine may not be the only neurotransmitter involved in the illness, it is leading to an investigation of the interconnection between dopamine and other transmitters which may be more directly involved in the pathology of the illness.

Genetic factors

Schizophrenia is a psychotic disorder of complex inheritance. The risk of developing the disorder is 1% in the general population but rises to 50% for monozygotic twins of an affected proband and approximately 10% for a sibling of a parent.

Schizophrenia does not fit into a pattern of inheritance seen for a single dominant gene but does fit the pattern of oligogenic inheritance. One of the main problems that arises in trying to summarize the evidence in favour of a specific genetic loci has been the difficulty in replicating the evidence. Thus conflicting results for the link between loci on chromosomes 5, 8, 11 and 22 and schizophrenia are apparent. Perhaps the most robust finding, and even this has not been universally replicated, has been the identification of a gene on the short arm of chromosome 6 which involves several markers in the region 6p21–24.

Because of the hypothesized abnormality in the dopaminergic system and schizophrenia, genes for the five types of dopamine receptor genes were the first to be studied in detail. Neither the D_1 or D_5 receptor gene would appear to be linked or to have polymorphisms associated with the disorder. Despite the apparent link between the D_2 receptor and the action of antipsychotic drugs, no evidence of a genetic link has been found. Similarly, the observation that the D_4 receptor was located primarily in the mesocortical limbic region of the brain, and for which many atypical antipsychotics had an affinity, led to a study of the polymorphic forms of the gene. Despite the initial success that showed a link between the D_4 receptor and schizophrenia, the findings could not be replicated. No link with D_3 or 5-HT_2 receptor genes has been observed.

Neuropathological aspects

Variable patchy gliosis and neuronal loss have been reported to occur in the schizophrenic brain, but such changes would not appear to be specific to the disease. It has been suggested that these changes are a manifestation of an inflammatory reaction, possibly due to a virus infection; cytomegalovirus has been specifically implicated. However, there would now appear to be little support for the virus hypothesis of schizophrenia. More recently, detailed analysis of the neuronal architecture of the hippocampal and cortical regions of the schizophrenic brain suggests that a region of the parahippocampal gyrus is abnormal, possibly due to a disturbance of

Table 11.1   Histological findings in schizophrenia

	Weight of evidence
Lack of neurodegenerative lesions (e.g. Alzheimer changes)	+++++
Lack of gliosis	++++
Smaller cortical and hippocampal pyramidal neurons	+++
Decreased cortical and hippocampal synaptic markers	+++
Decreased dendritic spine density	++
Loss of neurons from dorsal thalamus	++
Abnormalities of white matter neurons	+
Entorhinal cortex dysplasia	+
Disarray of hippocampal neuron orientation	+/−
Loss of hippocampal or cortical neurons	0

0: no good evidence; +/−: equivocal data: + to +++++: increasing amounts of supportive data.

neuronal migration in a late phase of cortical development. Varying degrees of pyramidal cell disorientation in the hippocampus and reduced parahippocampal width suggest structural abnormalities in the basal cortical regions of the temporal lobe. A summary of the histological changes reported to occur in the brains of schizophrenic patients is given in Tabel 11.1.

Computed axial tomography (CAT) scan studies of the brains of schizophrenics have led to a renewed interest in the possibility that neuronal loss is causally connected with the disease. Most studies have implied that the ventricular size is increased, particularly in older patients, such structural changes being associated with neuropsychological impairment and negative symptoms of the disease, but not all investigators have found such correlations. Other CAT studies have shown that in right-handed patients there may be a lesion of the left hemisphere which correlates with the degree of psychological defect and with the occurrence of delusions. PET studies also suggest that the rate of glucose utilization by the left pre-frontal cortical lobe is slightly diminished in the schizophrenic patient. It is of interest that neurochemical studies of transmitters and their synthesizing enzymes also show asymmetry, with a higher concentration of dopamine and a higher activity of choline acetyltransferase in the left basal ganglia of the normal brain. The concentration of dopamine would appear to be greater in the left amygdala of the schizophrenic brain. A summary of the risk factors for schizophrenia is shown in Table 11.2.

Neurotransmitters and the pathogenesis of schizophrenia

In its original form, the dopamine hypothesis of schizophrenia postulated that the positive symptoms of the illness arose as a consequence of the

Table 11.2.   Risk factors for schizophrenia

1. Genetic factors – polygenic inheritance
2. Pre- and perinatal events, e.g. maternal viral infection during second trimester; toxaemia and/or hypoxia at birth
3. Environmental factors, e.g. the use of cannabis, brain trauma

hyperactivity of the dopaminergic system, particularly in the mesocortico-limbic region of the brain that originated in the ventral tegmental area. It is now realized that this is a gross over-simplification and recently attempts have been made to develop the dopamine hypothesis to take into account the neurochemical changes that may underlie both the positive and negative symptoms of the condition.

It is well known that typical neuroleptics, all of which have a high affinity for dopamine receptors (particularly D_2 receptors), do not effectively treat all schizophrenic patients and have only limited beneficial effects on the negative symptoms of the illness. Furthermore, neither typical nor atypical neuroleptics have an immediate effect on the positive symptoms even though it can be shown by both experimental studies in animals and by imaging methods in schizophrenic patients that neuroleptics rapidly bind to dopamine receptors. Thus factors other than an overactive dopaminergic system are probably operative in this disorder. The question is which of the numerous neurotransmitters and modulatory neuropeptides are responsible for both the negative symptoms and the delay in onset of the therapeutic effects of neuroleptics on the positive symptoms?

The deficit syndrome of schizophrenia, characterized by prominent negative symptoms, is presumed to be due to diminished prefrontal cortical activity. In experimental studies in patients, these symptoms often show response to dopaminergic agonists. As there are no dopamine autoreceptors on dopamine terminals in the cortex of the brain, it must be assumed that such agonists are acting on postsynaptic dopamine receptors to alleviate the negative symptoms. A diminished frontal cortical activity, as shown by PET studies for example, appears to be a characteristic feature of the untreated schizophrenic patient which would support the view that, at least in some patients, cortical dopaminergic activity is lower than normal and is not globally increased as was postulated by the original dopamine hypothesis.

Recently, attempts have been made to reconcile the deficiencies in the dopamine hypothesis by focusing on other neurotransmitters that may interact with dopamine in discrete cortical and subcortical neural circuits. In particular, the involvement of the glutamatergic system has received considerable attention. This possibility has arisen from the finding that dissociation anaesthetics such as ketamine and phencyclidine (PCP) can cause a schizophreniform psychosis in normal individuals. Such effects bear a much closer resemblance to the positive and negative symptoms of schizophreniform psychosis than the changes elicited by amphetamine which produced changes that more closely resemble the positive symptoms of the condition. In schizophrenic patients, PCP has also been shown to exacerbate a psychotic episode.

As will be discussed in detail later (see Chapter 15) PCP is a non-competitive inhibitor of the N-methyl-D-aspartate (NMDA) subtype of the glutamate receptor. This has led to the suggestion that schizophrenia may be associated with a decreased glutamatergic activity particularly in cortical regions of the brain.

Glutamate is the most important excitatory neurotransmitter in the brain, probably influencing more than 50% of all synapses. The major glutamatergic system involves a projection from the cortex to the striatum. Thus the hypofunctioning of the cortex may be a reflection of the diminished glutamatergic and dopaminergic activity in that area of the brain. It has been suggested that dopamine hetero receptors may regulate the release of glutamate in the striatum which could help to verify the hypothesis implicating both glutamate and dopamine in the aetiology of schizophrenia. This forms the basis of the hypothesis proposed by Arvid Carlsson that schizophrenia arises due to an abnormality in the dopamine–glutamate systems in the corticostriatal pallido-thalamic circuit (Figure 11.2).

In addition to an abnormality in the corticostriatal system, it is also possible that a disorder in the dopamine–glutamate system occurs in other subcortical regions which could account for some of the symptoms seen in schizophrenia. The hippocampus and the associated entorhinal cortex are important areas of the brain concerned in memory formation, information

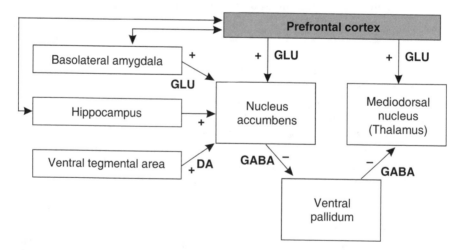

Figure 11.2. Schematic representation of ventral limbic circuits implicated in the positive symptoms of schizophrenia.

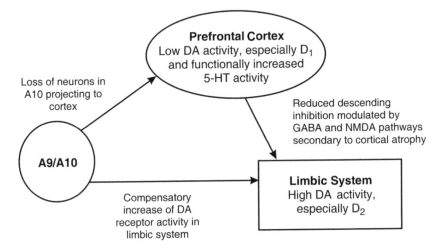

Figure 11.3.   Integrated model of schizophrenia.

processing and the generation of specimen-specific behaviours. Neuro-psychological tests in schizophrenic patients have occasionally been shown to be abnormal and the cytoarchitecture and other morphological changes in the hippocampus and entorhinal cortex suggest that the positive symptoms of the illness may originate within the hippocampus. These regions of the brain are innervated by the dopaminergic system while glutamate is the predominant intrinsic excitatory transmitter in the hippocampus. Thus a dysfunction of the hippocampal dopamine–glutamate system in these areas could also account for the positive symptoms of the illness. This forms the basis of the integrated model of schizophrenia (Figure 11.3). The role of a dysfunctional dopaminergic system in the development of the disorder is shown in Figure 11.4.

In Chapter 15, the complexity of the glutamatergic system is briefly outlined. Four distinct families of glutamate receptors were described of which the alpha-amino-3-hydroxy-5-methyl-4-isoxazole proprionic acid (AMPA) and the NMDA glutamate receptors have been most extensively studied. Recently the cloning of both NMDA and non-NMDA (for example, AMPA) receptor genes has enabled receptor expression at the transcriptional level to be made. Such techniques are much more sensitive than those used previously that relied on the binding of a radioactive ligand to a glutamatic receptor. Using this technique of *in situ* hybridization it has been shown that after 2 weeks of treatment of rats with either haloperidol or clozapine (representing a typical and an atypical neuroleptic respectively) substantial alteration occurs in non-NMDA receptors in the hippocampus. It has been postulated that one of the functions of neuroleptics is to "up-regulate" some

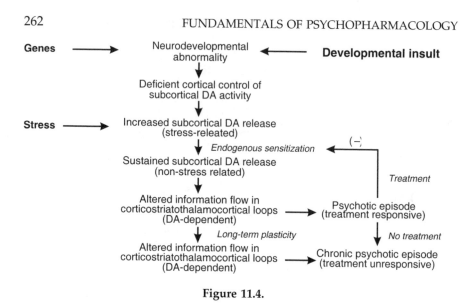

Figure 11.4.

types of non-NMDA glutamate receptors in the cortex and hippocampus, thereby leading to an amelioration of the symptoms of schizophrenia. It is of interest that there were some subtle differences in the changes in the glutamate receptor subtypes between haloperidol and clozapine which may account for the greater efficacy of clozapine in the treatment of the negative features of schizophrenia. It now remains to be shown that similar changes occur in the schizophrenic patient following therapeutically effective doses of typical and atypical neuroleptics. Nevertheless such studies do help to extend the dopamine hypothesis to explain the neurochemical basis of the positive and negative symptoms, the selectivity of the atypical neuroleptics in ameliorating the negative symptoms and, partly, the reason why it is necessary to administer neuroleptics for several weeks before optimal therapeutic benefit is obtained by the patient. A summary of the evidence implicating changes in dopamine, glutamate 5-HT and GABA in schizo-phrenia is shown in Table 11.3.

Effects of neuroleptics on dopaminergic and other neurotransmitter systems

Because of the discovery that all neuroleptics in clinical use are dopamine receptor antagonists, and that an abnormality in the dopaminergic system might underlie the pathology of the condition, the action of neuroleptics on the dopaminergic system has been extensively studied over the past two decades. Four major anatomical divisions of the dopaminergic system have been described:

Table 11.3. Key post-mortem findings concerning the major transmitter systems implicated in schizophrenia

Transmitter	Main post-mortem findings	Other supporting evidence
Dopamine	Increased density of D_2 receptors Increased cortical DA innervation Increased D_4-like receptor binding Alterations in D_3 receptor binding	DA-releasing agents produce psychosis All antipsychotics are D_2 receptor antagonists Increased striatal release *in vivo*
Glutamate	Decreased presynaptic markers Decreased HC AMPA and kainate receptor expression Minor changes in FC NMDA R sub-units Altered glutamate fibres in cingulate cortex	NMDA receptor antagonists produce schizophrenia-like psychosis Roles of NMDA receptors in development and neurotoxicity Partial NMDA receptor agonists have some therapeutic benefits
5-HT	Decreased FC $5-HT_{2A}$ receptor expression Increased FC $5-HT_{1A}$ receptors Increased 5-HT transporter affinity Developmental and trophic roles of 5-HT	$5-HT_2$ agonists (e.g. LSD) are psychotomimetics $5-HT_2$ receptor polymorphisms associated with schizophrenia and clozapine response Atypical antipsychotics have high affinity for several 5-HT receptors
GABA	Increased density of FC GABAergic terminals Increased $GABA_A$ receptor binding in limbic areas Altered expression of FC $GABA_A$ receptor sub-units Decreased FC expression of glutamic acid decarboxylase Altered density of cingulate GABAergic cells	Roles of GABA in stress and neurotoxicity

AMPA: amino-3-hydroxy-5-methyl-4-isoxazole propionic acid; DA: dopamine; FC: frontal cortex; GABA: γ-aminobutyric acid; HC: hippocampus; 5-HT: serotonin; LSD: lysergic acid diethylamide; NMDA: *N*-methyl-D-aspartate.

1. *The nigrostriatal system,* in which fibres originate from the A9 region of the pars compacta and project rostrally to become widely distributed in the caudate nucleus and the putamen.
2. *The mesolimbic system,* where the dopaminergic projections originate in the ventral tegmental area, the A10 region, and then spread to the amygdala, pyriform cortex, lateral septal nuclei and the nucleus accumbens.
3. *The mesocortical system,* in which the dopaminergic fibres also arise from the A10 region (the ventral tegmental area) and project to the frontal cortex and septohippocampal regions.
4. *The tuberoinfundibular system,* which originates in the arcuate nucleus of the hypothalamus and projects to the median eminence.

Following its release, dopamine produces its physiological effects by activating postsynaptic receptors which have been classified into the D_1 and D_2 families. The D_1 *receptors* are linked to adenylate cyclase which, when activated, produces cyclic AMP as a secondary messenger. The D_2 *receptors* are not positively linked to adenylate cyclase and may owe their physiological effects to their ability to inhibit this enzyme. The D_2 receptors are probably the most important postsynaptic receptors mediating behavioural and extrapyramidal activity. Most therapeutically effective neuroleptics block the D_2 receptors, while drugs like bromocriptine, which is a dopamine receptor agonist used in the treatment of parkinsonism, activate them. The correlation between the antagonist effect of a series of neuroleptics on brain D_2 receptors and their appropriate therapeutic potency is shown in Figure 11.5. It should be emphasized that recent studies on the effects of atypical neuroleptics on the D_2, D_3 and D_4 *receptors* show an even better correlation between dopamine receptor antagonism and the therapeutic dose.

Agonist stimulation of D_1 receptors results in cyclic adenosine monophosphate (cyclic AMP) synthesis followed by phosphorylation of intracellular proteins, including dopamine- and AMP-regulated phospho-protein (DARPP-32). The receptor binding affinity of a dopamine agonist is dependent on the degree of association of the receptor and the guanine nucleotide binding regulatory protein, which is regulated by guanosine triphosphate (GTP) and calcium or magnesium ions. Thus the D_1 receptor may exist in a high or low agonist affinity state depending on the balance between GTP (which favours low affinity) and the divalent cations (which favour high affinity). The high affinity D_1 receptor is classified as a D_5 receptor.

The D_3 and D_4 receptors appear to be largely restricted to the limbic areas of the rat and human brain. These receptors are of particular interest as they have a high affinity for such atypical neuroleptics as clozapine. Such

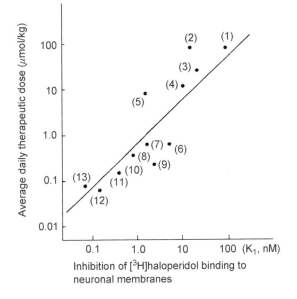

Figure 11.5. Correlation between the average daily dose of various neuroleptics and their affinity for D_2 receptors. (1)=promazine; (2)=chlorpromazine; (3)=thioridazine; (4)=clozapine; (5)=triflupromazine; (6)=penfluridol; (7)=trifluoperazine; (8)=fluphenazine; (9)=haloperidol; (10)=pimozide; (11)=fluspirilene; (12)=benperidol; (13)=spiroperidol (spiperone).

findings suggest that the D_3 and D_4 receptors in the human brain may mediate the antipsychotic actions of many typical and atypical neuroleptics. The restriction of these receptors to the limbic regions may lead to the development of neuroleptics which are specifically targeted to these areas but so far the results have been disappointing. This may assist in the development of drugs that combine antipsychotic potency with reduced extrapyramidal side effects.

In the mammalian brain, the D_1 receptors are located postsynaptically in the striatum, nucleus accumbens, olfactory tubercle, substantia nigra, etc., but their precise physiological function in the brain is currently unclear. The partial D_1 receptor agonist SKF 38393 stimulates grooming and stereotypic motor behaviour in rodents, effects that are blocked by the D_1 antagonist SCH 23390. This antagonist also blocks the behaviour initiated by the selective D_2 receptor agonist quinpirole (LY 171555), which suggests that there is a functional interaction between the D_1 and the D_2 receptors.

Unlike the D_1 receptor, the function of the D_2 receptor in the brain is at least partially understood. The anterior lobe mammotrophs of the pituitary control lactation via prolactin release, and dopamine acting on the D_2 receptor in this area acts as the *prolactin release inhibitory factor*. In the intermediate lobe of the rat, dopamine inhibits alpha melanocyte-stimulating hormone release. In the striatum, D_2 receptors inhibit acetylcholine release, while on the dopaminergic nerve terminals the D_2 receptors function as autoreceptors and inhibit the release of dopamine. D_2 receptors occur on the dopaminergic neurons in the substantia nigra where they inhibit the firing of the neurons. In man, these receptors stimulate growth hormone release. Lastly, in the *chemoreceptor trigger zone*, stimulation of the D_2 receptors elicits emesis. The selective agonist for D_2 receptors is quinpirole (LY171555), while the selective antagonist is spiroperidol (spiperone).

Increased motor activity and stereotypic behaviour arises as a result of the activation of central D_2 receptors in rodents, while in man psychosis, stereotypic behaviour and thought disorders occur. Conversely, neuroleptic drugs with selective D_2 antagonist properties (e.g. the benzamides such as sulpiride) are antipsychotic and can lead to Parkinsonism in man or catalepsy in rodents, although the propensity of the benzamide neuroleptics to cause these effects is much less than the phenothiazine neuroleptics that have mixed D_1 and D_2 receptor antagonist properties. The butyrophenone neuroleptics such as haloperidol are approximately 100 times more potent in acting as D_2 receptor antagonists than as D_1 antagonists.

The results of such studies suggest that the major classes of neuroleptics in therapeutic use owe their activity to their ability to block D_2 and/or D_1 receptors, particularly in the mesocortical and mesolimbic regions of the brain. Side effects, such as parkinsonism and increased prolactin release, would seem to be associated with the antagonistic effects of these drugs on D_2 and/or D_1 receptors in the nigrostriatal and tuberoinfundibular systems.

While the precise importance of D_1 and D_2 receptors in the clinical effects of neuroleptics is still uncertain, there is experimental evidence from studies in primates that oral dyskinesia (which may be equivalent to tardive dyskinesia in man) is related to an imbalance in D_1 and D_2 receptor function, the dyskinesia arising from a relative overactivity of the D_1 receptors. Thus the elucidation of the precise function of these receptor subtypes may be important not only in determining the mode of action of neuroleptics but also in understanding their side effects.

The relationship between pre- and postsynaptic receptors and a summary of the suspected sites of action of the different classes of drugs that modulate the functioning of the dopaminergic system in the striatum are shown in Figure 11.6.

While there is extensive experimental evidence showing that all clinically effective neuroleptic drugs block dopamine receptors, and a general agreement that blockade of the D_2 receptors in the mesocortical regions is particularly important for antipsychotic activity, only with the advent of

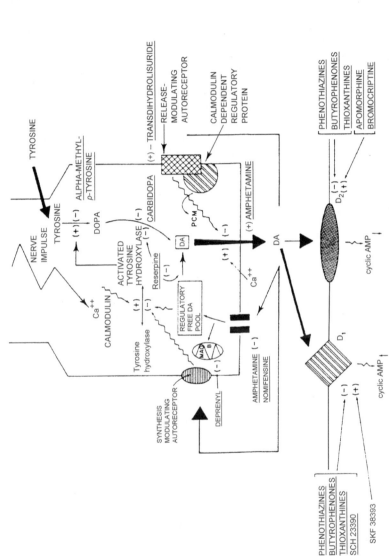

Figure 11.6. Schematic diagram of the possible sites of action of drugs that modify dopaminergic function in striatal and other non-mesocortical regions of the mammalian brain. PCM=protein;O-methyltransferase, which catalyses the transfer of methyl groups from S-adenosylmethionine to the calmodulin-dependent regulatory protein and may regulate calcium–calmodulin dependent transmitter synthesis and release. (−)=inhibition; (+)=stimulation; DA=dopamine. Sites of action of drugs are underlined.

PET has it been possible to determine the relative importance of these receptor subtypes in schizophrenic patients on neuroleptic therapy. Using PET the occupancy of D_2 receptors in the cortical regions of the brains of schizophrenics treated with phenothiazines (chlorpromazine, trifluoperazine or perphenazine), a thioxanthine (flupenthixol), butyrophenones (haloperidol or melperone), a diphenylbutylpiperazine (pimozide) or the atypical neuroleptics sulpiride, raclopride or clozapine has been calculated. The results of this study with this structurally disparate group of drugs showed that 65–89% of the D_2 receptors were occupied. Other investigators have also shown that over 70% of D_2 receptors are occupied in the brains of schizophrenics following effective treatment with melperone. In contrast, no D_1 receptors were occupied by sulpiride or perphenazine, while 42% of these receptors were occupied by clozapine. From such a study it may be speculated that a D_2 receptor antagonist action may be essential for the therapeutic effect of neuroleptics.

A summary of the new families of dopamine receptors and their distribution and properties is shown in Table 11.4.

Mechanism of action of neuroleptics

Laborit in the early 1950s is credited with the observation that chlorpromazine had a "calming" effect in disturbed schizophrenic patients and since that time psychopharmacologists have sought to explain the mechanism of action of neuroleptic drugs. Carlsson and Linquist in 1963 demonstrated a link between the therapeutic effects of the phenothiazine neuroleptics and an inhibition of dopamine receptor function. This led to

Table 11.4. New families of dopamine receptor subtypes

Family	Relevance for antipsychotic drug action
"D_1-like"	
D_{1A}	The classical "D_1" receptor; selective antagonists neglected as putative antipsychotics
D_{1B}/D_5	Novel site with low density, corticolimbic localization; no specific function(s) or selective antagonist yet known
"D_2-like"	
$D_{2long/short}$	The classical "D_2" isomorphs; reliable correlation between D_2 affinity and neuroleptic potency
D_3	Novel site with low density, corticolimbic localization; no specific function(s) or selective antagonist yet known
D_4	Novel site with low density, corticolimbic localization; no specific function(s) or selective antagonist yet known, but blocked "preferentially" by clozapine

the dopamine hypothesis of schizophrenia which postulated that psychosis was associated with an increase in dopaminergic function in the brain and that neuroleptics alleviate the symptoms of the illness by blocking the receptors that are specifically activated by dopamine. Later, during the 1970s, it was shown that the antipsychotic action of neuroleptics was correlated with their affinity to block dopamine receptors *in vitro*. It was discovered, by Kebabian and Calne in 1979, that dopamine receptors could be classified into two specific types, D_1 and D_2, and that there was a good correlation between the therapeutic potency of the phenothiazine neuroleptics and haloperidol and their affinity for the D_2 receptors. With the introduction of molecular cloning techniques it has now been possible to define at least five distinct subtypes of the dopamine receptor in the human brain as well as two variants (termed isoforms) of the original D_2 receptor. These different subtypes of the dopamine receptor may be broadly classified into those resembling the original D_1 receptor (D_1 and D_5) and those resembling the D_2 receptor (D_2, D_3 and D_4).

The neuroleptics that are widely available may be divided into two general categories, those with low potency (such as chlorpromazine and thioridazine) and those with high potency (exemplified by haloperidol, trifluoperazine and pimozide). The former groups have a lower propensity to cause extrapyramidal side effects but are more sedative and likely to cause postural hypotension and have anticholinergic side effects. *In vitro* studies have shown that chlorpromazine has an affinity for all five types of dopamine receptor and has some preference for D_2 and D_3 receptors. By contrast, haloperidol is more potent than chlorpromazine for the D_2, D_3 and D_4 receptors with a low affinity for the D_1 and D_5 receptors.

In addition to their affinity for dopamine receptors, which appears to be essential for their therapeutic activity, all neuroleptics in current clinical use have affinities for other types of neurotransmitter receptor. Mention has already been made of the side effects of the weaker neuroleptics such as chlorpromazine for histamine-1, muscarinic and alpha-1 adrenoceptors. However, it is now apparent that many of the newer, atypical, neuroleptics have an affinity for subtypes of 5-HT (particularly 5-HT_{2A}) receptors which may be beneficial in reducing the frequency of extrapyramidal side effects. Thus neuroleptics may now be broadly classified into those which are selective antagonists of D_2 receptors, those that are D_2 and D_3 receptor antagonists, those blocking both D_1 and D_2 receptors and, a most important group of novel neuroleptics, those that are antagonists of 5-HT_2 and D_2 receptors.

Despite the efficacy of the typical neuroleptics such as chlorpromazine and haloperidol in treating the acute symptoms of schizophrenia, their side effects and failure to treat the negative symptoms emphasized the need to develop atypical antipsychotics. The desirable features of a new antipsychotic are shown in Table 11.5.

Table 11.5. Desirable features of a new antipsychotic

- Improve positive symptoms in partial and non-responders
- Benefit negative symptoms
- Reduce relapse rates
- Few/no extrapyramidal side effects
- Few adverse effects
- Patient acceptability

Atypical neuroleptics

An important breakthrough in the development of novel neuroleptics arose over 25 years ago with the discovery of the dibenzazepine neuroleptic clozapine. This neuroleptic was novel because it attenuated both the positive and negative symptoms of schizophrenia without causing extrapyramidal side effects or elevating serum prolactin concentrations, effects which characterize most typical neuroleptics such as chlorpromazine and haloperidol.

Despite its novel therapeutic profile, it was soon evident that clozapine occasionally caused agranulocytosis, a potentially fatal immune condition, in approximately 3% of patients. The use of clozapine was therefore restricted largely to patients who suffered severe side effects with the typical neuroleptics, who were resistant to conventional neuroleptics or who had a high proportion of negative symptoms. Thus, clozapine has served as a useful prototype for the development of new neuroleptics and these will be briefly described.

Clozapine binds with a high affinity (in the nanomolar range) to D_4 and D_2 receptors and with lower affinity for the D_1, D_3 and D_5 receptors. The finding that clozapine had a high affinity for the D_4 receptors was particularly exciting when it was discovered that an elevated expression of D_4 receptors occurred in the brains of schizophrenic patients. However, more recent studies have shown that clozapine also binds with a high affinity to the short form of the D_2 receptor. Further evidence for the relative lack of specificity of clozapine, not only for different types of dopamine receptors but also for 5-HT, muscarinic, adrenergic and histaminergic receptors, suggests that it is a neuroleptic with a very broad basis of action. However, the beneficial effects of clozapine (and other atypical neuroleptics such as risperidone, seroquel and sertindole) may be due to its selective effects on mesolimbic and mesocortical dopaminergic neurons. Clinical and experimental studies suggest that such atypical neuroleptics decrease the negative symptoms of schizophrenia by enhancing prefrontal dopaminergic activity while decreasing the activity of this transmitter in the mesolimbic

Table 11.6. Antipsychotic drugs: *in vitro* receptor binding (affinity values K_i in nmol)

	Hal	Cloz	Risp	Olanz	Quet	Zip
D_1	210	85	430	31	460	525
D_2	1	160	2	44	580	4
D_3	2	170	10	50	940	7
D_4	3	50	10	50	1900	32
5-HT_{1A}	1100	200	210	>10 000	720	3
5-HT_{1D}	>10 000	1900	170	800	6200	2
5-HT_{2A}	45	16	0.5	5	300	0.4
5-HT_{2C}	>10 000	10	25	11	5100	1
5-HT_6	9600	14	2200	10	33	130
5-HT_7	1200	100	2	150	130	23
5-HT reuptake	1700	5000	1300	–	–	50
NA reuptake	4700	500	>1000	–	–	50
$NA_{\alpha 1}$	6	7	1	19	7	10
$NA_{\alpha 2}$	360	8	1	230	90	200
H_1	440	1	20	3	1	50
Muscarinic	5500	2	>1000	2	>1000	>1000

The lower the number, the stronger the affinity for the specific neuroreceptor.
K_i, inhibitory constant; NA, noradrenaline.

system, thereby attenuating the psychotic symptoms of schizophrenia. Experimental studies also show that clozapine, and other novel atypical neuroleptics, have little effect on the activity of the nigrostriatal dopaminergic system which probably accounts for the low incidence of extrapyramidal side effects seen with these drugs. Clozapine and several other atypical neuroleptics are also potent inhibitors of 5-HT_2 type receptors, particularly the 5-HT_{2A} and 5-HT_{2C} subtypes (see Table 11.6) and it has been postulated that their antipsychotic action combined with a low propensity to cause extrapyramidal side effects may be attributable to the antagonism of 5-HT_{2A} receptors combined with an inhibition of mesocortical D_2 receptors. The experimental evidence to support this view arises from findings that stimulation of 5-HT_{2A} receptors enhances the synthesis and release of dopamine in the rat brain. Conversely 5-HT_{2A} receptor antagonists reduce the stimulant effects of amphetamine, a drug that in high doses can produce symptoms not unlike paranoid schizophrenia, possibly due to its ability to release dopamine in the mesocortical and mesolimbic regions of the brain.

Partly as a result of the extensive experimental and clinical studies which have been carried out on clozapine in recent years there have been two major approaches to the development of atypical neuroleptics. The first approach has been to develop drugs which broadly simulate the pharmacological profile of clozapine but which lack the adverse haematological effects. Olanzapine is an example of a drug recently marketed in Europe and North America which is based on this principle. The second approach has involved targeting specific dopamine receptors located in the forebrain. Clearly the aim of such developments is to produce neuroleptics that attenuate both the positive and negative symptoms of schizophrenia without causing extrapyramidal side effects. This has largely been achieved with the introduction of several atypical antipsychotics.

Pharmacological profiles of some atypical antipsychotics

The atypical antipsychotics are divided into two major pharamacological groups, namely the multiple receptor antagonists, such as clozapine, olanzapine and quetiapine, and the more selective 5-HT_2/D_2 antagonists as exemplified by risperidone, sertindole, ziprasidone and zotepine. The benzamide antipsychotic amisulpride is the most selective antagonist for the D_2/D_3 receptors which presumably gives it the mesocortical selectivity of action with a minimal effect on the dopamine receptors in the basal ganglia.

Olanzapine, like clozapine, has a broad spectrum of action on dopamine, 5-HT, adrenergic, histamine$_1$ and muscarinic receptors (see Table 11.6). While the precise significance is presently unclear, it is of interest that whereas clozapine binds with a high affinity to 5-HT_6 and 5-HT_7 receptors, olanzapine only shows a high affinity for 5-HT_6 receptors.

Clinical studies have demonstrated that olanzapine has a similar profile to clozapine without causing agranulocytosis; preliminary studies also show that it does not cause extrapyramidal side effects or increase prolactin release. Olanzapine has recently been introduced for the treatment of mania.

Risperidone has been developed as a combined D_2/5-HT_{2A} receptor antagonist. In addition, it has a high affinity for 5-HT_{1A} and 5-HT_7 receptors. Whether such an effect has any relevance to its beneficial effects on the negative symptoms of schizophrenia, and lack of extrapyramidal side effects at moderate therapeutic doses, is unknown. An important advantage of risperidone over clozapine lies in its lack of antagonism of muscarinic receptors.

Remoxipride is a selective D_2 antagonist with higher affinity for the D_{2S} subtype of receptors. It has no affinity for 5-HT, adrenergic, muscarinic or histamine receptors but, unlike the other atypical neuroleptics, does bind to sigma receptors (see p. 453 for possible importance of sigma receptors).

In clinical studies, remoxipride has been shown to improve both positive and negative symptoms of schizophrenia and may have a place in the treatment of resistant schizophrenic patients. In addition such side effects as the neuroleptic-induced deficit syndrome, sedation and extrapyramidal side effects are apparently absent in patients treated with the drug.

Unfortunately, a few cases of aplastic anaemia have been reported which may be drug related. This has led to the untimely withdrawal of the drug from the European market.

Amisulpride. The ability of amisulpride to reduce the negative symptoms of schizophrenia has been explained in terms of its selective antagonism of the dopamine (D_2) autoreceptors in the prefrontal cortex that results in an increased release of dopamine in that region. This effect is most pronounced in low therapeutic doses. Higher doses reduce the subcortical dopaminergic system thereby reducing the positive symptoms of the disorder, an effect that is similar to that seen with the typical neuroleptics. In clinical studies, the frequency of extrapyramidal side effects is significantly lower than with any of the traditional neuroleptics which may be explained by the fact that less than 70% of the D_2 receptors in the basal ganglia are occupied even at the higher therapeutic doses.

Quetiapine. This has a somewhat similar pharmacological profile to clozapine and olanzapine due to its multiple receptor antagonists action. It has been shown to reduce both the positive and negative symptoms of schizophrenia and has a low frequency of extrapyramidal side effects.

Sertindole. This is structurally unique among the atypical neuroleptics in that it is an indole derivative with a high affinity for $5\text{-}HT_{2A}$, D_2-like (D_2, D_3, D_4) and also alpha-1 receptors. The antagonistic action on the $5\text{-}HT_2$ receptors probably accounts for its beneficial effects on negative symptoms. Sertindole was suspended from marketing a few years ago because of the rare occurrence of cardiac conduction defects. As the causal relationship of this adverse effect to the drug was never firmly established it is likely to be relaunched in the near future.

Ziprasidone is a high potency antagonist of $5\text{-}HT_2$ receptors and to a lesser extent to D_2-like receptors. It also acts as an agonist at $5\text{-}HT_{1A}$ receptors and blocks the reuptake of noradrenaline which gives it a potential anti-depressant as well as an antipsychotic profile. It has a slight antagonistic action on both histamine1 and alpha-1 receptors which might be associated with a sedative profile and also a possible hypotensive effect. Like the other atypical antipsychotics, ziprasidone has little action on the basal ganglia.

Zotepine, like ziprasidone, is a potent $5\text{-}HT_2$ antagonist which also reduces the reuptake of noradrenaline. Its side effects, sedation and postural hypotension, are attributable to its antagonistic action on histamine1 and alpha-1 receptors. Zotepine, which has not yet been marketed in Europe, may have a similar profile to ziprasidone and could be useful in the treatment of depression associated with schizophrenia. Because of the evident clinical superiority of the atypical antipsychotics over the traditional neuroleptics, the World Psychiatric Association Task Force has

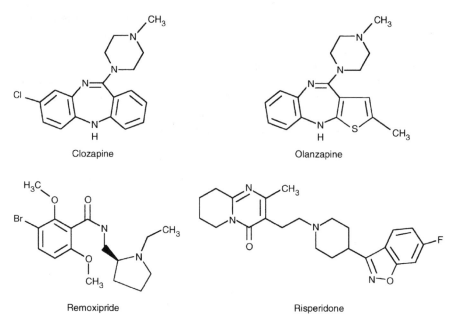

Figure 11.7. Chemical structure of selected atypical antipsychotics.

recently recommended that these drugs should be the first-line treatment for schizophrenia.

The chemical structures of some of these atypical antipsychotics are shown in Figure 11.7. A comparison of the sites of action and clinical effects of typical neuroleptics and atypical antipsychotics is shown in Table 11.7.

Atypical neuroleptics and their effects on serotonin and dopamine receptors: relevance to clinical action

Imaging techniques such as CAT have shown that enlargement of the lateral ventricles is a frequent feature of schizophrenia. Such structural changes do not appear to be associated with the nature or duration of neuroleptic therapy and are found in affective disorders. The changes found in the schizophrenic brain may be triggered by environmental factors such as birth complications. In addition, selective reduction in the size of the temporal lobe commonly occurs in schizophrenics and such changes appear to be lateralized in the left hemisphere. Regional blood flow studies, and the measurement of regional glucose metabolism, has provided evidence of reduced frontal lobe function (hypofunctionality).

Table 11.7.   Activity profile of typical and atypical antipsychotic drugs

Brain region	Influence of DA system	Antipsychotic activity		
		Ideal	Typical	Atypical
A10 Prefrontal cortex	Negative symptoms	↓	–	↓
A10 Limbic system	Positive symptoms	↓	↓	↓
A9 Striatum	Extrapyramidal effects	–	↑	–

Atypical neuroleptics such as clozapine and risperidone have been developed because it was found that up to 20% of schizophrenic patients did not respond to "classical" neuroleptics of the phenothiazine or butyrophenone type, while those patients who do initially respond to such medication frequently relapse during the first 2 years of treatment. Another reason for developing novel neuroleptics has been motivated by the finding that the "classical" neuroleptics have little beneficial effect either on the chronic course of the illness or on the negative symptoms. The negative symptoms of schizophrenia are frequently problematic to the patient and tend to be persistent, disabling and difficult to treat. In addition, the side effects of the "classical" neuroleptics which are associated with the sedative, anticholinergic and extrapyramidal effects of these drugs often result in poor compliance.

The potential advantage of the atypical antipsychotics arises from their ability to act on both positive and negative symptoms, to have a reduced tendency to cause extrapyramidal side effects, to be less sedative and to have little antimuscarinic activity. In terms of their actions on central neurotransmitters, the atypical neuroleptics can be divided into broad classes, namely those drugs such as remoxipride and amisulpride which are highly selective as D_2 receptor antagonists and those that have a relatively weak D_2 antagonistic action but which are potent inhibitors of 5-HT_{2A} receptors. This latter group includes clozapine, risperidone, zotepine, sertindole, olanzapine and amperozide.

It has been postulated that the 5-HT_2 antagonistic action of the atypical neuroleptics plays an important role in their efficacy in reducing the negative symptoms. There is evidence from PET studies in man that atypical neuroleptics such as clozapine occupy 80–90% of 5-HT_2 receptors whereas the "classical" neuroleptics, such as haloperidol, occupy hardly any 5-HT_2 receptors even at high therapeutic doses. The precise mechanism whereby such a high affinity of the atypical neuroleptics leads to a reduction in the negative symptoms of schizophrenia is uncertain. It is hypothesized that hypofrontality is associated with the negative symptoms and that the blockade of 5-HT_2 receptors in the corticolimbic region of the brain reduces such symptoms. Experimental studies in rats have shown that serotonin modifies the pattern of dopamine release. When treated with the psychotomimetic drug phencyclidine, which can induce both positive and negative symptoms of schizophrenia in man under experimental conditions, the activity of the dopaminergic terminals in the frontal cortex is reduced. This hypofunctioning dopaminergic system can be normalized by treatment with 5-HT_2 antagonists. It therefore appears that 5-HT_2 antagonists cause an indirect activation of midbrain dopaminergic cell activity, together with an increase in dopamine release in the frontal cortex.

The consequence of the combination of D_2 and 5-HT_2 receptor antagonism is therefore the selective enhancement of dopaminergic activity in the prefrontal cortex and, as a consequence, a correction of the regional imbalance between the cortical and midbrain dopaminergic systems.

Regarding the extrapyramidal side effects commonly found after treatment with the "classical" neuroleptics, PET studies of schizophrenia patients have shown that such drugs occupy 70–80% of D_2 receptors in the basal ganglia at therapeutic doses. It has been calculated that a D_2 receptor occupancy in the basal ganglia of approximately 80% carries a high risk that the patient will develop extrapyramidal side effects. Furthermore, Canadian studies have shown that the occurrence of extrapyramidal side effects was a major predictor for the subsequent development of tardive dyskinesia.

Thus the atypical neuroleptics with their lower affinity for D_2 receptors in the basal ganglia, and their high affinity for 5-HT_2 receptors in the frontal cortex, appear to combine therapeutic efficacy with a reduced tendency to cause neurological side effects.

Tardive dyskinesia

This syndrome was first described by Schonecker within 5 years of the introduction of the neuroleptics. It comprises involuntary movements of the tongue, lips and face (such as protrusion or twisting of the tongue, lip smacking, puffing of the cheeks, sucking of the lips and chewing) often combined with abnormal involuntary movements of the trunk and limbs, termed choreiform or choreoathetoid movements. Despite the association of tardive dyskinesia with the introduction of neuroleptics, it is evident that 5–15% of elderly people who have never received neuroleptics also show an orofacial dyskinesia, the prevalence rate of the condition in schizophrenic patients on neuroleptics being variously reported to be between 0.5 and 56% (mean of 20%).

Factors predisposing a patient to tardive dyskinesia include age, sex (female patients show a greater prevalence), presence of brain damage, early susceptibility to drug-induced extrapyramidal side effects and the presence of a primary affective disorder. In patients with such predisposing factors, the presence of neuroleptics may precipitate the onset of the syndrome. In addition, the schizophrenic illness itself may be a risk factor as there is evidence from clinical reports published long before the advent of neuroleptics that abnormal movements similar to tardive dyskinesia occurred. Recent evidence further suggests that schizophrenic patients with pronounced negative symptoms (e.g. blunting of affect and social withdrawal) are more likely to develop the syndrome than those with primarily positive symptoms (hallucinations, delusions, etc.). Clearly the somewhat simplistic view advanced some years ago that tardive dyskinesia was due to dopamine receptor supersensitivity resulting from prolonged dopamine receptor blockade by a neuroleptic is now redundant. Table 11.8 summarizes the risk factors for tardive dyskinesia.

Despite the diversity of drugs which have been tried for the *treatment of tardive dyskinesia*, no satisfactory drug therapy exists to date. In some cases the short-acting reserpine analogue tetrabenazine has been used with limited success. More recently, some success has been claimed for the calcium channel blockers verapamil and diltiazem, and for the antioxidant alpha-tocopherol (vitamin E), but double-blind controlled studies are still needed to validate the efficacy of such treatments. Clearly, since neuroleptics may precipitate this syndrome, it is essential that such drugs be prescribed only when clearly indicated, at a minimum effective dose and for only as long as their beneficial effects are clearly needed. Concurrent anticholinergic drug administration leads to a worsening of the symptoms of tardive dyskinesia, and the possibility of the syndrome arising is much greater in patients over the age of 50.

Akathisia, considered to be one of the leading causes of non-compliance with typical neuroleptics, is not thought to be linked to dopamine receptor

Table 11.8.   Tardive dyskinesia: risk factors

- Age
- Gender
- Duration of treatment
- Organicity
- Diagnosis
- Extrapyramidal side effects
- Antiparkinsonian medications
- Drug-free intervals
- Alcohol
- Smoking
- Familial
- Diabetes
- Neuroleptic: dose, potency

function. Treatment with propranolol or a benzodiazepine, which may be effective, would suggest a disorder of the sympathetic or GABAergic systems. There is no evidence that a sedative antipsychotic is beneficial in the symptomatic relief of akathisia.

Recently it has been found that haloperidol and several putative atypical neuroleptics such as rimcazole, BMY 14802 and HR 375 have a high affinity for sigma receptors in the mammalian brain. It is now established that the sigma receptors (see p. 453) are different from the phencyclidine receptors which are located in the ion channel of the NMDA receptor complex. Drugs like N-allylnormetazocine (NANM) and (+) pentazocine for example, bind specifically to sigma sites but not to the phencyclidine sites thereby enabling the two receptor sites to be distinguished. However, it must be emphasized that not all neuroleptics have an affinity for the sigma receptors and furthermore drugs such as rimcazole and BMY 14802 have questionable antipsychotic activity. Nevertheless it is possible that some atypical neuroleptics may owe some of their therapeutic activity to their action on sigma receptors. The possible significance of sigma receptors to the action of different classes of psychotropic drugs is discussed in Chapter 19.

It may be concluded that despite the importance of the dopamine hypothesis of schizophrenia in serving to unify the mechanism of action of both typical and atypical neuroleptics, it is apparent that some serotonin receptor subtypes, and glutamate receptors of the NMDA subtype, may also play a crucial role.

Novel antipsychotics in development

Serotonin receptor antagonists as antipsychotics

The improvement of the secondary negative symptoms, and the symptoms of depression often associated with schizophrenia, has been an important feature of the atypical antipsychotics. Such pharmacological features may reside in the actions of the atypical antipsychotics on 5-HT_2 receptors in addition to their actions on dopamine receptors. For example, all these drugs have a high affinity for 5-HT_{2A} and $_{2C}$ receptors, and to a lesser extent 5-HT_6 and 5-HT_7 receptors. For these reasons, several compounds have been developed with a high affinity for 5-HT_2 receptors. Of these, pipamerone, a highly selective $5\text{-HT}_2/D_2$ antagonist, has been shown to have an anti-autistic, disinhibiting and resocializing effect and a low frequency of extrapyramidal side effects. By contrast, MDL 100 907, a compound largely lacking D_2 antagonism but a potent 5-HT_{2A} antagonist, while showing promising antipsychotic properties in pre-clinical studies, was not found to be as effective as haloperidol in the treatment of schizophrenia. Similarly, the $D_4/5\text{-HT}_{2A}$ antagonist fananserin lacked clinical efficacy despite a promising experimental profile. It is not without interest that several selective D_4 antagonists have failed to show clinical efficacy in the treatment of schizophrenia despite the evidence that some typical (e.g. haloperidol) and atypical (e.g. clozapine) agents increase the density of these receptors following chronic treatment. Thus it would appear that the $5-HT_{2A}$ antagonism, together with D_2 antagonism, may contribute to the atypical profile of the new antipsychotics but the $5-HT_{2A}$ antagonism alone would not appear to confer antipsychotic effects.

Adrenergic receptors and antipsychotic action

While most schizophrenia research has focused on the importance of dopamine, there is evidence that hyperactivity of the noradrenergic system also occurs in these patients. There is clinical evidence that the alpha-2 adrenoceptor antagonists can improve memory in schizophrenic patients and that atypical antipsychotics are more effective than typical neuroleptics in normalizing the cognitive deficits in these patients presumably due to their actions on alpha-2 receptors. There is also evidence that both alpha-1 adrenoceptors and $5-HT_{2A}$ receptor stimulation of the prefrontal cortex can cause cortical dysfunction. As many of the atypical antipsychotics are antagonists of both alpha-1 and $5-HT_{2A}$ receptors, such actions could help to explain the improved cognitive function seen with these drugs. So far such clinical and experimental findings have not been extended to the development of novel antipsychotics with a view to enhancing their improved cognitive action.

Glutamatergic receptors and antipsychotic action

Recent experimental and clinical evidence suggests that the glutamatergic system plays a vital role in the pathophysiology of schizophrenia and may also contribute to the efficacy of atypical antipsychotics. In post-mortem schizophrenic brains, messenger RNA expression of the main glutamate receptor subtypes has shown that the kainate and AMPA metabotropic receptors, and subtypes of the NMDA ionotropic receptor, are decreased. Most studies have concentrated on the NMDA receptors where it has been shown that atypical antipsychotics such as clozapine decrease some subtypes of this receptor: the densities of the kainate and AMPA receptors have been shown to increase. Such findings underpin the application of drugs which activate the NMDA receptors as possible novel antipsychotics. Thus glycine and D-serine, as NMDA receptor agonists, have been studied for their potential antipsychotic effects. High doses of glycine (30–60 g/day) have been shown to improve the negative symptoms in schizophrenia. D-serine, a full agonist at the NMDA receptor glycine site, was also reported to improve the negative symptoms, psychosis and cognitive function of schizophrenic patients while D-cycloserine, a partial agonist of the glycine site, was also shown to improve the negative symptoms when added to conventional neuroleptics without improving the cognitive function. These preliminary clinical findings would support the possible value of drugs that enhance glycine receptor function at least in the treatment of the negative symptoms of schizophrenia.

Several compounds that act as positive modulators of the AMPA receptors have also been studied. Of these, CX516 was shown to improve the attention, memory and distractability of patients together with a significant improvement of cognitive function. Thus it would appear that agonists of the glycine site on the NMDA receptor, and modulators of the AMPA receptors, may prove to be novel antipsychotics in the future.

Sigma receptors and antipsychotic action

Since the discovery that the psychotomimetic benzomorphans act on sigma receptors in the brain, while some antipsychotics such as haloperidol and remoxipride act as sigma receptor antagonists, attention has been directed towards the development of sigma receptor antagonists as potential antipsychotic agents (see p. 453). Several sigma antagonists have been clinically tested over the past 17 years. However, most trials to date involve few patients, few studies have been replicated and many of the first sigma agents to be tested were also antagonists of $5-HT_2$ receptors (e.g. rimcazole, tiosperone). Of the more specific sigma antagonists, panamesine (EMD 57445) has been the subject of three trials involving a small number of patients. Panamesine was found to exert acute antipsychotic effects at least in some patients. Eliprodil (SL 820715) is also a sigma ligand but in addition has NMDA antagonistic properties which could limit its efficacy. In an open trial, eliprodil was shown to improve the negative symptoms in a small number of patients. A potent selective sigma antagonist, SR-31742, is also currently undergoing clinical trials in schizophrenia, the results of which may provide conclusive evidence regarding the antipsychotic potential of such drugs. Thus it would appear that there is some evidence that sigma antagonists may have antipsychotic potential but more detailed clinical studies are required to substantiate this.

GABAergic receptors and antipsychotic action

Experimental studies have demonstrated that the GABA-A receptors have an inhibitory action on the dopaminergic system while the GABA-B receptors have an indirect stimulatory action on these receptors. Thus it would be anticipated that GABA-A receptor agonists might be of some value in the treatment of schizophrenia. Of the drugs available, the benzodiazepines have been reasonably well studied and shown to be beneficial in the treatment of both positive and negative symptoms. However, such drugs are limited by their abuse potential and because tolerance develops to their therapeutic effects. Valproate acts as a GABAmimetic by inhibiting the metabolizing enzyme GABA trans-aminase thereby enhancing central GABAergic tone. The evidence for the efficacy of valproate has been reviewed and suggests that valproate is of limited value as the sole therapy for the treatment of schizophrenia but could be an effective drug for adjunctive treatment. Thus anticonvulsants with GABAergic properties may be promising candidates for the future.

Polyunsaturated fatty acids and antipsychotic action

There is evidence that schizophrenic patients have a deficiency in omega 3 fatty acids in their neuronal membranes while clozapine has been shown to increase the concentration of such fatty acids in red blood cell membranes, thereby suggesting that atypical antipsychotics may con-tribute to the normalization of neuronal membrane function by increasing their polyunsaturated fatty acid content. This forms the basis of the membrane hypothesis of schizophrenia. Two open studies in which fish oils rich in omega 3 fatty acids were given over a period of 6 weeks showed an improvement in both positive and negative symptoms and a marked reduction in the Abnormal Voluntary Movement scores; there was a strong correlation between the clinical improvement and the increase in the omega 3 fatty acids in the red blood cell membranes. These studies have been extended to show a marked and sustained response to treatment over a 1-year period. Thus omega 3 fatty acids may provide an important and novel approach to the development of antipsychotics in the future.

Action of neuroleptics on different types of neurotransmitter receptor: relevance to side effects

In recent years traditional neuroleptics, as exemplified by chlorpromazine, have been structurally modified to produce drugs with greater affinity for dopamine receptors while retaining some of their activity on other receptor systems (e.g. on $alpha_1$ adrenoceptors, $5-HT_2$ receptors and histamine$_1$ receptors). In the non-phenothiazine series, a high degree of specificity for the D_2 receptors has been achieved with sulpiride and pimozide, with haloperidol showing antagonistic effects on the $5-HT_2$ and alpha$_1$ adrenoceptors in addition to its selectivity for D_2 receptors. The *cis*-(Z) isomers of the thioxanthines are potent neuroleptics that, in addition to their selectivity for D_2 receptors, also show antagonistic effects on D_1, 5-HT_2 and alpha$_1$ adrenergic receptors; *cis*(Z)-flupenthixol has a greater effect on D_1 receptors than *cis*-(Z)-clopenthixol. It should be emphasised that the effect of such drugs on 5-HT_2 receptors is weak.

In the phenothiazine series of neuroleptics, thioridazine has less antimuscarinic potency than chlorpromazine, but appears to be equally active as an antagonist of 5-HT_2 and D_2 receptors; like chlorpromazine, however, it is a potent alpha$_1$ adrenoceptor antagonist. In contrast, the potent phenothiazine neuroleptic perphenazine is only slightly less selective in blocking D_2 receptors than haloperidol but, unlike the latter, has a greater antagonistic effect on histamine receptors.

With the *typical neuroleptics* in wide clinical use (e.g. chlorpromazine, thioridazine, haloperidol, pimozide, flupenthixol and clopenthixol), there would appear to be a correlation between their D_2 antagonistic potency and their clinical potency; presumably the ability of these drugs to block 5-HT_2 receptors to varying extents is also evidence that the serotonergic system is involved in their clinical activity in some way.

The actions of neuroleptics on histamine, muscarinic and alpha$_1$ adrenergic receptors explain the side effects of these drugs, i.e. sedation, anticholinergic effects and hypotensive effects, respectively, which are generally considered to be undesirable and can lead to poor patient compliance. Table 11.9 summarises the main side effects of the typical neuroleptics.

Table 11.9.   Main side effects of typical neuroleptics

Side effect	Possible cause
Parkinsonism, dystonias, akathisia	Dopamine blockade of basal ganglia *All potent typical neuroleptics*
Hypotension	Due to α_1 receptor blockade *All less potent neuroleptics*
Sedation	Due to histamine$_1$ blockade *All less potent neuroleptics*
Tachycardia and other anticholinergic effects	Due to muscarinic receptor blockade *All less potent neuroleptics*
Seizures	?Due to muscarinic receptor blockade *Most neuroleptics*
Agranulocytosis, skin rashes	Allergic reactions *Many neuroleptics; clozapine*
Skin pigmentation	Dopamine–melanin conversion *All less potent neuroleptics*
Jaundice	Bile duct obstruction? *Chlorpromazine*
Cardiac conduction defects	Muscarinic blockade, Na^+ channel blockade *Thioridazine, chlorpromazine, sertindole?*

Clinical pharmacology of the typical ("classical") neuroleptics

Despite the wide differences in the potency of the neuroleptics in current use, and the differences in specificity regarding their effects on various neurotransmitter systems in the mammalian brain, there is little evidence to suggest that their overall efficacy in treating the symptoms of schizophrenia, mania and other psychoses markedly differs. Thus the "classical" neuroleptics appear to be effective in attenuating the positive symptoms of schizophrenia (e.g. hallucinations and delusions) without affecting appreciably the negative symptoms of the illness (lethargy and social withdrawal), although a critical analysis of the actions of neuroleptics on the positive and negative symptoms suggests that both types of symptoms, which may coexist in the patient simultaneously or occur at different times during the course of the illness, may be favourably influenced by those drugs. Whether these effects on the positive and negative symptoms can be explained in terms of changes in the functional activity of different subtypes of dopamine and other neurotransmitter receptors is presently uncertain.

Dopamine receptor adaptation occurs in response to chronic neuroleptic treatment, and this may be important in understanding both the efficacy and side effects of the drugs. Thus while the blockade of dopamine receptor functions is quite rapid, the clinical response does not occur for several days. Further, the extrapyramidal side effects which occur as a consequence of dopamine receptor blockade in the basal ganglia cause a sequence of changes beginning with *dystonia* and followed by *akathisia* and *parkinsonism-like* movements after several weeks or months of treatment. *Tardive dyskinesia*, should it occur, may take months or even years to be manifest. While attempts have been made to explain the complexity of these adverse neurological effects in terms of changes in dopamine receptor sensitivity arising as a consequence of prolonged dopamine receptor blockade in the basal ganglia, knowledge that the commonly used neuroleptics also interact with many other neurotransmitter systems in that region of the brain makes such an explanation implausible. Furthermore, orofacial dyskinesias occur to a significant extent in untreated schizophrenic patients and it is now well established that neuroleptics combined with the ageing process increase the prevalence of such disorders. Nevertheless, there is clear evidence from clinical studies on schizophrenic patients being treated with neuroleptics that changes in central dopaminergic function are related to the clinical response to treatment. Thus it has been shown that the free plasma concentration of homovanillic acid (HVA), the main metabolite of dopamine, correlates significantly with the antipsychotic effect of the phenothiazines. Undoubtedly the increased use of PET techniques to study neurotransmitter receptors in schizophrenic patients during neuroleptic treatment will provide invaluable information regarding the precise sites of action of these drugs in the patient's brain.

The *serum concentrations* of "classical" neuroleptics and their metabolites vary considerably in patients, even when the dose of drug administered has been standardized. Such interindividual variation may account for the differences in the therapeutic and side effects. High interindividual variations in the steady-state plasma levels have been reported for pimozide, fluphenazine, flupenthixol and haloperidol, some of these differences being attributed to differences in absorption and metabolism between patients.

Various factors may account for the *variability in response* to neuroleptics. These include differences in the diagnostic criteria, concurrent administration of drugs which may affect the absorption and metabolism of the neuroleptics (e.g. tricyclic antidepressants), different times of blood sampling, and variations due to the different type of assay method used. In some cases, the failure to obtain consistent relationships between the plasma neuroleptic concentration and the clinical response may be explained by the contribution of active metabolites to the therapeutic effects. Thus chlorpromazine, thioridazine, levomepromazine (methotrimeprazine) and loxapine have active metabolites which reach peak plasma concentrations within the same range as those of the parent compounds. As these metabolites often have pharmacodynamic and pharmacokinetic activities which differ from those of the parent compound, it is essential to determine the plasma concentrations of both the parent compound and its metabolites in order to establish whether or not a relationship exists between the plasma concentration and the therapeutic outcome.

Even in the case of drugs like haloperidol which do not have active metabolites, an unequivocal relationship cannot be found between the clinical effects and the plasma concentrations.

Fluphenazine enanthate, fluphenazine decanoate and haloperidol decanoate were developed as *depot* preparations to overcome many of the problems of oral neuroleptic administration, particularly lack of compliance, which has been estimated to be as high as 60% in outpatients. Depot neuroleptics produce a fairly predictable and constant plasma level and have the advantage of not being metabolized in the gastrointestinal tract or liver before reaching the brain. Despite the clear advantages of depot over oral preparations, the relapse rate among schizophrenic patients on such preparations over a 2-year period approaches 30%. The incidence of extrapyramidal side effects would also appear to be similar, but the longer half-life of the depot neuroleptic means that there is a longer delay before such symptoms may be controlled.

The relationship between plasma levels, drug doses and clinical response gives no clear guidelines for clinical practice. There is no convincing evidence that a "therapeutic window" exists for neuroleptics. Furthermore, there is little evidence to show that very high doses of neuroleptics improve the overall level of response or speed of resolution of an acute psychosis. High doses of neuroleptics may benefit those patients who fail to achieve optimal plasma concentrations on standard doses. Regarding the depot preparations, in a study in which patients treated with a low dose of fluphenazine decanoate (range 1.25–5.0 mg every 2 weeks) were compared with a group on a standard dose (range 12.5–50.0 mg every 2 weeks) over a 12-month period, the relapse rates were significantly higher in the low dose group (56% versus 7%). Furthermore, there was no clear advantage in the lower dose regarding the frequency of side effects or improved social functioning. It would seem that depot neuroleptics may be the appropriate method of drug administration for short-term treatment, just as orally administered neuroleptics have a place in long-term maintenance treatment.

Classification of the typical neuroleptics

In addition to their well-established antipsychotic properties, the neuroleptics have a number of clinically important properties that include their antiemetic and antinauseant actions, their antihistaminic effects and their ability to potentiate the actions of analgesics and general anaesthetics.

Reserpine is unique among the neuroleptics in that it is a naturally occurring alkaloid obtained from the snake plant *Rauwolfia serpentina*. The use of aqueous extracts of the root of this plant for the treatment of "hysteria" was known to the native practitioners in the Indian subcontinent for centuries before the main active principal, reserpine, was isolated in the early 1950s. The marked antihypertensive effect of the drug, combined with its tranquillizing activity, led to its use in the treatment of schizophrenia. However, as has already been discussed in an earlier chapter, reserpine depletes all transmitters that are contained in storage vesicles in nerve terminals by selectively blocking their uptake by the magnesium-dependent adenosine triphosphatase (ATPase) linked transport site on the vesicle membrane. This renders the transmitter susceptible to intraneuronal catabolism. However, the side effects of long-term reserpine administration in schizophrenic patients were so numerous that its use has been largely discontinued. These side effects, which can be predicted from the action of reserpine on the storage vesicles for noradrenaline, 5-HT, dopamine and acetylcholine, include sedation, Parkinsonism, predisposition to seizures, hypotension and a general impairment of peripheral sympathetic activity associated with parasympathetic hyperactivity (e.g. nausea, diarrhoea, gastric hypersecretion with susceptibility to gastric ulceration, bradycardia and hypersalivation).

Of the *phenothiazines*, chlorpromazine was the first drug to be introduced for the treatment of schizophrenia and is still the most widely used worldwide. All phenothiazines have antihistaminic, anticholinergic, anti-dopaminergic and adrenolytic properties, the potencies of the drugs for these different types of receptors depending upon the structure of the side chain which is attached to the tricyclic ring system. In general terms, it appears that the substitution of a halogen atom in the tricyclic ring (position "R" in Figure 11.8) is essential for neuroleptic activity. Thus *promazine*, which lacks a halogen substituent, has weak neuroleptic properties but it is a potent antihistaminic and anticholinergic agent. The side chain (position "B" in Figure 11.8) is important for the neuroleptic potency and also the anticholinergic, antihistaminic and adrenolytic side effects. Of the three main chemical classes of phenothiazines in clinical use, the *aliphatic* type are the least potent neuroleptics but are the most sedative, with pronounced anticholinergic, antihistaminic and adrenolytic properties. These effects are related to the structure of aliphatic side chain. The *piperidine* type are slightly more potent as neuroleptics and also have anticholinergic and adrenolytic side effects. The most potent, and least sedative, phenothiazines are in the *piperazine* group. This type of neuroleptic largely lacks anticholinergic, antihistaminic and adrenolytic activity.

The aliphatic phenothiazine chlorpromazine is the prototype neuroleptic with a wide range of pharmacological effects. Its antipsychotic and antiemetic properties are attributed to its antagonist action at central dopamine receptors in the mesocortical and vomiting centres, respectively, while the hypotensive action of chlorpromazine and related phenothiazines is associated with their alpha$_1$ adrenoceptor antagonist properties combined with their ability to reduce hypothalamic and central vasomotor function. The depression of hypothalamic activity also accounts for the hypothermia which may occur at therapeutic doses, particularly in the elderly patient. The antimuscarinic and antihistaminic activity, which can be predicted from the structure of the aliphatic side chain, accounts for the sedative and peripheral anticholinergic effects of this group of drugs. The aliphatic phenothiazine *triflupromazine* is a more potent neuroleptic than chlorpromazine due to substitution of $-CF_3$ for the $-Cl$ group in the ring.

The piperidine phenothiazines, as exemplified by the most widely used member of this series *thioridazine*, are approximately equivalent to the aliphatic phenothiazines but tend to be more sedative. Members of this series are therefore widely used for the more agitated, anxious psychotic patient. As their ability to cause parkinsonism appears to be less than with the other phenothiazines, possibly because of their potent central anticholinergic effects and slightly greater selectivity for mesocortical dopamine receptors, they are widely used to treat elderly psychotic patients.

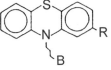

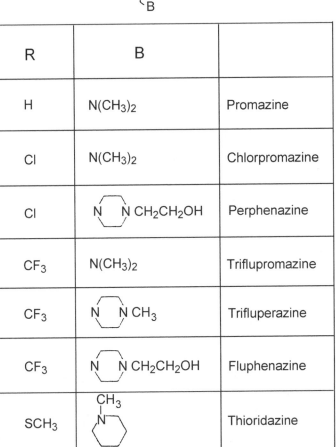

R	B	
H	N(CH₃)₂	Promazine
Cl	N(CH₃)₂	Chlorpromazine
Cl	N⎯N CH₂CH₂OH	Perphenazine
CF₃	N(CH₃)₂	Triflupromazine
CF₃	N⎯N CH₃	Trifluperazine
CF₃	N⎯N CH₂CH₂OH	Fluphenazine
SCH₃	(CH₃-N piperidine)	Thioridazine

Figure 11.8. Chemical structure of the phenothiazine series of neuroleptics.

The *piperazine* phenothiazines, as exemplified by *fluphenazine*, are the most potent members of the phenothiazine group, being at least 50 times more potent than chlorpromazine. Because of the structure of their side chain, members of this series lack anticholinergic, antihistaminic, adrenolytic and sedative effects. However, they are more likely to cause extrapyramidal side effects.

The *thioxanthines* are structurally closely related to the phenothiazines (see Figure 11.9) and may be divided into three separate series of

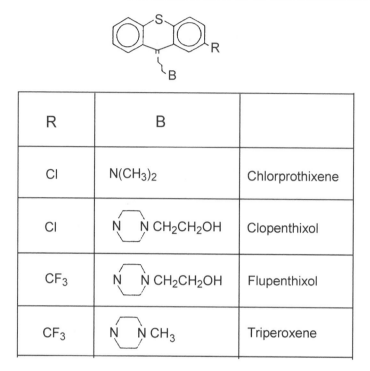

R	B	
Cl	N(CH₃)₂	Chlorprothixene
Cl	N N CH₂CH₂OH	Clopenthixol
CF₃	N N CH₂CH₂OH	Flupenthixol
CF₃	N N CH₃	Triperoxene

Figure 11.9. Chemical structure of the thioxanthine series of neuroleptics.

compounds with aliphatic (e.g. *chlorprothixene*), piperazine (e.g. *clopenthixol, flupenthixol*) or piperidine side chains. Their potency and side effects are essentially similar to the corresponding phenothiazine neuroleptics.

The *butyrophenones* and *diphenylbutylpiperidines* differ from the phenothiazines and thioxanthines in that they are not tricyclic structures. The first butyrophenone to be developed was *haloperidol*, and this is the most widely used, potent neuroleptic. Unlike many of the phenothiazines, these neuroleptics largely lack antihistaminic, anticholinergic and adrenolytic activity; they are also non-sedative in therapeutic doses. Their potent antidopaminergic activity renders them likely to cause extrapyramidal side effects. Of the various butyrophenones shown in Figure 11.10, *benperidol* has been selectively used to suppress asocial sexual behaviour.

The diphenylbutylpiperidines are structurally related to the butyrophenones and have essentially similar properties. *Pimozide* is the most well-established member of this series and is a potent neuroleptic that, like other potent neuroleptics, is likely to cause extrapyramidal side effects.

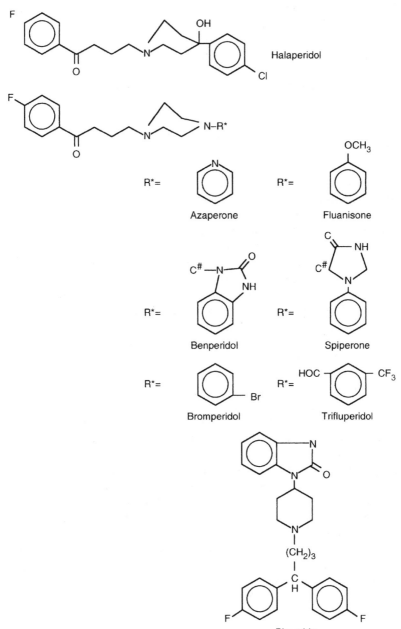

Figure 11.10. Chemical structure of the butyrophenone and diphenylbutylpiperidine series of neuroleptics indicates that N has been replaced by C.

Sulpiride is a member of a series of neuroleptics, the benzamides, of which the antiemetic drug metoclopramide is another example. The benzamides have a lower propensity to cause extrapyramidal side effects, probably because they show a high degree of selectivity for the D_2 dopamine receptors.

The chemical structure of sulpiride is shown in Figure 11.11.

Efficacy of high doses of "classical" neuroleptics in the treatment-resistant patient

There is no published evidence for the efficacy of high dose medication as an effective strategy either to accelerate therapeutic response or to increase the number of patients who respond to medication. Neither is there any objective evidence to show that escalating the dose of a "classical" neuroleptic is likely to produce a beneficial response in chronically resistant patients. Furthermore, there are anecdotal reports that high dose neuroleptics can cause sudden death (due to cardiotoxicity), severe Parkinsonism and/or akathisia with the possibility of paradoxical and violent behaviour (possibly associated with akathisia). The possibility of the neuroleptic malignant syndrome occurring following high dose neuroleptics is more closely related to the rate of dose escalation than to the quantity of neuroleptic administered.

However, despite the absence of firm evidence for efficacy because of the real dangers that may arise, it is occasionally justified to consider administering a high therapeutic dose of a "classical" neuroleptic to a patient who is responding poorly to a normal dose of the drug. It is well established that the blood concentration of a neuroleptic varies considerably between patients given the same oral dose. Such variation probably arises from differences in compliance, in first-pass metabolism and in the rate of elimination. Where possible, the plasma concentrations should be determined before proceeding with the dose escalation of a standard neuroleptic. Assuming that pharmacologically active concentrations of the drug have been achieved, it is possible that poor therapeutic response is due to an insufficient population of the D_2 receptors in the mesocortical areas of the brain being blocked by the neuroleptics. However, it must be emphasized that the use of high doses of neuroleptics should be the last resort for carefully selected and supervised patients. It may be argued that as the new atypical neuroleptics are equi-effective with the "classical" antipsychotics, and certainly superior in their tolerability and side-effect profile, such drugs (despite their high unit cost) should be considered before escalating the dose of a non-response patient on a "classical" neuroleptic.

Treatment decisions for schizophrenia are shown in Table 11.10.

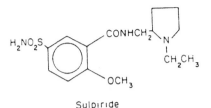

Sulpiride

Figure 11.11. Chemical structure of the benzamide neuroleptic sulpiride.

Hormonal changes resulting from neuroleptic treatment

Acute dopamine receptor blockade by neuroleptics has long been known to induce a dose-dependent increase in *prolactin* as a consequence of the decreased activity of the inhibitory D_2 receptors that govern the release of this hormone from the anterior pituitary. However, dose–response studies show that the dose of a neuroleptic required to raise the plasma prolactin concentration is lower than that necessary to have an optimal therapeutic effect. Furthermore, the time of onset of the rise in prolactin is short (hours), whereas the antipsychotic effect of a neuroleptic takes many days or even weeks. There is also evidence that raised serum prolactin levels persist throughout drug treatment, which suggests that tolerance of the tubero-infundibular dopaminergic system to the action of neuroleptics does not occur; it should be noted that not all investigators agree with such a view. There is little evidence to suggest that a relationship exists between the symptoms of schizophrenia, or the response to drug therapy, and changes in plasma prolactin concentrations.

The secretion of *growth hormone* is under the control of the dopaminergic, noradrenergic, serotonergic and possibly other neurotransmitter systems. The acute apomorphine growth hormone challenge test has been used to assess D_2 receptor function in untreated schizophrenics and in patients during neuroleptic treatment. Apomorphine-stimulated growth hormone secretion is reported to be higher in untreated schizophrenics and to be

Table 11.10. Treatment decisions for schizophrenia

- First choice – atypical antipsychotic (e.g. risperidone, olanzepine, quetiapine, amisulpride, clozapine)
- Switching – alternative atypical antipsychotic to that previously used
- Augmentation – mood stabilizer, high potency first-generation neuroleptic (e.g. flupenthixol), possibly a benzodiazepine
- Other options – i.m. formulations

---

blunted following both acute and chronic neuroleptic treatment, returning to control values within a few weeks of drug withdrawal.

Sexual dysfunction in schizophrenic patients on long-term neuroleptic therapy is well established and may result from hyperprolactinaemia. Menstrual cycle disruption is a common feature of neuroleptic treatment which may be complicated in hyperprolactinaemia. However, it seems unlikely that the changes in gonadotrophin secretion are a unique feature of schizophrenia, as patients with depression and anorexia nervosa also show such abnormalities. Furthermore, detailed studies of the luteinizing hormone and follicle-stimulating hormone levels in a group of male and female patients on very long-term neuroleptic therapy could not confirm an abnormality in sex hormone dysfunction due to drug treatment. Thus it must be concluded that unequivocal evidence showing that prolonged neuroleptic treatment results in sexual dysfunction due to a defect in gonadotrophin release is not yet available.

Changes in cognitive function during neuroleptic treatment

The effects of long-term neuroleptic administration on cognitive and psychomotor function have been the subject of many studies. Some of the early studies undertaken during the 1960s reported that acute doses of phenothiazine neuroleptics caused cognitive impairment in schizophrenic patients, whereas chronic treatment led to improvement. More recent studies, however, have reported improvement in attention and in cognitive function following short-term administration. Detailed studies revealed that memory and fine motor coordination were impaired by many neuroleptics, the amnesic effects probably being related to the central anticholinergic effects of the drugs while the effects on motor control may be ascribed to the blockade of dopamine receptors. In general, it would appear that the hyperarousal state that occurs in schizophrenia is reduced by neuroleptics, thereby leading to an improvement in attention. However, the consensus would now appear to be that a general decrease in brainstem arousal does not account for the beneficial effect of neuroleptics, and it seems more probable that these drugs correct a frontal lobe dysfunction. It should be noted that tardive dyskinesia is almost invariably associated with a deterioration of intellectual function.

Thus it would appear that neuroleptics have little effect on higher cognitive functioning in schizophrenic patients and that the improvement in attention is facilitated by a non-mesocortical–mesolimbic mechanism. There is also evidence that neuroleptics improve asymmetry in hippo-campal function which may be deranged in the illness. It is generally agreed that studies of the effects of neuroleptics on normal subjects, which frequently show impaired cognitive and psychomotor function, are of only limited relevance to our understanding of the beneficial effects which these drugs produce in schizophrenic patients.

Potential cardiotoxicity of antipsychotic drugs

Most antipsychotic drugs have effects on the heart as a consequence of their pharmacological actions. Recently, thioridazine has been subjected to a restricted indication notice and the atypical antipsychotic sertindole had its licence withdrawn because of concerns about its potential cardiotoxicity.

It has been known since the 1960s that ECG abnormalities are relatively common in those patients on antipsychotics, occurring in approximately 25% of all cases. The most commonly reported changes are the prolonged QT interval, suggestive of repolarization disturbances, depressed ST segments and abnormal T waves. A prolongation of the corrected QT interval (cQT) greater than 420 msec was found to be more frequent in chronic schizophrenic patients than in controls (23% versus 2%). This increase was more pronounced in patients treated with high doses of typical neuroleptics (greater than 200 mg chlorpromazine equivalents a day). TCAs, thioridazine and droperidol were most likely to be associated with this cardiac effect. At therapeutic doses, it has been reported that 75% of all cases of sudden death in schizophrenic patients are associated with thioridazine.

In the development of new antipsychotics, cQT intervals are routinely evaluated but it is currently unclear how predictive these are of clinically significant cardiotoxicity or sudden death. For this reason, the heart rate variability (HRV) index has been developed. It has been shown that the HRV decreases after TCAs and clozapine. In a comparison of the acute effects of olanzapine, risperidone and thioridazine in healthy male volunteers, olanzapine was shown to increase, thioridazine to decrease while risperidone was without effect on the HRV. A decrease in the HRV is an established predictor of poor cardiac outcome. The cardiac changes were unrelated to the degree of sedation caused by the drugs.

Other factors which predispose to the cardiotoxicity of antipsychotic drugs include raised triglyceride and low density lipoprotein concentrations, diabetes and weight gain. The latter is a frequent side effect of many psychotropic drugs including the TCA antidepressants, and mianserin and mirtazepine, clozapine, olanzapine and to a lesser extent quetiapine and risperidone. Clearly the long-term cardiotoxicity of antipsychotic medications is a cause for concern, particularly in the case of patients on long-term treatment with typical neuroleptics.

In CONCLUSION, the use of the "classical" neuroleptics, as exemplified by the phenothiazines, thioxanthines, butyrophenones and diphenylbutyl-piperidines, has been a landmark in the pharmacotherapy of schizophrenia and psychotic disorders. The efficacy of such drugs in the alleviation of the symptoms of schizophrenia is universally accepted. However, it is also evident that they have a spectrum of adverse effects that frequently renders their long-term use problematic. Side effects such as akathisia, Parkinson-ism, tardive dyskinesia and the all too frequent changes in peripheral autonomic activity are largely predictable from the structure of the molecules and the basic animal pharmacology data. Such adverse effects, and the difficulties encountered when attempting to reduce their frequency and severity by concurrent medication, has stimulated the development of "atypical" neuroleptics such as clozapine and risperidone which, hopefully, will combine efficacy with a reduction in side effects.

12 Drug Treatment of the Epilepsies

Introduction

Hughlings Jackson, reputed to be the "father" of the modern concept of epilepsy, defined epilepsy about 100 years ago as "an episodic disorder of the nervous system arising from the excessively synchronous and sustained discharge of a group of neurons". Such a definition implies that, in addition to the seizure, there are disturbances in both motor and cognitive function. Hughlings Jackson also noted that a single seizure is not indicative of epilepsy, but he did not exclude seizures that are secondary to systemic metabolic disorders – such seizures would not be included in the classification of epilepsy today. The main importance of this definition is that it emphasized for the first time that epilepsy has a neuropathological basis and suggested that excitatory and inhibitory neurotransmitter processes are probably involved in the causation of the symptoms.

The term "epilepsy" applies to a group of disorders that are characterized by sudden and transient episodes (seizures) of motor (convulsions), sensory, autonomic or psychic origin. The seizures are usually correlated with abnormal and excessive discharges in the brain and can be visualized on the electroencephalogram (EEG).

The epilepsies are estimated to affect 20–40 million individuals worldwide and are more common in children than in adults. They are classified into two broad groups: *primary* or *idiopathic* epilepsy is the term applied to those types for which no specific cause can be identified, and *secondary* or *symptomatic* epilepsy arises when the symptoms are associated with trauma, neoplasm, infection, cerebrovascular disease or some other physically induced lesion of the brain. Seizures that accompany severe metabolic disturbances are not classified as epilepsy.

For the purpose of drug treatment, the epilepsies are classified according to the seizure type. The classification generally used is based on that proposed by the Commission on Classification and Terminology of the International League against Epilepsy. The main groups are:

Fundamentals of Psychopharmacology. Third Edition. By Brian E. Leonard
© 2003 John Wiley & Sons, Ltd. ISBN 0 471 52178 7

1. *Partial (focal) seizures*, or seizures initiated locally in the brain. These include:
   (a) Simple partial seizures, which encompass focal motor attacks and seizures with somatosensory signs or psychic symptoms.
   (b) Complex partial seizures, including temporal lobe or psychomotor seizures where consciousness is impaired; these may begin as simple partial seizures.
   (c) Secondary generalized seizures, which commence as (a) or (b) but later develop into generalized tonic–clonic, clonic or tonic seizures.
2. *Generalized seizures*, including bilateral symmetrical seizures or seizures without local onset. This group includes:
   (a) Clonic, tonic and tonic–clonic seizures
   (b) Myoclonic seizures.
   (c) Absence and atypical absence seizures.
   (d) Atonic seizures.

This classification does not take into account the frequency, duration or causes of precipitation of the seizure. Any type of attack that is maintained for more than 1 hour is termed *status epilepticus*, which may be qualified as focal or generalized.

The changes in the cortical EEG of patients with different types of epilepsy are illustrated in Figures 12.1, 12.2 and 12.3.

Pathological basis of the epilepsies

The pathophysiology of epilepsy is poorly understood and so far there is no clear association between the abnormal function of a specific group of neurons and the genesis of seizures. It is generally agreed that epileptogenesis involves the complex interaction of multiple factors. In some cases lesions such as those arising from traumatic haemorrhage can cause secondary seizures, whereas other forms of brain damage, for example that caused by ischaemic stroke, are less likely to cause seizures. Microscopic changes involving glial proliferation and loss of neurons have been identified in epileptic patients, and a loss of those neurons containing inhibitory neurotransmitters has been particularly implicated in the aetiology of the disease. Whether such changes are the cause or the consequence of the seizures is uncertain.

There is considerable controversy regarding the possible *genetic* basis of the epilepsies. It has been calculated that there are at least 100 different trait markers that may predispose some individuals to the disease, and it has been shown that identical seizure disorders may be present in patients who

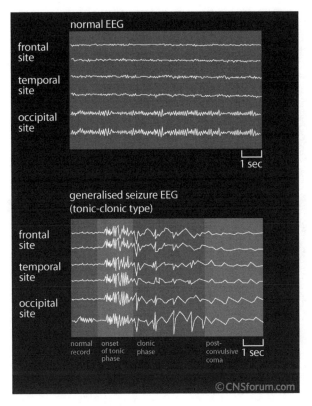

Figure 12.1. Changes in the cortical EEG of a patient showing tonic–clonic type generalized seizures.

either have, or do not have, a particular genetic marker. Clearly this is an important area of research for the future.

Animal models

Animal models have been developed not only in an attempt to screen potential antiepileptic drugs but also to define more precisely the possible aetiology of the condition. In mice, there are at least 12 single locus mutations that produce neurological syndromes with spontaneous seizures. One particular species, the "tottering mouse", shows spontaneous seizures which resemble absence attacks both in terms of the behavioural and the EEG changes. The only specific cellular pathology which has been found in this model is a selective outgrowth of axons from the locus coeruleus which results in an increase in the noradrenaline content of the neocortex,

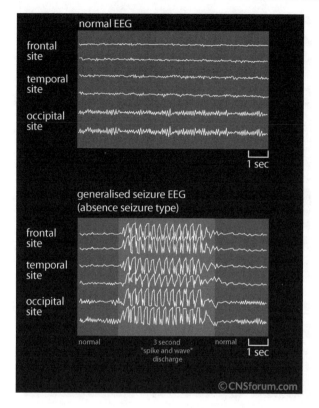

Figure 12.2. Changes in the cortical EEG of a patient showing absence seizures.

hippocampus, cerebellum and thalamus. The seizures are attenuated in this species by the local injection of the neurotoxin 6-hydroxydopamine, which destroys the noradrenergic terminals. However, it should be noted that this neurotoxin usually results in the lowering of the seizure threshold in most species of animal, so the precise relevance of these findings in the "tottering mouse" to the human condition is unclear.

Strong sensory stimuli (e.g. 90 dB sound) can precipitate tonic–clonic seizures in some strains of mice, the DBA/2 strain being particularly susceptible, while posturally induced seizures in "epileptic-like" mice have been extensively studied and have been shown to be associated with abnormalities in both the adenosine triphosphatases (ATPases) and various biogenic amine neurotransmitters.

Beagle dogs show a high incidence of epileptic seizures, including those of the secondary type; complex partial and generalized tonic–clonic seizures frequently occur in this species. However, the nearest model to

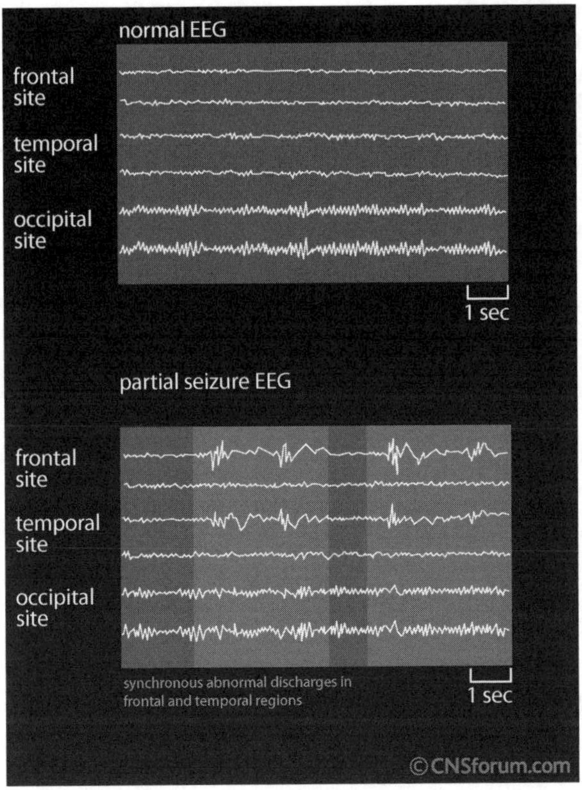

Figure 12.3. Changes in the EEG of a patient showing partial seizures.

human epilepsy is undoubtedly photically induced seizures in the Senegalese baboon.

Chronic focal epilepsy can be induced in rats, cats and monkeys by the topical application of metals such as aluminium, cobalt and iron. Alumina paste applied to the motor cortex of the monkey initiates spontaneous convulsive seizures that eventually generalize to the rest of the brain. It has been shown that neurons in the vicinity of the seizure focus have a reduced glutamate decarboxylase activity, which suggests that gamma-aminobutyric acid (GABA) synthesis in this area is impaired. Not all animal models of epilepsy show such changes in GABA content, however. Some strains of Mongolian gerbil exhibit myoclonic and clonic–tonic seizures in early adulthood, but in such species the GABA content of the hippocampus has been shown to increase, which suggests that a process of disinhibition of inhibitory transmitter pathways may occur in this model.

Recently there has been much interest in the *kindling* of epileptic seizures in rodents. This occurs following focal electrical stimulation of cortical regions, usually the temporal region, by a current that is sufficient to cause an after-discharge but insufficient to cause a direct seizure. When such stimuli are repeated at regular intervals for several days, a stage is reached whereby a subthreshold stimulus results in a full seizure. This suggests that kindling is associated with the lowering of the seizure threshold consequent upon the induction of enhanced neurotransmitter receptor sensitivity. There is no evidence that brain damage is responsible for such changes but it has been suggested that the alterations in receptor sensitivity are similar to those occurring in long-term potentiation, a phenomenon produced by high frequency stimulation of afferent inputs to the hippocampus that leads to enhancement of excitatory synaptic potentials and increased memory formation.

Whereas the genetic and kindling models have been widely used to investigate possible neurotransmitter defects that cause different types of epilepsy, rodent models in which seizures are induced by electroshock, or by convulsant drugs such as pentylenetetrazol (also called pentetrazol, leptazol), picrotoxin or bicuculline, are mainly used in screening procedures to identify potential anticonvulsants.

Biochemical changes in human epilepsy

Membrane-bound enzymes, particularly the ATPases involved in the ionic pumps for calcium, sodium and potassium, have been found to function abnormally in the brains of epileptic patients and animals. A reduction in Na^+K^+-ATPase activity has been reported in human focal epileptogenic tissue, but it is uncertain whether such changes are due to the disease itself or a reflection of drug treatment. Similar changes have, however, been reported in experimental animals following the localized application of alumina cream and in DBA/2 mice that exhibit sound-induced seizures; a reduction in calcium-dependent ATPase has also been found in the brain of DBA/2 mice. Such findings are consistent with the hypothesis that a defect in ion channels may occur in epilepsy.

Another possibility is that endogenous epileptogenic compounds may be produced in the brain of the epileptic patient. Both tetrahydroisoquinolines and beta-carbolines have been detected in the human brain, as has the tryptophan analogue quinolinic acid, which all have convulsant and excitotoxic properties. The enzymes that synthesize quinolinic acid have also been identified in human brain tissue.

Of the various amino acid neurotransmitters which have been implicated in epilepsy, the inhibitory transmitter glycine has been shown to be present in normal concentrations, or even slightly elevated, in the vicinity of the epileptic focus. Conversely, the concentration of GABA has been found to be reduced in the cerebrospinal fluid (CSF) of chronic epileptics and in patients with febrile seizures. The central role of GABA in epilepsy is further suggested by the observation that drugs that reduce the GABA concentration are epileptogenic, while those that raise the GABA concentration are generally anticonvulsants. The observation that the concentration of glutamate may be reduced in the epileptic focus lends further support to the view that there may be a defect in GABA synthesis which predisposes the individual to the disease.

Despite early studies suggesting that the acetylcholine concentration was raised in epileptogenic foci, which would be consistent with the finding that anticholinesterases cause seizures in both animals and man, it now appears that overactivity of the central cholinergic system is unlikely to be the cause of seizures in the human epileptic. Other candidates that have been implicated in the aetiology of epilepsy include adenosine and the enkephalins, but conclusive evidence for their involvement is presently lacking.

Treatment of epilepsies

Pharmacokinetic considerations when prescribing antiepileptic drugs

Generic formulations of antiepileptic drugs

The regulatory authorities in most industrialized countries require that the generic equivalent of a standard antiepileptic drug has a bioavailability which is similar to that of a proprietary drug. Rates of absorption, however, do vary even if the extent of absorption does not. With few exceptions, generic formulations are acceptable despite the claims often made by commercial companies which purport to show otherwise. Only in the case of phenytoin, at tissue concentrations that approach saturation, do generic formulations pose particular problems. Even then the serum concentration can be monitored to provide a guide to the appropriate dosage for a particular patient.

Measurement of the serum concentration of antiepileptic drugs

Once the steady state of the drug has been reached, there is a fairly consistent relationship between the plasma and the brain concentrations. It should therefore be possible to define those plasma concentrations that are associated with the optimal clinical effects (i.e. the optimal balance between the effectiveness and the side effects). Because of the biological variation, however, such concentrations may vary from one individual to another but it is possible to develop a range of drug concentrations which are based on statistical or population parameters. The therapeutic range for some of the commonly used antiepileptic drugs is shown below:

Drug	Therapeutic range (μmol/L)
Carbamazepine	20–50
Ethosuximide	300–700
Felbamate	200–460
Lamotrigine	4–60
Oxacarbamazepine	50–125
Phenobarbitone	40–170
Phenytoin	40–80
Primidone	<60 primidone; 40–170 for phenobarbitone
Topiramate	300–600

Regarding the usefulness in measuring the serum concentrations of antiepileptic drugs, it is often of value to do so with those drugs that are liable to cause toxic side effects such as carbamazepine, ethosuximide, phenobarbitone and phenytoin. In general, there seems to be little advantage in determining the serum concentrations of the newer, and better tolerated, antiepileptics.

Factors which influence the serum concentrations of the antiepileptic drugs depend on the chemical nature of the drug, the drug formulation and drug interactions and the time at which the blood sample is taken (usually at the trough concentration before the daily dose). In addition, the individual patient can cause changes in the drug concentration. Such factors include genetic and constitutional factors, such as the age and gender, the absorption of the drug (which is influenced by food and gastrointestinal function), the metabolism (which is affected by the hepatic enzyme status), the distribution of the drug (which is influenced by the serum protein concentration, nutritional status and pregnancy), and lastly the excretion (which is affected by renal disease).

In practice, the monitoring of the serum drug concentration is generally unnecessary but there are criteria which may help the clinician to decide when monitoring is appropriate. These include:

- Poor therapeutic response in spite of an adequate dose of the drug.
- Physiological or pathological conditions that are known to affect the kinetics of the drug (e.g. renal or liver disease, pregnancy)
- Minimizing the problems caused by the non-linear kinetics of the drug (e.g. phenytoin).
- Minimizing the problems caused by drug interactions.
- To assess the changes in bioavailability caused by changes in drug formulation.

It should be emphasized that the outcome of therapy in newly diagnosed patients is generally good. In about 70–80% of these patients, seizures will cease usually within a few years of treatment. In the case of such patients, the risk of subsequent recurrence is low (approximately 10% after a 5-year period without an attack) and most patients will be able to discontinue medication. The prognosis is worse if there is structural brain damage, severe epilepsy syndromes, a family history of epilepsy, a high frequency of tonic–clonic seizures before the start of therapy or in those patients with psychiatric or neurological disorders. EEG analyses have, in general, been shown to be a poor indicator of prognosis.

Limitations of current antiepileptic drug therapy

It has been estimated that drug therapy will fail in 10–20% of patients. In this situation the epilepsy is described as intractable and the goal of therapy should be changed to defining the best compromise between inadequate seizure control and drug-induced side effects. The concept of intractability is invariably fairly arbitrary. There are over 10 widely used antiepileptic drugs and far more combinations. The chances of a new drug controlling the seizures after five appropriate drugs have failed to do so has been estimated to be less than 5%. Thus from the practical point of view one may categorize a patient as intractable when at least five of the major antiepileptics have been shown to be ineffective.

Summary of the antiepileptic drugs used for different types of seizures

There is a dearth of good comparative data on the appropriate drugs to be used for different seizure types. The following table is based upon summaries published in standard monographs, several of which are mentioned in the references to this chapter:

For simple and complex partial seizures and secondary generalized tonic–clonic seizures, the first line drugs are – carbamazepine, valproate and phenytoin. Second line drugs include – acetazolamide, clobazam, clonazepam, ethosuximide, felbamate, gabapentin, lamotrigine, levetiracetam, oxacarbamazepine, primidone, tiagabine, topiramate and vigabactin.

For generalized absence seizures, first line treatment is with valproate or ethosuximide and second line treatment with acetazolamide, clobazam, clonazepam, lamotrigine, phenobarbitone and primidone.

For atypical absence, tonic and clonic seizures, first line treatment is with valproate and second line with acetazolamide, carbamazepine, clobazam, clonazepam, ethosuximide, felbamate, lamotrigine, oxacarbamazepine, phenobarbitone, phenytoin, primidone or topiramate.

Myoclonic seizures are best treated with valproate but, as a second choice, with clobazam, clonazepam, ethosuximide, lamotrigine, phenobarbitone, piracetam or primidone.

Action of anticonvulsants on central neurotransmitters

The anticonvulsants in clinical use may be divided into eight major groups. These are:

1. The *barbiturates*, such as phenobarbitone and primidone.
2. The *hydantoins*, such as diphenylhydantoin (phenytoin) and ethytoin.
3. The *dibenzazepines*, such as carbamazepine.
4. The *oxazolidinediones*, such as trimethadione (troxidone).
5. The *succinimides*, such as ethosuximide.
6. The *benzodiazepines*, such as diazepam, clobazam and clonazepam.
7. The *sulphonamides*, such as acetazolamide and sulthiame.
8. The *short chain fatty acids*, such as sodium valproate.

The chemical structure of representative drugs from each of these groups is shown in Figure 12.4.

Of the various animal models of epilepsy that have been developed to screen compounds for their potential therapeutic activity, antagonism of maximal electroshock seizures is generally indicative of the drug being useful in the control of partial seizures; drugs such as diphenylhydantoin and carbamazepine are active in such tests. Conversely, antagonism of pentylenetetrazol seizures is usually associated with the effective control of absence (petit mal) seizures, the succinimides and oxazolidinediones being particularly effective in antagonizing such seizures. Drugs such as sodium valproate and the benzodiazepines have a broad spectrum of action and are effective against primary generalized seizures (including petit mal) as well as partial seizures (including temporal lobe epilepsy).

The actions of anticonvulsants at the cellular level are complex and include facilitation of inhibitory feedback mechanisms, membrane stabilization and changes in synaptic transmission to reduce excitatory transmission. Of these various possibilities, it is widely accepted that anticonvulsants enhance GABA-mediated inhibitory processes. Such a mechanism has been clearly demonstrated for the benzodiazepines, barbiturates, diphenylhydantoin and sodium valproate.

Enhanced GABAergic transmission

Electrophysiological studies show that benzodiazepines, barbiturates and sodium valproate facilitate GABAergic transmission in the animal brain. Further evidence comes from studies on the GABA-benzodiazepine receptor complex, the order of potency of a series of benzodiazepines to displace [^{3}H] diazepam from its receptor site being clearly correlated with the antagonism of pentylenetetrazol seizures, but not with electroconvulsive seizures. However, most classes of anticonvulsants appear to facilitate

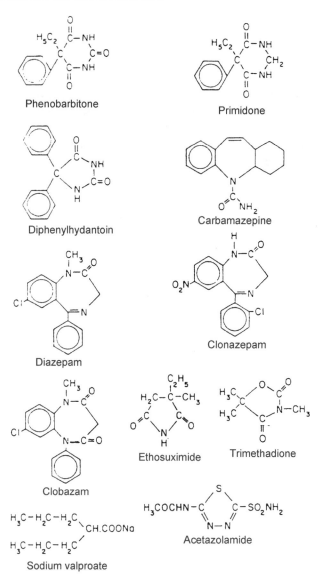

Figure 12.4. Chemical structure of the principal anticonvulsant drugs.

GABAergic transmission via the picrotoxin-binding site on the GABA-benzodiazepine receptor complex (see p. 56).

The precise mechanism of action of valproate in facilitating GABA transmission is still uncertain. There is evidence that the drug can facilitate

GABA synthesis, probably by inhibiting GABA transaminase activity, but the dose of drug necessary to achieve this effect is very high and not relevant to the clinical situation. One possibility is that valproate desensitizes GABA autoreceptors and thereby facilitates the release of the transmitter.

A reduction in the activity of excitatory neurotransmitters as a possible mechanism of action is largely confined to experimental studies on the barbiturates and benzodiazepines. *In vitro* studies have shown that drugs such as phenobarbitone can reduce the release of glutamate and acetylcholine, probably by impairing the entry of calcium ions into presynaptic terminals.

Membrane and ionic effects

The hydantoins have been most widely studied for their effects on ion movements across neuronal membranes. In the brain, these drugs have been shown to decrease the rise in intracellular sodium that normally occurs following the passage of an action potential; a reduction in calcium flux across excitable membranes also occurs.

In cell culture preparations, diphenylhydantoin, carbamazepine and valproate have been shown to reduce membrane excitability at therapeutically relevant concentrations. This membrane-stabilizing effect is probably due to a block in the sodium channels. High concentrations of diazepam also have similar effects, and the membrane-stabilizing action correlates with the action of these anticonvulsants in inhibiting maximal electroshock seizures. Intracellular studies have shown that, in synaptosomes, most anticonvulsants inhibit calcium-dependent calmodulin protein kinase, an effect which would contribute to a reduction in neurotransmitter release. This action of anticonvulsants would appear to correlate with the potency of the drugs in inhibiting electroshock seizures. The result of all these disparate actions of anticonvulsants would be to diminish synaptic efficacy and thereby reduce seizure spread from an epileptic focus.

Pharmacokinetic aspects

Unlike most classes of psychotropic drugs where there is no direct correlation between the blood concentration and the therapeutic effect, for most of the commonly used anticonvulsants there is a high degree of correlation between the blood and brain concentrations and the therapeutic effect. A knowledge of the pharmacokinetic properties of the anticonvulsant drugs is therefore essential if their therapeutic efficacy is to be maximized and side effects minimized.

The anticonvulsants are metabolized in the liver by the microsomal oxidative pathway, although some drugs, such as phenobarbitone and ethosuximide, are partially eliminated unchanged. Most anticonvulsants act as inducers of the liver microsomal enzyme system and thereby enhance their own rate of destruction. In patients on a combination of anti-convulsants, this can result in shorter elimination half-lives for some of the drugs and a corresponding wide fluctuation in the plasma drug concentrations. Sodium valproate is an exception in that it does not act as a microsomal enzyme inducer.

Some anticonvulsants are metabolized in the liver to pharmacologically active metabolites which, if they have long half-lives, may accumulate and have neurotoxic effects. The following commonly used anticonvulsants are known to produce active metabolites:

Primidone   – Phenobarbitone and phenylethylmalonamide
Carbamazepine – Carbamazepine 10,11-epoxide
Trimethadione   – Dimethadione (long half-life)
Methsuximide   – N-Desmethylmethsuximide (long half-life)

Most anticonvulsants have relatively long half-lives, which is clearly a major therapeutic advantage in achieving steady blood levels. Sodium valproate is exceptional in that it has a relatively short half-life, while phenobarbitone has the longest half-life of those drugs in general use. As with most psychotropic drugs, the half-life varies with the age of the patient; the older the patient, the longer the half-life. Slow absorption of a drug generally favours stable blood levels and to achieve this several anticonvulsants have been formulated into slowly absorbed formulations. Clearly it is important that the patient is treated with the same formulation of the drug. For patients being treated with diphenylhy-dantoin for example, changing formulations can lead to a sudden change in the steady-state drug concentration due to differences in the bioavailability of the preparations. This can lead to large fluctuations in the tissue drug concentrations with an increasing possibility of neurotoxicity and lack of seizure control despite similar peak blood concentrations being reached.

Most anticonvulsants have linear elimination kinetics, which means that an increase in the dose of drug administered leads to a proportional increase in the blood concentration and pharmacological activity. However, diphenylhydantoin and valproate are exceptions; the former does not follow linear kinetics so that the blood concentration is not directly related to the dose administered, while valproate is highly bound to serum proteins so that the total blood concentration may not directly reflect the quantity of drug available to the brain.

Drugs used in the treatment of epilepsy

The clinical applications of some of the most widely available anti-convulsants may be summarized as follows:

Febrile seizures	Phenobarbitone, benzodiazepines
Idiopathic Lennox–Gastaut syndrome	Valproate, benzodiazepines, adreno-corticotrophic hormone
Absence seizures (petit mal)	Ethosuximide, valproate, benzodiazepines, acetazolamide
Generalized tonic–clonic seizures (grand mal)	Valproate, phenobarbitone, carbamazepine, diphenylhydantoin
Juvenile myoclonic epilepsy	Valproate, ethosuximide, primidone
Reflex epilepsy	Benzodiazepines, valproate, phenobarbitone, methsuximide
Status epilepticus	Benzodiazepines, diphenylhydantoin

Benzodiazepines

Benzodiazepines used to treat epilepsy include diazepam, clonazepam, clobazam and lorazepam. Of these, diazepam and lorazepam have been most widely used to control status epilepticus, while use of clonazepam is usually restricted to the chronic treatment of severe mixed types of seizures (e.g. Lennox–Gastaut syndrome and infantile spasm). The major problem with most of the benzodiazepines, with the possible exception of clobazam, is sedation.

Lorazepam is less lipophilic than diazepam and there is evidence that it has a longer duration of anticonvulsant action than diazepam after intravenous administration. This could be due to the fact that diazepam is more rapidly removed from the brain compartment than lorazepam, which limits its duration of antiepileptic activity. In practice, when diazepam is used to control status epilepticus it is often necessary to continue treatment with diphenylhydantoin, which has a longer duration of action in the brain. The principal hazards of benzodiazepines when given intravenously include respiratory depression and hypotension. Diazepam may be administered rectally, its ease of absorption leading to peak plasma levels within about 10 minutes.

Clonazepam is the most potent of the benzodiazepine anticonvulsants and is particularly indicated in the treatment of the more difficult cases of epilepsy, especially those of the multiple seizure type. More recently, *clobazam*, which at therapeutic doses has the advantage of causing little sedation, has been advocated as an "add-on" anticonvulsant in those cases where the seizures cannot be readily controlled by more conventional drug treatment.

Carbamazepine

Mode of action. The precise mode of action of carbamazepine has not been fully established. It has been shown to stabilize both pre- and postsynaptic neurons by blocking the use and frequency-dependent sodium channels. While this is probably its main action, the blockade of the glutamate NMDA ionotropic receptors also leads to a reduction in the influx of sodium and calcium ions into the neuron. The net effect of these changes is a reduction in the sustained high-frequency repetitive firing of the action potentials which characterize epileptic activity. There is also evidence that carbamazepine blocks purine, noradrenaline, serotonin and muscarinic acetylcholine receptors which probably accounts for the use of carbamazepine as a mood stabilizing agent.

Oxacarbamazepine is a major metabolite of carbamazepine and has a mechanism of action which is identical to that of the parent compound.

Side effects. Sedation, weight gain, nystagmus, gastrointestinal distress, tremor and a change in the mood of the patient in that order are the most frequently observed side effects. There is evidence that carbamazepine can exacerbate atypical absence, tonic and myoclonic seizures. Between 30 and 50% of patients on carbamazepine experience some side effects, although these are generally mild and less than 5% of patients are estimated to withdraw from the drug because of the severity of the side effects.

Carbamazepine is a hepatic microsomal enzyme inducer and therefore will lower the serum concentration of a wide variety of drugs given concurrently. These include the antiepileptic drugs phenytoin, primidone, valproate, ethosuximide and clonazepam. In addition, carbamazepine can compromise the therapeutic effects of oral contraceptives, oral anti-coagulants, beta-blockers, haloperidol and theophylline.

The side-effect profile of oxacarbamazepine is qualitatively similar to that of the parent compound. However, the frequency of the side effects is lower which is one of the major reasons why oxacarbamazepine has been developed as an antiepileptic drug in its own right.

Succinimides

Of the succinimide anticonvulsants, *ethosuximide* is particularly effective in the control of absence seizures. The main side effects of this drug are singultus (hiccups) and sedation at high doses. Hallucinations have also been reputed to occur. Ethosuximide has no beneficial effect in generalized tonic–clonic seizures. A close analogue of ethosuximide, *methsuximide*, has largely been reserved as a "second-line" drug and as a useful adjunct to the treatment of refractory partial complex seizures. It is, however, more sedative than ethosuximide.

Diphenylhydantoin

Diphenylhydantoin is the most widely used drug in the treatment of all types of partial seizures, generalized tonic–clonic seizures and status epilepticus. It is relatively non-sedative. There is a good correlation between the increase in the blood levels of the drug and the occurrence of neurotoxicity, concentrations about $25 \mu g/ml$ usually being associated with such symptoms.

The well-known dose-related side effects include gingival hyperplasia (due to altered collagen metabolism), cerebellar-vestibular effects (nystagmus, vertigo, ataxia), behavioural changes (confusion, drowsiness, hallucinations), increased seizure frequency, gastrointestinal disturbances (nausea, anorexia), osteomalacia (due to reduced calcium absorption and increased vitamin D metabolism) and megaloblastic anaemia (due to reduced folate absorption).

The main problem arising from the routine use of diphenylhydantoin relates to its non-linear elimination kinetics. This means that as the blood concentration is increased the apparent half-life is progressively prolonged. Thus at the therapeutic range of $10–20 \mu g/ml$ blood, the half-life is in the range of 6 to 24 hours, but it increases to 20–60 hours when the blood concentration exceeds $20–25 \mu g/ml$. Furthermore, significant differences in the bioavailability of the oral preparations of the drug have been found, leading to a variation in the time of peak drug concentration from 3 to 12 hours. Because of the non-linearity of the drug elimination kinetics, formulations of the drug with different absorption rates are not bioequivalent, so it is important that the patient should always be maintained on the same form of the drug. About 90% of the drug is bound to serum proteins (mainly serum albumin) which is an important consideration if the patient is given other drugs concurrently that may compete for the protein binding sites. The main metabolite of diphenylhydantoin is inactive.

Phenobarbitone and primidone

Phenobarbitone is the oldest anticonvulsant in common use but suffers from a high incidence of behavioural and cognitive effects, particularly in children. While tolerance may develop to the sedative effects of the drug, high blood levels are associated with a measurable deterioration in motor performance, and learning difficulties are likely to occur in children as a consequence of the central depressant properties of the drug. Phenobarbitone has the longest half-life of all the anticonvulsants in common use (30–150 hours).

Primidone has a relatively short half-life (4–15 hours), but it is metabolized to phenobarbitone and phenylethylmalonamide, which prolongs the duration of the anticonvulsant effect.

Sodium valproate

Sodium valproate is useful in the control of most seizure types and has the shortest half-life of the commonly used anticonvulsants (4–15 hours); a slowly absorbed form of the drug, divalproex sodium, is sometimes preferred. Valproate is relatively free from cognitive and behavioural side effects, but alopecia and weight gain frequently occur. The most severe side effect is idiosyncratic hepatotoxicity and pancreatitis, particularly in younger patients. However, these side effects are more frequent in patients taking valproate as a co-medication with other anticonvulsants.

Some novel anticonvulsant drugs

The chemical structure of some of the novel antiepileptic drugs is shown in Figure 12.5.

Clobazam

Mode of action. Clobazam, like most of the benzodiazepines in clinical use, acts as an agonist on the benzodiazepine receptor site and thereby enhances GABAergic transmission. It is uncertain why the action of clobazam differs from the conventional benzodiazepines but it is possible that it could reflect differential binding to the GABA-A receptor sub-units. In addition to its action on GABA receptors, clobazam also reduced voltage-sensitive calcium ion conductance and sodium channel conductance.

Side effects. Because clobazam has been widely used as an anxiolytic, its side effects are well known and essentially similar to those of the other benzodiazepines. Thus sedation, dizziness, ataxia, blurred vision and diplopia are the most commonly reported in epileptic patients. One of the most problematic features of clobazam is its tendency to produce tolerance, an effect which may occur more frequently with clobazam than with the other widely used benzodiazepine, clonazepam. It has been estimated that at least 50% of patients develop tolerance. Tolerance to the sedative effects of the drug develop more rapidly than those to the antiepileptic effect. Clobazam should be considered as adjunctive therapy whenever treatment with a single first-line drug has proven to be ineffective.

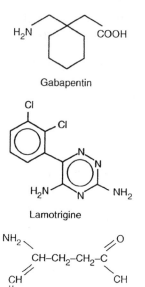

Gabapentin

Lamotrigine

Vigabatrin; gamma-vinyl GABA

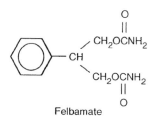

Felbamate

Figure 12.5.   Chemical structure of some novel anticonvulsants.

Felbamate

Mode of action. The specific site of action of felbamate is unknown. There is experimental evidence that felbamate blocks NMDA receptors, but less potently than carbamazepine, ethosuximide, phenytoin or valproate. It also modulates sodium channel conductance but does not enhance GABAergic function. In addition to its protective action against chemically induced seizures felbamate has also been shown to have a neuroprotective action in models of hypoxic ischaemia as induced by bilateral carotid ligation.

Side effects. The most common side effects are insomnia, weight loss, nausea, anorexia, dizziness, fatigue and lethargy. Approximately 12% of patients in the clinical trials of felbamate were reported to discontinue treatment due to such side effects. Cases of aplastic anaemia and hepatic failure have been reported: 14 cases of fatal hepatic failure and 31 cases of aplastic anaemia resulting in 10 deaths. The use of felbamate has been restricted to Lennox–Gastaut syndrome or patients with severe partial epilepsy who have not responded to the first-line medication.

Gabapentin

Mode of action. This drug, which is a cyclohexone analogue of GABA, was originally synthesized in the hope that it would act as a central agonist of GABA receptors which could readily cross the blood–brain barrier. Its efficacy in the treatment of drug-resistant partial and secondary generalized epilepsy clearly points to its brain penetration but there is no evidence that it directly affects GABA receptors. There is evidence that it increases the concentration of GABA in the brain of epileptic patients and some experimental evidence that it is a weak inhibitor of GABA transaminase and that it slightly enhances GAD, the main synthesizing enzyme of GABA. There is evidence of specific gabapentin binding sites within the brain; there is evidence that it binds to a calcium channel receptor in the neocortex and hippocampus.

More recently, clinical evidence has been obtained that gabapentin has analgesic activity in patients with neuropathic pain states of varying origin. These include postherpetic neuralgia and diabetic neuropathic pain. The mechanism whereby gabapentin acts as an analgesic is unknown but it seems possible that its action on N-type calcium channels could be responsible as behavioural and electrophysiological studies have shown that drugs blocking these channels reduce the effects of sensory stimuli after nerve injury and tissue damage.

Side effects. These include somnolence, dizziness, ataxia, nystagmus, headache, tremor, fatigue, diplopia and nausea. However, few potentially serious side effects have been reported.

Gabapentin is a useful drug in the treatment of partial and secondary generalized tonic–clonic seizures. Unlike most of the other antiepileptic agents in current use, gabapentin has an excellent pharmacokinetic profile due to its lack of protein binding, and lack of metabolic drug interactions. However, its absorption is erratic and it has only relatively modest efficacy at least in lower doses. It is ineffective in generalized seizure disorders and in myoclonus.

Lamotrigine

Mode of action. One unwanted side effect of phenytoin is its antifolate action. This stimulated research into the development of pyrimethium compounds which lacked the antifolate action of phenytoin but maintained its antiepileptic potential. This resulted in the synthesis of lamotrigine which was subsequently found to be effective in the treatment of partial and generalized epilepsy and in absence seizures.

Experimental studies showed that lamotrigine reduced the release of glutamate, and to a lesser extent GABA, which could be induced in brain slices by the sodium channel activator veratridine. It would now appear that the primary action of lamotrigine is in blocking the sodium channels in a use-dependent manner in a somewhat similar fashion to phenytoin. However recent experimental studies have shown that phenytoin is particularly effective in reducing repetitive firing of neurons induced by a direct current and in reducing the EPSPs induced by the direct application of glutamate, whereas lamotrigine was active against those EPSPs induced by corticostriatal tract stimulation. This suggests that lamotrigine may act *in vivo* by reducing the release of glutamate. In experimental seizure models, lamotrigine has a similar profile to phenytoin and carbamazepine.

Side effects. The most common side effects are headache, nausea and vomiting, diplopia, dizziness, ataxia and tremor. There are also reports that lamotrigine can cause such psychiatric side effects as aggression, agitation, confusion, hallucinations and psychosis, some of these effects possibly being associated with a reduction in the glutamatergic system. Rashes are a frequent side effect, occurring in up to 5% of patients. Usually rashes are mild but occasionally can be severe and amount to a Stevens–Johnson syndrome. The severe rash occurs more commonly in children.

Levetiracetam

Mode of action. Initially the experimental studies were undertaken on the racemic mixture which contained the R- and the S-enantiomers of etiracetam. Only the S-enantiomer was shown to have antiepileptic potential in a wide range of animal models of epilepsy. It was shown to be particularly active in the kindling models but the precise action of this drug at the cellular level is uncertain.

Side effects. Detailed safety studies show that levetiracetam is well tolerated, the most frequent side effects reported being somnolence, asthenia and dizziness. To date, levetiracetam would appear to be a highly effective new antiepileptic drug with an excellent safety and tolerability profile. Few drug interactions have been reported so far. The efficacy and safety of the drug have been established as add-on therapy for refractory partial onset seizures with or without secondary generalization and there is now evidence of its efficacy in monotherapy.

Piracetam

Mode of action. Piracetam is a drug with an unusual history. It was initially developed as a memory enhancing drug for use in age associated memory impairment and in the early stages of dementia. However, the efficacy of piracetam has proven to be contentious and it has not been licensed for such indications in either the UK or the USA. In 1978 the antimyoclonic effect of piracetam was demonstrated. This property has since been verified in several clinical trials. Levetiracetam is closely related chemically to the L-isomer of piracetam, but unlike piracetam it has a broader spectrum of action. The precise mode of action of piracetam is uncertain but there is experimental evidence that it acts as a metabolic stimulant that increases cerebral metabolism and the synthesis of ATP. How this relates to its antimyoclonic action, if at all, is unknown.

Side effects. Piracetam is well tolerated and there is a low incidence of reported side effects. Those that do occur, at a frequency of less than 10%, include dizziness, insomnia, nausea, gastrointestinal discomfort, weight gain, drowsiness and agitation. Piracetam is indicated only for the treatment of myoclonus, particularly cortical myoclonus. It is used as a second-line drug for patients who are resistant to valproate or the benzodiazepines.

Tiagabine

Mode of action. Tiagabine increases the brain GABA concentration by inhibiting the GABA transporter-1, one of at least four different types of specific transporters which are responsible for the reuptake of the inhibitory transmitter into neurons and glia. The action of tiagabine on the GABA transporter is reversible and its affinity for the glial transporter is greater than for the neuronal transporter. Tiagabine has little effect on other neurotransmitter transporters or receptors, neither does it appear to have an effect on sodium or calcium channels.

Side effects. Probably as a consequence of its potent action on the GABAergic system, tiagabine has been shown to cause dizziness, asthenia, tremor, depressed mood and emotional lability. Diarrhoea is also a frequent occurrence. Most of these symptoms are of relatively mild intensity.

Tiagabine is used as a second line add-on therapy in refractory patients with partial or secondary generalized seizures.

Topiramate

Mode of action. Topiramate has multiple actions which contribute to its antiepileptic potential. It appears that its most important action is its inhibitory effect on sodium conductance in neuronal membranes, an action which it shares with phenytoin and carbamazepine. It reduces the frequency of action potentials and the duration of spontaneous bursts of neuronal firing. Topiramate also enhances GABA function and, like the conventional benzodiazepines, increases the GABA mediated influx of chloride into neurons. However, unlike the benzodiazepines topiramate does not activate the benzodiazepine site on the GABA-A receptor. Topiramate is unique as an antiepileptic drug in that it inhibits the metabotropic glutamate receptors of the AMPA type. There is also evidence that topiramate has a weak carbonic anhydrase inhibitory action. While this is several orders of magnitude less than that due to acetazolamide, it may contribute to its antiepileptic profile. Probably as a result of its numerous effects on excitatory and inhibitory mechanisms within the brain, topiramate has been shown to be effective in a wide range of experimental models of epilepsy. In addition, no tolerance to the antiepileptic effects of the drug has been reported. It also has some neuroprotective effects as shown in some animal studies.

Side effects. Many of the side effects reported to occur with topiramate have been found in patients receiving other antiepileptic drugs concurrently. Such side effects as ataxia, confusion, dizziness, fatigue, somnolence, memory disturbance, depression and agitation appear to be less frequent in those patients receiving topiramate as a monotherapy. Weight loss has been reported in many patients; this effect may be due to drug induced anorexia. Topiramate has proven efficacious in the treatment of severe epilepsy.

Valproate

Mode of action. Valproate enhances GABA function, particularly at high doses in animal experiments. It also potentiates GABA mediated postsynaptic inhibition and inhibits GABA transaminase and succinic semialdehyde dehydrogenase, thereby reducing the metabolism of GABA. There is some experimental evidence that valproate increases GABA synthesis by stimulating glutamate decarboxylase and reduces excitatory transmission initiated by the amino acid transmitters aspartate, glutamate and gamma hydroxybutyrate by unknown mechanisms. In hippocampal slices, valproate reduces the threshold for calciuim and potassium conductance. However, the relative importance of these different mechanisms to its antiepileptic actions is uncertain.

Side effects. The common dose-related side effects of valproate include nausea, vomiting and gastrointestinal distress; weight gain is frequent (estimated as high as 30%) and may be associated with a drug-induced decrease in the beta oxidation of fatty acids. Sedation is also frequent. Alopecia is an unusual side effect of valproate, possibly caused by an abnormal metabolite. Valproate has a number of metabolically linked side effects due to its action on mitochondrial metabolism. Tĥse changes result in hypocarnitaemia, hyperglycinaemia and hyperammonaemia. Such metabolic effects may be exacerbated by genetically determined enzyme defects. When hyperammonaemia is severe, stupor and coma can occur; patients with existing urea cycle enzyme defects or those with hepatic disease are particularly at risk. Acute liver failure, though rare, can be fatal; it has been most frequently observed in children under the age of 2 years.

Valproate is now the most commonly used antiepileptic drug worldwide. It is the drug of choice in primary generalized epilepsy, particularly in the treatment of generalized absence, myoclonus and tonic–clonic seizures. Valproate is the drug of first choice in atypical absence and atonic seizures, for Lennox–Gastaut syndrome and myoclonic epilepsy.

Vigabactin

Mode of action. Structurally vigabactin is gamma-vinyl GABA and therefore it is not surprising to find that it increases GABA function by inhibiting the action of GABA transaminase in the synaptic cleft by binding irreversibly to the active site on the enzyme surface. The effect of vigabactin on brain GABA function is well established in animal studies and there is now evidence that both the CSF and brain concentrations of this inhibitory transmitter are raised in patients with epilepsy who have been effectively treated with vigabactin. It does not appear to have any actions on other neurotransmitter or ionic processes.

Side effects. Initial animal studies showed that vigabactin caused widespread intramelinic vacuolization but this side effect has not been reported in primate or human studies. Minor side effects include fatigue, drowsiness, headache, dizziness, weight increase, tremor, abnormal vision and double vision. Though rare, psychiatric side effects include depression, confusion and psychosis. A very important side effect of vigabactin is the development of visual field failure. This is usually asymptomatic although in some patients this is associated with a deterioration of the vision. The cause is unknown but there is evidence that the increase in retinal GABA may contribute to the visual defect; the retina has a high density of GABA-C receptors.

Vigabactin is indicated for second-line use in patients with refractory partial epilepsy but, unlike lamotrigine and topiramate, it does not appear to be useful in generalized epilepsies. It is the drug of choice for infantile spasms.

Which type of anticonvulsant should be used for which type of seizure?

This is often a question of clinical choice but the following summary may be of practical use. In the case of a child with infantile spasms the use of adrenocorticotrophic hormone (ACTH) or glucocorticoids would appear to be essential. Similarly ethosuximide has a high degree of specificity for the treatment of generalized absence seizures. However, in the majority of seizure types there is a considerable overlap between the various antiepileptic drugs. Apart from carbamazepine which may be superior to the other drugs for the treatment of complex partial seizures, the choice of drug will largely depend on the tolerance of the patient to the adverse side effects. For example, phenytoin is often unsuitable because of its frequent, and often intolerable, side effects. Teratogenic effects are common with most anticonvulsant drugs although there is some evidence that carbamazepine is less teratogenic than most of these drugs. It should also be emphasized that in pregnancy the metabolism of most anticonvulsants is increased so that the plasma drug concentrations should be monitored if the therapeutic efficacy of the drug is in doubt.

In CONCLUSION, epilepsy is a term used to describe a variety of recurrent symptoms which result from the synchronous or sustained discharge of a group of neurons. It is not clear which specific abnormality in synaptic function is associated with epilepsy, but there is some evidence that an impairment of inhibitory transmission in the neocortex and hippocampus may be primarily involved. The possible causative role of GABA is supported by the fact that many clinically useful anticonvulsants facilitate GABA transmission. Other anticonvulsants may owe their efficacy to their ability to stabilize cation movements across neuronal membranes and/or to affect the phosphorylation of membrane proteins.

With regard to the antiepileptic drugs that are currently available, no attempt has been made to be entirely comprehensive. There are a number of exciting developments in the search for novel anticonvulsants, of which the selective GABA transaminase inhibitor *gamma-vinyl GABA* (vigabatrin) is particularly interesting. However, we must await the outcome of the extensive clinical trials before a proper assessment may be made of its efficacy and lack of toxicity. Another novel approach to the treatment of epilepsy has been to reduce the functional activity of the glutaminergic pathway in the cortical and limbic regions of the brain. *Lamotrigine* has recently been introduced for the treatment of partial seizures and generalized tonic–clonic seizures that are not satisfactorily controlled by standard medication. *Lamotrigine* acts by reducing the excitatory effects of glutamate by acting as an NMDA receptor antagonist. Perhaps the most unique antiepileptic drug to be developed so far is *gabapentin*, the mechanism of action of which still remains elusive.

13 Drug Treatment of Parkinson's Disease

Introduction

Idiopathic Parkinson's disease was first described by James Parkinson in 1817 as paralysis agitans, or the "shaking palsy". It is a relatively common neurodegenerative disease afflicting approximately 1% of all adults over the age of 65. The primary neurological features of the disease include difficulty in walking, a mask-like facial expression, and impairment of speech and of skilled acts such as writing. Without effective treatment, these symptoms progress to a rigid akinetic state in which the patients are incapable of caring for themselves and which inevitably ends in death due to complications of immobility such as pneumonia. There have been major advances in the drug therapy of parkinsonism in recent years which have markedly reduced the morbidity from this disease. A brief history of the treatment of Parkinson's disease is shown in Table 13.1.

Parkinsonism is a clinical syndrome that comprises four main features: *bradykinesia* (a slowness and poverty of movement), *muscular rigidity* (increased resistance of muscles to passive movement), *resting tremor*, which usually disappears during voluntary movement, and *abnormalities in posture and gait*.

It is now widely accepted that the term *Parkinson's syndrome* refers to a collection of neurodegenerative diseases, all of which are characterized by movement disorders. It also applies to drug-induced disorders of the parkinsonian type. A schematic representation of this syndrome is shown in Figure 13.1.

Most of these disorders are related to degenerative processes that are confined to the neuromelanin-pigmented nuclei of the basal ganglia (the substantia nigra), the locus coeruleus and parts of the dorsal vagal nucleus and reticular formation. While the cause of idiopathic Parkinsonism is unknown, neuroleptics, viral infections and metals such as manganese are

Fundamentals of Psychopharmacology. Third Edition. By Brian E. Leonard
2003 John Wiley & Sons, Ltd. ISBN 0 471 52178 7

Table 13.1.   Treatment of Parkinson's disease

- Parkinsonian syndromes described in ancient Egyptian and Indian texts in 1200 BC and 2500 BC respectively. Latter describe the beneficial effect of a herb rich in L-dopa

- 1817 – John Parkinson described the essential symptoms of the disease

- Later Charcot described the beneficial effects of Belladona alkaloids

---

known to precipitate non-degenerative forms of the disorder. In addition to defects of movement, Parkinsonian patients often show symptoms such as depression and lack of concentration, an inability to associate ideas, a tendency to perseveration and a general slowness of thought which may progress to a true dementia. Abnormal endocrine function, involving for example prolactin and growth hormone secretion, has also been reported to occur in this disorder. A summary of the possible causes of Parkinson's disease is shown in Table 13.2.

Idiopathic Parkinsonism is distinguished from the other syndromes by the presence of Lewy bodies in the substantia nigra and locus coeruleus, and to a lesser extent in the substantia innominata, hypothalamus, dorsal medulla and sympathetic ganglia (Figure 13.2).

While the aetiology of idiopathic Parkinsonism is unknown, the underlying pathology is established. In 1960, Hornykiewicz demonstrated that patients with the disease showed a deficit in the concentration of dopamine in the zona compacta and substantia nigra, the reduction in the concentration of this transmitter correlating with the severity of the symptoms. Genetic factors do not appear to play an important role, although familial forms of the disease have been described. The lack of genetic factors that predispose patients to the disease has prompted research into possible environmental causes. So far no specific environmental toxins have been identified, but there has been considerable interest in the discovery that N-methyl-4-phenyl-1,2,4,6-tetrahydropyridine (MPTP), a toxic metabolite formed during the synthesis of pethidine, can

Table 13.2.   Causes of Parkinson's syndromes

- Neurodegenerative changes in basal ganglia as in Parkinson's disease, Huntington's chorea, Wilson's disease

- Toxic damage as in manganese, cyanide, carbon monoxide, ethanol, MPTP induced changes

- Infections as in Jakob–Creutzfeldt disease and HIV

- Brain trauma as in head injury

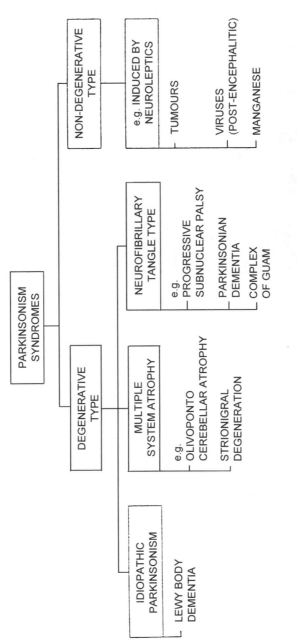

Figure 13.1. Neurobiological diseases in which Parkinsonian symptoms occur.

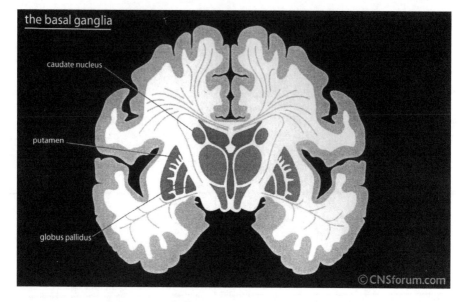

Figure 13.2. Section through the brain showing the location of the areas of the basal ganglia that are dysfunctional in Parkinson's disease.

cause a syndrome in man and primates which is indistinguishable from true Parkinsonism. This experimentally induced form of the disease responds to anti-parkinsonian therapy and has been of considerable importance in the development of a useful animal model of the disease. It has been speculated that substances that are structurally related to MPTP may occur in the environment (e.g. some herbicides can produce such compounds), and the possibility arises that repeated exposure to small quantities of such toxins, combined with the effects of ageing, may be sufficient to cause the disease.

While there is little evidence to suggest that endogenous excitotoxic mechanisms play a role in the neuronal degeneration found in parkinsonism, there is experimental evidence that the excitotoxic action of methamphetamine against dopaminergic nigrostriatal neurons is blocked by the N-methyl-D-aspartate (NMDA) receptor antagonist MK-801. As these neurons degenerate selectively in Parkinsonism it may be postulated that an endogenous excitotoxin is instrumental in causing the disease. Thus it may be speculated that nigrostriatal neurons are sensitive to a sequence of events in which either physical trauma or some toxic agent induces oxidative stress resulting in the release of excitatory amino acids that damage the nigrostriatal dopaminergic cells.

Aetiology of Parkinson's disease

Symptoms of Parkinson's disease only arise when more than 50% of the nigrostriatal dopaminergic cells are lost. By contrast, drug-induced parkinsonism, arising from the chronic administration of classical neuro-leptics such as haloperidol, occurs when about 80% of the dopaminergic receptors (D_2) are blocked. Normal ageing is also associated with loss of cells from the basal ganglia but the rate of cell loss is only about 10% of that found in patients with Parkinson's disease. Thus Parkinson's disease, like any of the dementias, is not an inevitable product of ageing.

The familial form of the disease, in which the age of onset may be as early as 20 years, is rare but studies of the genetic basis have enabled genetic markers to be described. Thus the gene for the protein parkin has been iocated on chromosome 6 and alpha-synuclein on chromosome 4. Locomotor deficits have been found in mice in which alpha-synuclein is dysfunctional but the precise physiological role of this protein is unclear. With regard to parkin, which appears to be abnormal in most patients with juvenile onset Parkinson's disease, it has been shown that this protein is located in the substantia nigra and locus coeruleus where it plays a role in protein degradation. This suggests that a mutation of parkin leads to an abnormal accumulation of proteins in the substantia nigra leading to early apoptosis of these cells.

With regard to the late onset, and common, form of the disease, one of the most popular theories suggests that free radicals accumulate and cause cellular injury leading to neuronal degeneration. This is known as the oxidative stress hypothesis and postulates that as the major pathway leading to the oxidative deamination of dopamine is via MAO-B, hydrogen peroxide is an essential end-product. Hydrogen peroxide then reacts with ferrous or cuprous ions which are present in the substantia nigra to form highly reactive hydroxyl radicals. Dopamine can also react non-enzymati-cally with oxygen to form quinines and semiquinones together with O_2^*, OH^* and hydrogen peroxide. The substantia nigra is a rich source of neuromelanin (the black pigment which gives it the name) which is formed from the auto-oxidation of dopamine. This process also generates the toxic quinines and reactive oxygen species. These three processes may therefore contribute to the destruction of the dopamine-rich cells in the striatum and therefore be responsible for the common form of Parkinson's disease that occurs in the elderly.

The striatal dopaminergic system and Parkinsonism

The classical studies of Hornykiewicz and colleagues in the early 1960s clearly established that the symptoms of Parkinsonism were correlated with a defect in the dopamine content of the striatum. The pigmented neurons of the substantia nigra contain dopamine as the major neurotransmitter, accounting for 80% of the total dopamine content of the brain, and the principal motor abnormalities of the disease occur when the transmitter has been depleted by about 80%. While it is now established that acetylcholine, gamma-aminobutyric acid (GABA), glutamate and a number of neuropeptides (e.g. somatostatin, the enkephalins and substance P) also occur in the basal ganglia, so far only dopamine and acetylcholine appear to be of significance with regard to the drug treatment of this disorder. A simple, but useful, model of basal ganglia function suggests that the neostriatum, containing the caudate nucleus and the putamen, normally contains a balance between the inhibitory dopaminergic and the excitatory cholinergic components. As the cholinergic neurons in the basal ganglia do not appear to be damaged in Parkinsonism, it is postulated that the symptoms of the disease arise as a consequence of the lack of inhibitory control of the excitatory cholinergic neurons. This provides a rational basis for the use of L-dopa (levodopa), the precursor amino acid of dopamine, and of anticholinergic drugs for the symptomatic relief of this disorder. The inter-relationship between the numerous transmitters that play a role in the function of the basal ganglia is shown diagrammatically in Figure 13.3.

Patients with Parkinson's disease show changes in the pre- and postsynaptic dopaminergic neurons which try to compensate for the progressive disappearance of the transmitter. Thus the surviving pre-synaptic terminals become hyperactive, while the postsynaptic D_2 receptors become hypersensitive in an attempt to compensate for the reduced dopaminergic function. These compensatory changes probably account for the relative lack of symptoms of the disease until the dopamine content has been depleted by more than 80%.

In addition to changes in the basal ganglia, a disruption of the mesocortical limbic dopaminergic system also occurs. Thus in Parkinsonism the ventral tegmental area, a dopamine-rich region of the mesocortical system, has been shown to have a reduced dopamine content, as have the terminals that project to the cortex from this region. However, there is no evidence to show that the D_2 receptors in the limbic region become hypersensitive as a consequence of dopamine cell loss. The impaired dopaminergic transmission in the limbic and cortical regions may play a crucial role in the psychiatric symptoms (e.g. perseveration, slowness of thought) that occur in the advanced stage of the illness. Similarly, the hallucinations which occasionally occur in patients on long-term L-dopa therapy may be a consequence of overstimulation of D_2 receptors in these regions of the brain.

Selective degeneration of dopamine neurons in the hypothalamus also occurs, which probably accounts for the rise in the release of prolactin, growth

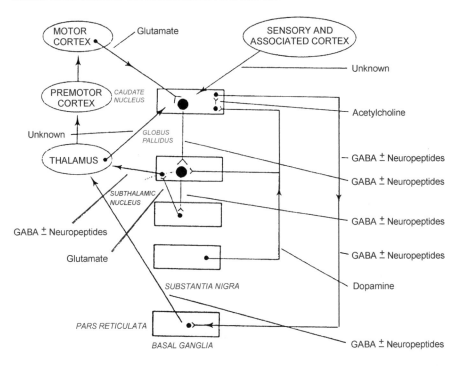

Figure 13.3. Relationship between neurotransmitters in the basal ganglia and the cortex.

hormone and melanocyte-stimulating hormone; dopamine is known to inhibit the release of these hormones under normal physiological conditions.

In addition to the well-established degenerative changes in the dopaminergic system which are the main neuropathological features of Parkinson's disease, it is now known that aminergic and cholinergic ascending subcortical neurons, and peptidergic pathways, are also affected in this disease. Thus lesions of the locus coeruleus occur, with a loss of noradrenaline and its main synthesizing enzyme, dopamine beta-oxidase, in both cortical and subcortical regions of the brain. It would appear that the dorsal bundle from the locus coeruleus is most severely damaged, while the ascending pathways are largely unaffected. In patients at an advanced stage of the disease, cortical alpha$_1$ and beta adrenoceptors show an increase which may be correlated with the onset of some of the symptoms of dementia in these patients. Similarly, a defect in serotonergic transmission has been reported in Parkinsonism, a change that may contribute to the depressive symptoms that often occur in the advanced stage of the disease.

Regarding the cholinergic system, there is evidence that the pathway from the substantia innominata to the cortex degenerates in Parkinsonism, and that the septohippocampal pathway is also functioning suboptimally. As more than 30% of Parkinsonian patients exhibit intellectual deterioration with deficits in cognitive function and memory, it is possible that these cholinergic deficits may account for at least some of the symptoms of parkinsonian dementia.

The enkephalins, somatostatin and substance P all appear to be depleted in idiopathic Parkinsonism, which may be a consequence of neuronal degeneration rather than a cause of any of the symptoms of the disease. Thus these changes do not correlate with the severity of the motor symptoms, although there is some indication that the loss of somatostatin may be associated with intellectual impairment.

Neuroanatomy of the basal ganglia: relevance to Parkinson's disease

There are two main efferent pathways from the striatum to the globus pallidus, the direct pathway, which is a monosynaptic pathway making contact with the internal globus pallidus and to a lesser extent the substantia nigra, and the indirect pathway that indirectly connects to these brain regions via the lateral globus pallidus and the subthalamic nuclei. The internal globus pallidus and, to a lesser extent, the substantia nigra modulate the activity of the circuits via the thalamocortical motor pathways; these pathways are mainly inhibitory in nature.

With regard to the neurotransmitters involved in these circuits, the striatal neurons are mainly GABAergic and they also contain met-enkephalin as a co-transmitter as part of the indirect pathway; D_2 receptors are also present. In the direct pathway, in addition to GABA, dynorphin and substance P act as co-transmitters; D_1 receptors are predominant in the direct pathway.

Activation of the D_2 receptors inhibits the GABA/enkephalin neurons of the indirect pathway, and possibly also the direct pathway. It appears that D_1 receptors could play an excitatory role in the direct pathway.

Normally, dopamine inhibits the indirect pathway to the external globus pallidus which then inhibits the subthalamic nuclei. This system can therefore no longer stimulate the substantia nigra and globus pallidus, therefore leading to a reduction in the inhibitory output from these regions. Under these conditions, it is assumed that the thalamocortical pathway can function, leading to normal movement. The role of the direct pathway is less certain. It appears that dopamine stimulates the neurons of the direct pathway so that the globus pallidus is inhibited and the thalamocortical system facilitated. This view is supported by studies of patients with Huntington's disease in which the GABA/enkephalin neurons of the indirect pathway degenerate. As a consequence the direct pathway dominates, leading to the dyskinesias which characterize patients with the disease.

In Parkinson's disease, in which the deficiency in dopamine is predominant, the inhibitory effect of the indirect pathway is reduced. This leads to a greater inhibition of the external globus pallidus that results in the subthalamic nuclei increasing the activity of the substantia nigra and internal globus pallidus to inhibit the thalamocortical circuit and thereby cause the hypokinesia which characterizes Parkinson's disease.

Because of the key role which dopamine plays in basal ganglia function, and the evidence that its deficiency results in Parkinson's disease, there are three main approaches to the effective treatment of the symptoms of the disease:

(a) By augmenting the action of dopamine.
(b) By modifying the action of other transmitters such as acetylcholine which counteract dopaminergic function.
(c) By using brain grafts, stem cells or neurotrophic factors to replace the redundant dopaminergic neurons.

The relationship between the direct and indirect pathways that affect the striatal–globus pallidus network, together with the neurotransmitters involved, is shown in Figure 13.4.

In addition to dopamine and GABA, excitatory amino acids and adenosine are now known to play an important role in the functioning of the basal ganglia. This raises the possibility that drugs modulating the activities of these transmitters may be potentially useful therapeutic agents. With regard to the excitatory amino acids, the deficiency of dopamine leads to an increased release of glutamate from the corticostriatal tract to the striatum, which may contribute to the symptoms of the disease. Thus glutamate antagonists, acting on either NMDA or AMPA receptors, could provide novel types of anti-parkinsonism drugs. There is experimental evidence from both rodent and primate models of Parkinson's disease that such drugs can alleviate the motor symptoms of the disease.

Adenosine is known to be a neurotransmitter in the striatal–substantia nigra network. It has been shown that activation of the A_2 adenosine receptors increases the release of acetylcholine and reduces that of GABA from the striatum *in vitro*. This could lead to an increase in the activity of the striatal GABAergic neurons. Activation of the adenosine receptors has also been shown to reduce dopaminergic function in the striatum. Thus adenosine A_2 antagonists would be expected to augment dopaminergic inhibition of the GABA/enkephalin neurons and thereby reduce the motor

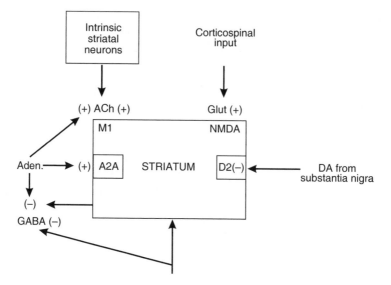

Figure 13.4. Neurotransmitters involved in the control of the striatum. Aden.= adenosine; A2A=adenosine type 2A receptor; M1=muscarinic type 1 receptor; NMDA=N-methyl-D-aspartate receptor.

symptoms. In support of this view, there is clinical evidence that the non-specific adenosine antagonist theophylline augments the effects of L-dopa in the treatment of parkinsonian symptoms. Figure 13.4 summarizes the inter-relationships between these neurotransmitters in the striatum.

In SUMMARY, the Parkinsonian syndromes all show a marked degeneration of the nigrostriatal dopaminergic system which Hornykiewicz has designated the "striatal dopaminergic deficiency syndromes". Nevertheless, other neurotransmitter systems, such as those involving the cortical noradrenergic, serotonergic, cholinergic and somatostatin-containing neurons have also been shown to be defective. Such systems may be responsible for the intellectual and cognitive deterioration which frequently occurs in the advanced stage of the disease.

Drugs used in Parkinson's disease

L-dopa

The discovery that dopamine was depleted in the basal ganglia of patients who suffered from Parkinsonism at the time of death led to the rational development of the therapeutic treatment, namely the use of L-dopa. Since dopamine does not cross the blood–brain barrier, and is rapidly catabolized in the wall of the intestinal tract by monoamine oxidase (MAO) the amine itself cannot be administered. However, L-dopa is rapidly decarboxylated in the brain to dopamine and it was found that high doses of the precursor could reverse many of the symptoms of the disease. Such high doses (up to 10 g were sometimes necessary) caused serious peripheral side effects because up to 95% of the drug was decarboxylated in the peripheral tissues and therefore never reached the brain. To prevent the peripheral catabolism of L-dopa, and to also reduce the dose of the drug that had to be given to produce a beneficial effect, a peripherally acting dopa decarboxylase inhibitor is now routinely combined with the drug. Decarboxylase inhibitors such as carbidopa or benserazide are structural analogues of L-dopa and thereby act as false substrates for dopa decarboxylase. Being charged molecules at physiological pH they cannot cross the blood–brain barrier and thereby permit parenterally administered dopa to reach the brain unchanged. The use of such inhibitors enables the dose of L-dopa to be reduced to a few grams or less, and thereby reduces the frequency and severity of the peripheral side effects which were so apparent in the early stages of its application. It should be noted, however, that an interaction occurs between dopa and pyridoxine due to the fact that pyridoxine is an essential cofactor for the enzyme metabolizing this drug. This can occasionally be a problem in patients who are concurrently taking a multi-vitamin preparation that contains pyridoxine. Despite the progress which has been made in recent years regarding the reduction in the effective dose of L-dopa that is administered, approximately 80% of patients have gastrointestinal disturbances on the drug. These take the form of

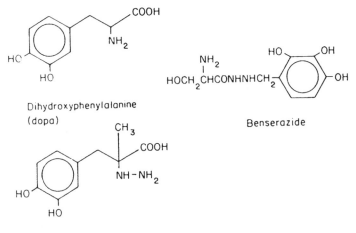

Figure 13.5.   Chemical structure of dopa and two peripheral dopa decarboxylase inhibitors.

nausea and occasionally vomiting. Orthostatic hypotension is also apparent in some patients. The structure of L-dopa and the peripheral dopa decarboxylase inhibitors is shown in Figure 13.5.

Approximately 75% of patients with idiopathic Parkinsonism respond satisfactorily to L-dopa therapy with a reduction in their symptoms of at least 50%. In addition to a beneficial change in their motor symptoms, the mood changes associated with the disease also improve. In some patients, L-dopa has an alerting effect and occasionally more disturbing mental symptoms arise. These take the form of hallucinations, paranoia, mania, insomnia, anxiety and nightmares. Older patients being treated with L-dopa appear to be more prone to these effects. In addition, enhanced libido may occur in male patients, which may be socially unacceptable! Approximately 15% of patients may show such symptoms, which are often controlled by lowering the dose of the drug. The more severe psychotic episodes appear to be more frequent in those patients who are dementing.

Abnormal involuntary movements appear in approximately 50% of patients within the first few months of the commencement of L-dopa therapy, these effects being correlated with the dose of the drug and the degree of clinical improvement. The frequency of the abnormal involuntary movements increases with the duration of administration and can reach 80% of patients after 1 year of therapy. Such abnormal movements are presumed to be due to postsynaptic dopamine receptor hyperactivity and include buccolingual movements, grimacing, head-bobbing, and various choreiform and dystonic movements of the extremities. Tolerance does not appear to develop to these effects and there is no known treatment apart from reducing the dose of L-dopa, a situation which inevitably leads to the likelihood of a return of the Parkinsonian symptoms.

Other side effects involve changes in gastrointestinal function, which may be reduced by increasing the dose of the decarboxylase inhibitor and/or giving the peripheral antiemetic drug domperidone. Postural hypotension arises as a consequence of the increase in the dopamine content of the sympathetic ganglia; in these ganglia dopamine acts as an inhibitory transmitter, so that the decreased ganglionic transmission inevitably leads to reduced peripheral sympathetic tone and a drop in blood pressure.

Figure 13.6 illustrates the relationship between the efficacy of L-dopa therapy and time.

Drug-induced Parkinsonism may arise following the long-term administration of neuroleptics that block central dopamine receptors or reserpine-like drugs that deplete dopamine stores. Because of their mode of action, neuroleptics should never be coadministered to patients being treated with L-dopa or vice versa.

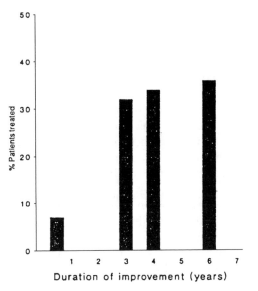

Figure 13.6. Relationship between the efficacy of L-dopa treatment and time. It should be noted that patients who fail to show any improvement (<50%) after short-term (<1 year) treatment with L-dopa are probably not suffering from idiopathic Parkinsonism.

Non-specific MAO inhibitors such as phenelzine, isocarboxazid or tranylcypromine are contraindicated in patients on L-dopa therapy as they are likely to precipitate hyperpyrexia and hypertension. However, recently the selective MAO-B inhibitor *deprenyl* (also called selegiline) has been shown to be a useful adjunct to L-dopa therapy. Deprenyl, by preventing the catabolism of dopamine in the basal ganglia, enables a lower dose of dopa to be administered and also appears to delay the onset of the more serious side effects of dopa. There is also experimental evidence to show that deprenyl can prevent the occurrence of the symptoms of Parkinsonism induced by the neurotoxin MPTP (see Chapter 15). There is evidence that MPTP is converted to its active metabolite the 1-methyl-4-phenylpyridinium ion (MPP$^+$) by MAO-B. By inhibiting MAO-B, deprenyl therefore protects the basal ganglia from the degenerative effects of MPP$^+$. The low incidence of the "cheese effect" and the synergistic interaction between deprenyl and L-dopa suggest that MAO-B type inhibitors will play an increasingly important role in the management of Parkinsonism in the future.

Dopamine receptor agonists

Because of the side effects commonly associated with L-dopa treatment, a number of directly acting dopamine receptor agonists have been tried in the hope that they may combine therapeutic efficacy with reduced adverse effects. *Apomorphine* was one of the first drugs to be tried and while it was shown to have some effect on the symptoms of Parkinsonism, its short duration of action and the frequency and severity of its side effects precluded its further use. Of the more recently developed dopamine agonists, the *ergolines* have received particular attention. These drugs include *bromocriptine, pergolide* and *lisuride*. Like apomorphine, these drugs are not specific agonists for the D_2 type receptors and all have side effects which are related to their ergot type of structure. Nausea and vomiting are particularly prominent side effects, even at low doses, while psychiatric reactions and postural hypotension of the type associated with L-dopa are also features of the ergolines.

Of the ergolines that have been developed, *bromocriptine* has received most attention. Since the first report in 1974 of its use as an adjunct to L-dopa therapy, more than a decade of clinical experience with bromocriptine has failed to establish a distinct role for the drug in the treatment of parkinsonism. Experience with the use of bromocriptine alone in newly diagnosed cases is even more limited. Unacceptable adverse reactions are frequent and even in those patients who can tolerate the gastrointestinal side effects the beneficial effects decline rapidly. It seems unlikely that the rapid onset of tolerance to the therapeutic effects is only due to changes in dopamine receptor sensitivity, as L-dopa is generally effective in patients who cease to respond to bromocriptine. It is also of interest that the abnormal involuntary movements which frequently occur following dopa therapy are seldom found after treatment with the ergolines. The reason for this is unknown but may be associated with differences in the action of these drugs on dopamine receptor subtypes. Bromocriptine, for example, acts as a partial agonist at D_1 receptors and as a full agonist at D_2 receptors. Whether the development of a specific D_2 agonist will combine therapeutic efficacy with a reduced frequency of side effects remains to be seen. The structure of some of the ergolines that have been used in the treatment of parkinsonism is shown in Figure 13.7.

Amantadine

This is an antiviral agent which was accidentally discovered to be of some value in the initial treatment of Parkinson's disease. While the precise mechanism of action of this drug is uncertain, there is experimental evidence to show that it increases the release and synthesis of dopamine and inhibits its reuptake, thereby facilitating the action of the neurotransmitter in those dopaminergic terminals that are still able to function. It has been found that patients soon develop a tolerance to the beneficial effects of the drug, which has largely precluded its long-term use.

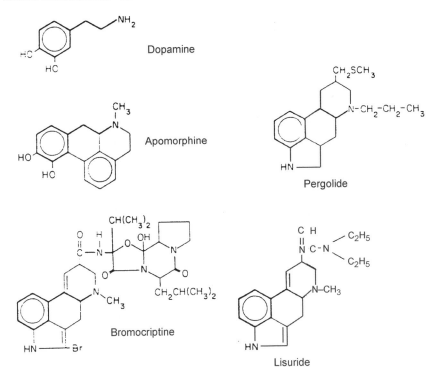

Figure 13.7. Chemical structure of some ergolines that have been or are currently used in the treatment of Parkinsonism. The outline structure of dopamine is also given to show why these drugs act as dopamine receptor agonists. The extended side chains in lisuride may also account for the action of the drug on 5-HT (particularly 5-HT$_2$) receptors. The hallucinogenic effects of lisuride may be attributed to its action on central 5-HT$_2$ receptors.

Anticholinergic drugs

These drugs, initially as the crude extract of *Atropa belladonna* and more recently as specific anticholinergic drugs such as *benztropine* or *biperiden*, have been used for over a century to reduce the tremor seen in patients with Parkinsonism. The mechanism of action of these drugs lies in their ability to reduce the functional activity of the excitatory cholinergic system in the basal ganglia; centrally acting anticholinesterases such as physostigmine are known to exacerbate the tremor associated with the disease.

In the past 40 years a wide variety of synthetic and semi-synthetic anticholinergic agents have been developed for their selectivity in blocking muscarinic receptors in the brain (see Figure 13.8 for the structure of some

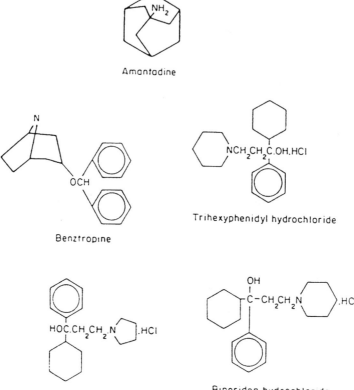

Figure 13.8. Chemical structure of amantadine and of centrally acting anti-cholinergic agents used in the treatment of Parkinsonism. The antiviral compound amantadine is a dopamine-releasing agent with some anticholinergic activity.

of those in current clinical use), but all are associated to some degree with the typical peripheral anticholinergic effects of blurred vision, dry mouth, urinary retention and constipation. The popularity of *benzhexol* lies in its additional ability to inhibit striatal dopamine reuptake.

The anticholinergic agents attenuate the tremor associated with Parkinsonism and relieve the muscular rigidity, but have no effect on the akinesia. This suggests that the features of increased tremor and rigidity are the result of disinhibited cholinergic efferent activity, whereas the negative symptoms of reduced motor function correlate with the dopamine deficiency. There is evidence of tolerance development after several years of treatment with these drugs, so that their use is largely restricted to the more acute phase of the disease.

Table 13.3. Drugs used in the treatment of Parkinson's disease

Mechanisms of action	Drugs
L-dopa	Levodopa, levodopa+carbidopa, levodopa+ benserazide, levodopa+carbidopa (controlled release formulation), levodopa infusion
Direct-acting dopamine receptor agonists	Apomorphine, bromocriptine, lisuride, pergolide
Dopamine releasing agent	Amantadine
Monoamine oxidase B inhibitor	Selegiline (deprenyl)
Centrally acting anticholinergic drugs	Benzotropine, trihexyphenidyl, procyclidine
Free radical scavengers (of doubtful clinical efficacy)	Ascorbate; tocopherol

In addition, antidepressants are sometimes necessary to reduce the depressive symptoms which frequently occur in these patients.

It must be stressed that elderly patients are particularly sensitive to the anticholinergic effects of drugs, whether they be tricyclic antidepressants, phenothiazine neuroleptics or central anticholinergics. Such drugs can cause toxic confusional states and impaired memory and intellectual function; these effects are particularly apparent following long-term therapy. For this reason, such drugs should only be used sparingly in the elderly and then only when other therapeutically effective agents cannot be used.

Table 13.3 summarizes the drugs which have been used to treat the symptoms of Parkinson's disease.

Limitations in the use of L-dopa in the treatment of parkinsonism: the "on-off" phenomenon

The combination of L-dopa with a peripheral dopa decarboxylase inhibitor is generally considered to be the most effective therapy for idiopathic parkinsonism. A major controversy concerns the timing of the initiation of drug treatment. Some investigators favour delaying treatment for as long as possible since there is evidence that drug-induced dyskinesias and fluctuations in response to treatment (the "on-off" phenomenon) are related to the early initiation of drug treatment. However, there is increasing clinical evidence that the dyskinesias and fluctuation in treatment response are a reflection of the degenerative changes caused by the disease. It has also been shown that there is a reduction in the mortality and a slower progression in the severity of the disease when treatment is initiated relatively soon after the disease has been diagnosed.

Two main phases of treatment with L-dopa have been distinguished. The initial induction phase lasts several weeks and is followed by the maintenance phase. During the induction phase the daily dose of L-dopa should be increased slowly to minimize the likelihood of side effects. However, following 2–5 years' successful therapeutic control of the symptoms, the dyskinesias and abnormal involuntary movements often occur. Such changes are attributed to striatal dopamine receptor super-sensitivity, possibly occurring as a consequence of denervation of the dopaminergic tracts in the nigrostriatal area. When they occur, the dyskinesias are superimposed on the waxing and waning of the response to treatment, and may be associated with the peak therapeutic effect (called "peak-dose" dyskinesia). Eventually the patient becomes unable to achieve any degree of mobility without experiencing some involuntary movement. Dietary factors and erratic gastric emptying may further complicate the picture so that the response to L-dopa may seem random and unrelated to the time of administration of the drug. At this stage, the patient may suddenly switch from a state of good therapeutic control to severe parkinsonism (the "on-off" effect); such a situation occurs in up to 50% of patients after 5 or more years of treatment and may eventually occur in 90% of patients after more than a decade of treatment.

The fluctuating motor performance can be partly explained by the pharmacokinetics of L-dopa. Most patients have a critical plasma dopa concentration above which the therapeutic effects are apparent. Presumably this reflects the dose necessary to raise the concentration of dopamine in the brain. However, as the degeneration of the nigrostriatal pathway continues, the capacity of dopaminergic neurons to synthesize and store the amine becomes progressively compromised so that the neurons that continue to function are increasingly dependent on the presence of L-dopa for immediate brain dopamine synthesis. Fluctuations in motor performance therefore reflect this dependency on plasma dopa. Thus the beneficial effects of L-dopa decrease with the increasing severity of the motor symptoms, despite the fact that the elimination half-life is relatively uniform throughout the period of treatment. This means that lowering the dose of L-dopa administered in an attempt to reduce the dyskinesia will inevitably lead to a shortened duration of therapeutic effect.

Management of the motor fluctuations has largely been concentrated on attempts to prolong the duration of action of the drug, either by the use of controlled release preparations to obtain "smooth" concentration–time curves or by combining dopa with deprenyl or bromocriptine. Long-term (about 16 years) follow-up studies of patients have shown that the mean "functional" status of the patient approaches pretreatment levels after 5 years, and by 16 years all surviving patients were functionally less well than at the initiation of therapy. From such studies it may be concluded that

L-dopa does not cure Parkinson's disease but does produce significant relief for many years and still remains the most effective treatment for the illness.

Use of brain transplants

Foetal mesencephalic tissue has been implanted in the striatum of patients with the juvenile form of Parkinson's disease and has been shown to develop functional axons; this has enabled the dose of L-dopa to be reduced. Both imaging and pharmacological studies have now shown that functional dopaminergic neurons can develop in the brain of the patient following tissue transplantation. However, a major ethical objection has been raised to such transplants as six to seven foetal brains are required to obtain sufficient tissue. In addition, only about 20% of neurons survive transplantation. The ethical problem may be overcome by using brain transplants from domestic animals such as pigs. Such xenotransplants have been shown to survive in the human brain but the main problem with the extensive use of such transplants is the possible spread of viruses and prion infections.

Other techniques which may overcome the need for foetal tissue or xenotransplants include the implantation of mesencephalic dopaminergic neurons grown in cell culture or, alternatively, the use of stem cells of human origin.

There is evidence that trophic factors, which are essential for the development of neurons and their maintenance in the adult brain, could play a role in delaying the degenerative changes in the brain of a patient with Parkinson's disease. Such trophic factors include the epidermal growth factor, basic fibroblast growth factor, brain-derived neurotrophic factor and the glia-derived neurotrophic factor. These factors have been shown to enhance the survival and growth of dopaminergic neurons in cell culture. The glia-derived neurotrophic factor appears to be particularly specific in stimulating the growth of dopaminergic neurons. It is now possible to add the appropriate factors to fetal dopaminergic cells prior to their transplantation to ensure their long-term viability and differentiation.

In CONCLUSION, the last 30 years have witnessed many important advances in our understanding of Parkinson's disease. Based on this understanding drugs have been developed that have led to a significant reduction in the mortality of patients with the disease. However, despite these advances there is no evidence that the drugs available prevent the progression of the disease. Perhaps the application of growth factors will provide the clinician with the means whereby this can be achieved.

Huntington's disease (also known as Huntington's chorea)

Huntington's disease is named after a 19th century New York neurologist who studied several families who suffered from a severe, and lethal, motor disorder which appeared to be inherited as an autosomal dominant gene. It was calculated that 50% of the offspring of an affected person have a probability of contracting the disease. The frequency in the general population is 0.01%.

Symptomatically, Huntington's disease is characterized by dyskinesias (choreoform movements) which start with the fingers and then spread to the rest of the body. Akinesia also occurs as a result of the basal ganglia dysfunction. However, unlike most types of Parkinson's disease, Huntington's disease develops during early middle age (30–40 years), it is progressive and results in death in approximately 20 years from the start of the symptoms. In the final years of the disease, the patient suffers severe motor impairment, emotional lability and dementia.

The main neurochemical deficit occurs in the GABA/enkephalin neurons in the striatum, particularly in the neurons that project to the external globus pallidus which forms part of the indirect striatal pathway. As a consequence, the direct pathway, in which the GABA/dynorphin-containing neurons predominate, becomes dominant which provides the neurochemical basis for the dyskinesia. Thus, unlike Parkinson's disease, there is no loss of dopaminergic neurons but a primary deficit in GABA, the opioid peptide and substance P. So far, it has not been possible to counteract the symptoms by replacing the defective neurotransmitters. In the early stages of the disease in which the dyskinesia predominates, antipsychotic drugs blocking the D_2 receptors may offer some relief by reducing the inhibitory input to the GABA/enkephalin neurons and thereby help to restore the balance between the direct and indirect pathways. However, such treatments are usually only marginally effective and there is a possibility that akinesia may be precipitated. Despite some interesting observations in the transgenic mouse model of Huntington's disease, in which such a diverse group of drugs as creatine, monocycline, remacemide (a glutamate antagonist) and co-enzyme Q were shown to slow the symptoms of the disorder, there is no evidence that they are effective in patients.

With regard to the pathological basis of Huntington's disease, research has been focused on the role of the mutant huntingtin protein. Huntingtin is associated with the cytoskeleton and the intracellular vesicles; it is enriched in the striatum. While the precise role of the mutant protein is uncertain, it has been hypothesized that it plays a role in the transcription and regulation of other proteins, abnormal transcription thereby resulting in premature apoptosis. Hopefully recent research into the transgenic mouse model, and the effects of subchronic interleukin-1 in the rat, may enable a better understanding of the pathology of the disorder to be obtained. It is not without interest that the polyunsaturated fatty acid eicosapentaenoic acid has been shown to attenuate the symptoms of the disorder not only in the animal models but also in patients. This finding, if replicated in controlled trials, could provide a new insight into the cause, and treatment, of Huntington's disease.

14 Alzheimer's Disease and Stroke: Possible Biochemical Causes and Treatment Strategies

Introduction

Alzheimer's disease is the most common dementing disease in the industrialized countries affecting approximately one in five persons over the age of 80 years. It is characterized by memory loss, personality changes and signs of cortical malfunction such as apraxia, aphasia and agnosia. Substantial pathological changes have been found in cortical and subcortical areas, including neurofibrillary tangles and amyloid-containing neuritic plaques. The hippocampus appears to be particularly vulnerable to such changes, which probably accounts for the gross disturbance in memory function that occurs early in the onset of the disease.

Alzheimer's disease was first described in 1907 by Alois Alzheimer who identified and described the presence of numerous *neurofibrillary tangles* in the brain of a 51-year-old woman who had suffered from progressive dementia over a number of years. These neurofibrillary tangles were predominantly found in the hippocampus, amygdala, nucleus basalis, hypothalamus and several other subcortical structures. Further studies clearly showed that the density of those tangles correlated with the degree of cognitive impairment shown by the patient prior to death. The other characteristic pathological feature of the brain of the patient with Alzheimer's disease is the presence of *senile* or *neuritic plaques*. Such structures are large, lie within the neurophil, and occur throughout the neocortex and hippocampus. The density of these plaques is also correlated with the degree of cognitive impairment shown by the patient at the time of death. In addition to the tangles and plaques, *Hirano bodies* are also a feature of the post-mortem brain of the Alzheimer patient. These bodies were first

Fundamentals of Psychopharmacology. Third Edition. By Brian E. Leonard
© 2003 John Wiley & Sons, Ltd. ISBN 0 471 52178 7

described in the brains of patients suffering from a rare dementing disease called amyotrophic lateral sclerosis of Guam (Figures 14.1, 14.2).

Gross changes are also apparent in the brain of an Alzheimer's patient, but do not appear to be specific for Alzheimer's disease. Thus the brain weight is reduced compared with age- and sex-matched non-demented indivi-duals, although it must be emphasized that there is considerable overlap

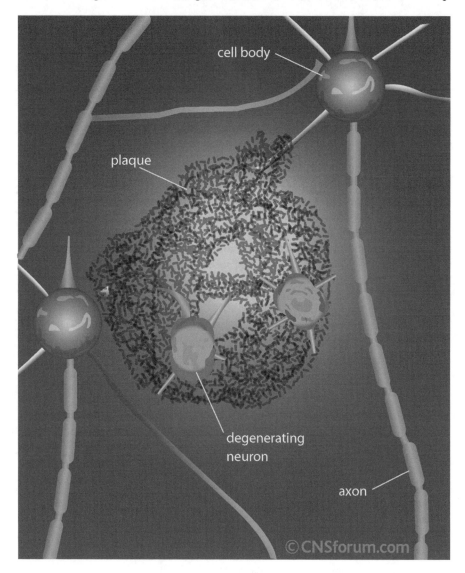

Figure 14.1. Diagrammatic representation of a β-amyloid protein plaque.

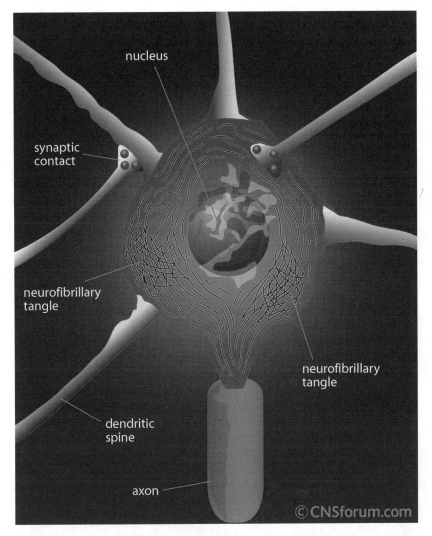

Figure 14.2. Diagrammatic representation of neurofibrillary tangles in neuron.

between the controls and demented patients. A moderate degree of lateral and third ventricular dilatation is also apparently associated with a thinning of the cortex. Loss of the underlying white matter also occurs in the brains of Alzheimer's patients. In contrast, the deeper subcortical nuclei of the basal ganglia and thalamus appear to retain their normal appearance (Figure 14.3).

Although it has been postulated that the presence of amyloid protein in the Alzheimer's brain could be specifically involved in the causation of the

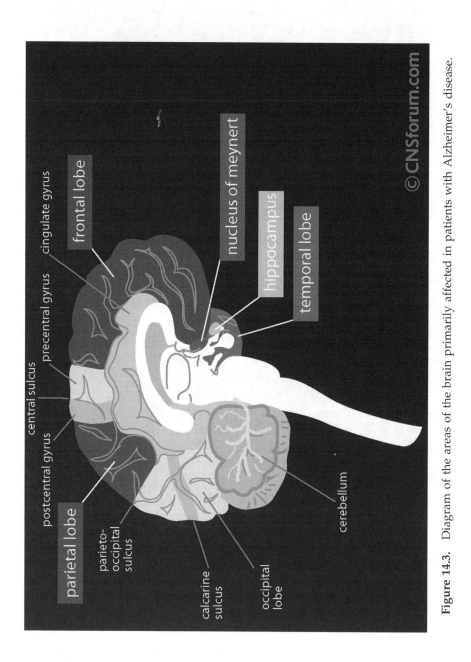

Figure 14.3. Diagram of the areas of the brain primarily affected in patients with Alzheimer's disease.

disease, there is now evidence that amyloid deposits also occur in the brains of patients with other types of neurological disorder and it is therefore doubtful whether amyloid protein alone is a primary pathogenetic factor for this illness. However, it is also possible that the structure of the amyloid protein in the brain of the Alzheimer patient differs from that in the brain of the aged individual.

By definition, Alzheimer's disease (AD) is a progressive, degenerative disease of the brain that is the most common cause of dementia in the elderly. Post-mortem studies have demonstrated that the most common pathological features of AD are neuritic plaques and neurofibrillary tangles. By definition, all patients with AD must have dementia, a progressive loss of memory and at least one other defect in cognitive function which is sufficient to impede daily functioning. A clinical diagnosis of AD can only be made with certainty when no other situation can account for the progressive cognitive impairment.

Neuropathological and genetic changes

As specific markers of AD have not so far been identified before post-mortem investigations have been undertaken, the accurate diagnosis can only be made retrospectively. However, even then no single neuropatho-logical lesion is definitive and the presence of multiple lesions, their density relative to the age of the patient and the absence of lesions characteristic of other types of dementia are essential for an accurate diagnosis. A gross decrease in brain weight and changes in gross brain structure (widening of the sulci and significant subcortical atrophy), while present to a greater extent than in elderly control subjects, are not considered to be specific for AD. However, atrophy of the cortex with a significant cell loss (40%+) together with a cell loss from subcortical structures such as the main cholinergic nuclei (the nucleus basalis of Meynert) are significantly correlated both with the major symptoms of dementia and with the cognitive deficits.

Neuronal loss and degeneration are associated with a significant decrease in markers of synaptic density. Thus the synaptophysin immunoreactivity in the frontal and parietal cortices and hippocampus is one of the strongest markers of the severity of dementia in AD. Such changes reflect neuronal degeneration but also the loss of presynaptic terminals together with the loss of neuropeptide and monoamine containing vesicles. The most prominent lesions associated with AD are the neuritic plaques (NPs) and the neurofibrillary tangles (NFTs) but it must be emphasized that these structures are not exclusively associated with AD as they frequently occur not only in elderly persons with normal brain function but also in other types of neurodegenerative disease.

NPs are extracellular protein deposits of varying size containing a core of amyloid beta peptide (Ab) together with neuritic inclusions. Ab is a 40–43 amino acid peptide formed from an amyloid precursor protein (APP) by two cleavage steps. The secretases (termed alpha, beta and gamma) are the enzymes involved in the cleavage of APP; gamma secretase is the enzyme primarily involved in the formation of Ab. There is evidence that presenilin-1 may be an essential component in the action of gamma secretase (Figure 14.4).

Evidence linking the abnormal breakdown of APP to the pathogenesis of AD has been provided by mutations of the APP gene and also the gene encoding the presenilins-1 and 2, these abnormalities inevitably being associated with AD. Furthermore, studies in transgenic mice have demonstrated that the introduction of such mutations leads to the deposition of Ab plaques that are associated with the memory deficits in the animals. With regard to the relationship between the accumulation of Ab and AD, it is now apparent that the increase in the density of NPs and Ab immunoreactivity that occurs even in the mildest cases of the disease are important; these changes are reported to occur before the patients meet the threshold criteria for the definitive diagnosis of the disease.

Insoluble clusters of misfolded ("sticky") proteins are a common feature of AD and related dementias but the link between the accumulation of such proteins and the symptoms of the disease has been uncertain. Recently, however, Walsh and coworkers have suggested that such protein aggregates are inherently neurotoxic. These investigators have shown that whereas natural proteins adopt a characteristic three-dimensional structure on the basis of their amino acid composition with the hydrophobic residues being hidden within the molecule, in some cases these groups are exposed on the surface of the protein where they assemble into insoluble aggregates. On reaching a certain size they become the Ab plaques seen in AD. However, it has long been established that the symptoms of dementia in AD do not correlate with the density of amyloid plaques but do correlate with the quantity of the soluble, neurotoxic form of Ab. Experimental studies have now shown that it is this form of Ab that inhibits long-term potentiation, the molecular basis of memory formation, in the hippocampus.

NFTs are the second most important pathological feature of AD. These consist of paired helical filaments that are abnormal aggregates of abnormally folded, or hyperphosphorylated, forms of the microtubule associated tau protein. The progressive increase in the distribution of NFTs throughout many regions of the brain is related to the stages in the development of the disease. Thus the NFTs first appear in the entorhinal

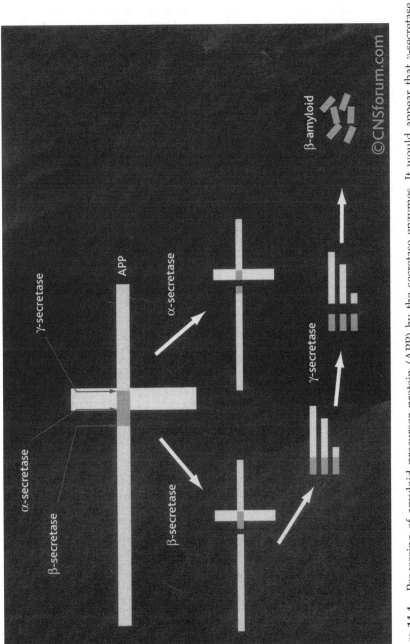

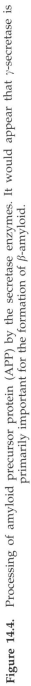

Figure 14.4. Processing of amyloid precursor protein (APP) by the secretase enzymes. It would appear that γ-secretase is primarily important for the formation of β-amyloid.

cortex followed by the hippocampus and eventually affect the complete cortex. Such changes reflect the duration and severity of the disease. Figure 14.5 illustrates the role of tau protein in the formation of NFTs in the axon and cell body.

As stated above, the main pathological features of Alzheimer's disease are the amyloid deposits around blood vessels and in many brain areas, intraneuronal neurofibrillary tangles, neuronal cell loss and brain atrophy. Recently four genes have been linked to Alzheimer's disease. Most of the cases of the familial, early onset, form are associated with mutations in genes on chromosomes 1, 14 and 21. The late onset and most common form of the disease which occurs in those of 55+ years, whether of the familial or sporadic type, is linked to a gene on chromosome 19.

Advances in the molecular biology of Alzheimer's disease reflect the application of genetics. The identification of the neuropathological changes in Down's syndrome with mutations on chromosome 21, and the mapping of the amyloid precursor protein (APP) gene, led to the discovery of several mutations of the APP gene in patients with Alzheimer's disease. However, it was found that mutations of the APP gene occurred in fewer than 5% of all familial forms of the disease. Subsequently it was found that the majority (70%) of the familial forms were associated with a gene on chromosome 14. This was subsequently found to be the presenilin-1 gene; a locus for the presenilin-2 gene was also found on chromosome 1.

The presenilins code for a seven-membrane protein, similar to G protein coupled receptors, but the precise function of these proteins is unknown. However, it is known that they resemble two proteins found in the nematode *Caenorhabditis elegans*. This is a microscopic organism containing about 100 neurons and a source of major interest to molecular biologists as it has enabled a functional link to be made between the genetic structure and the biochemical and behavioural changes. It would appear that the presenilin-type proteins in *C. elegans* play a role in intracellular protein trafficking and may therefore be important in apopotosis (programmed cell death) and in the processing of beta amyloid protein.

The mutation of APP and the presenilins account for most early onset, hereditary Alzheimer's disease. With regard to the common, late onset form of the disease, it appears to be highly associated with the apolipoprotein E_4 allele on the long arm of chromosome 19. The cholesterol binding protein $ApoE_4$ is however neither necessary nor adequate to develop Alzheimer's disease, but it does confer a greater risk for the development of the disease. ApoE is localized in senile plaques and binds to beta amyloid protein. This suggests that it is involved in the processing of APP and in the generation of amyloid plaques. The role of ApoE is summarized in Figure 14.6 and Figure 14.7 summarizes the inter-relationship between the various neuropathological changes associated with Alzheimer's disease.

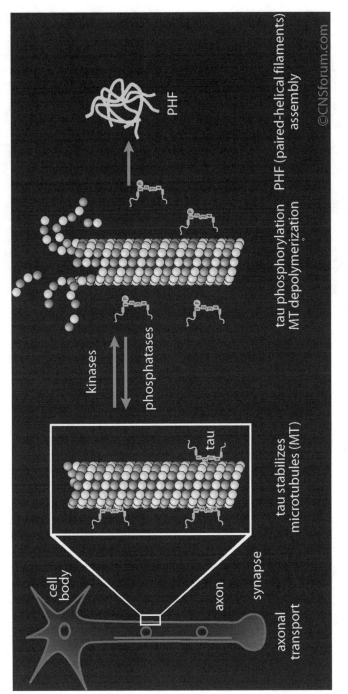

Figure 14.5. Diagrammatic representation of the role of tau protein (a) in the normal axon where it stabilizes the microtubules and (b) in the formation of neurofibrillary tangles (paired helical filaments) in the brain of patients with Alzheimer's disease.

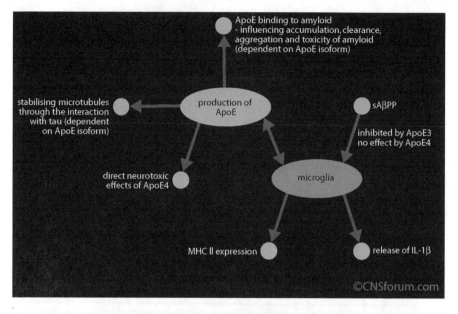

Figure 14.6. The role of apolipoprotein (Apo)E$_4$ in the genesis of plaque and neurofibrillary tangle formation. Note that ApoE$_3$ may have a protective effect against the activation of the microglia and the production of pro-inflammatory cytokines (such as interleukin-1).

Neurochemical changes associated with Alzheimer's disease

The pathological lesions seen in the brain of those with AD are inevitably associated with dysfunctions of the neurotransmitter systems. Of these, deficits in the neocortical cholinergic system have been well established for over a decade but more recently changes in the concentrations of the neuropeptides somatostatin and corticotrophin releasing factor (CRF) have been added to the list. Deficits in the biogenic amines noradrenaline and serotonin have also been reported to occur but a significant decrement in their concentrations in the brains of patients with AD has not been consistently reported. Nevertheless, a functional deficit in such mono-amines may contribute to mood and other psychological changes which are often associated with the condition. In regard to the cholinergic deficit, a decrease in the synthesizing enzyme, choline acetyltransferase, and the degradative enzyme acetylcholinesterase, would appear to play a key role. Such abnormalities have therefore become the most important neurotrans-mitter markers of AD. A compensatory increase in the activity of the choline transporter has also been reported, which presumably occurs in an attempt to compensate for the deficit in the cholinergic function.

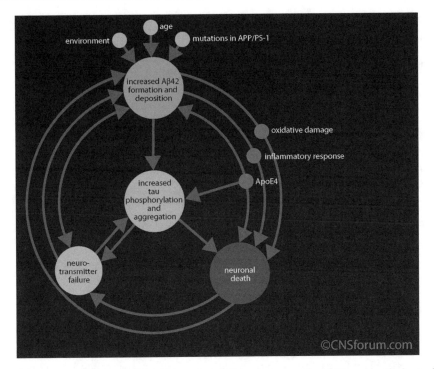

Figure 14.7. Summary of the inter-relationships between the different pathological factors and the cellular changes seen in Alzheimer's disease.

It was following the identification of the cell loss in the nucleus basalis of Meynert, from which the cortical and limbic regions receive their cholinergic inputs, together with the demonstration that the cholinergic system is involved in learning and memory, that the anticholinesterases were developed for the treatment of AD. However, it should not be overlooked that despite the presumed importance of the cholinergic deficit in the terminal stages of AD, there appears to be little change in this system in the mild to moderate stages of the disease.

Deficits in several neurotransmitters, in addition to somatostatin and CRF, have consistently been reported to occur in AD. In addition, the density of CRF receptors appears to be increased while those for somatostatin are either decreased or unchanged. The changes in both the brain and the CSF concentration of CRF would, unlike those in somatostatin, appear to occur relatively early in the disease and correlate with the severity of the condition. Such changes may be reflected in a dysfunctional hypothalamic–pituitary–adrenal (HPA) axis that may play an important role in the pathology of AD.

Table 14.1.   Changes in the neurotransmitters in the brain of an Alzheimer patient

Neurotransmitter system	Changes occurring in Alzheimer's disease
Cholinergic system	Decreased choline acetyltransferase and acetyl-cholinesterase activity in cortex. Reduced choline uptake and acetylcholine synthesis. Loss of cells in nucleus basalis and occurrence of tangles in remaining cells in the brain area
Noradrenergic system	Decreased dopamine beta-oxidase and reduced noradrenaline synthesis. Loss of cells in the locus coeruleus and occurrence of tangles in remaining cells
Dopaminergic system	Slight reduction in dopamine
Serotonergic system	Some reduction in 5-HT synthesis with a loss of cells in the raphé nuclei and the occurrences of tangles in remaining cells
Peptidergic system	Reduction in somatostatin and corticotrophin releasing factor immunoreactivity in cortex. No convincing evidence of change in the concentration of substance P, enkephalins, cholecystokinin, neuropeptide Y, glutamate, aspartate or GABA

There has been considerable interest in the involvement of the major neurotransmitters in the possible aetiology of Alzheimer's disease. Thus it is well established that the nucleus basalis of Meynert and related areas of the basal forebrain show a distinct loss of cholinergic cell bodies in patients with Alzheimer's disease. Similarly, serotonergic neurons of the midbrain raphé area and noradrenergic neurons of the locus coeruleus have been shown to be significantly diminished, particularly in early onset Alzheimer's disease. A summary of the pathological changes in the neurotransmitter systems in the brain of the Alzheimer patient is given in Table 14.1.

The finding that a gross deficit occurs in *central cholinergic transmission* in Alzheimer's disease, the degree of dementia being correlated with the relative deficit in central cholinergic transmission, has led to the suggestion that this is the primary cause of the dementia of Alzheimer's disease. However, it is now increasingly accepted that a cholinergic deficit is unlikely to be the only or indeed a major causative factor. Thus not all patients with the disease, and showing the typical neuropathological changes, show a reduction in the activity of choline acetyltransferase, the enzyme concerned in the synthesis of acetylcholine. Additionally, other patients show normal cholinergic cell numbers in the nucleus basalis of Meynert. More recently it has been shown that patients with a rare neurological disorder, olivopontocerebellar atrophy, exhibit a gross loss of cholinergic neurons in the basal forebrain and yet show no signs of dementia.

It might also be argued that if Alzheimer's disease was primarily due to a cholinergic deficit, it should be possible to correct the deficit by suitable centrally acting cholinomimetic drugs. Despite the numerous studies in which different types of cholinomimetic drugs have been administered, there is no overwhelming evidence to suggest that these drugs have any substantial benefit to the patient (see below). Thus it would appear that, despite the widely confirmed findings that various "classical", peptide and amino acid neurotransmitters are defective in Alzheimer's disease, it is debatable whether a defect in one specific neurotransmitter system is responsible for the clinical signs and symptoms of the disease. There is also some debate about whether the site of the lesion is primarily cortical or subcortical.

The involvement of the excitatory amino acid neurotransmitters, particularly *glutamate*, in post-stroke epilepsy and possibly multi-infarct dementia has led to the suggestion that they may also be involved in the aetiology of Alzheimer's disease. Glutamate is the principal excitatory amino acid neurotransmitter in cortical and hippocampal neurons. In the hippocampus, glutamate has been implicated in memory; it is widely believed that its ability to elicit long-term potentiation is of fundamental importance in memory formation. One of the major excitatory amino acid receptors activated by glutamate is the N-methyl-D-aspartate (NMDA) receptor. Antagonists of the NMDA receptor block the action of glutamate and impair spatial discrimination learning in animals and also memory formation. A disruption in the pre- and postsynaptic excitatory amino acid pathways has been found in patients with Alzheimer's disease. It has been suggested that initial hyperactivity of the glutaminergic input to the hippocampus results in excessive hyperexcitability of the hippocampal cells, leading eventually to cell death.

The primary mechanism whereby glutamate can cause excessive cellular hyperactivity, and ultimately cell death, is via a loss of calcium homeostasis. Calcium ions serve as an intracellular signal that mediates the actions of neurotransmitters and growth factors. The increase in intracellular free calcium is normally transient and is rapidly restored to resting levels by membrane extrusion mechanisms and calcium-binding proteins such as calmodulin. Sustained increases in intracellular calcium, as could occur following excessive glutamate release, result in cytoskeletal disruption, axonal degeneration and cell death.

In addition to glutamate, various growth factors and amyloid have also been shown to destabilize the intracellular calcium concentration and to induce neurofibrillary-like degeneration in cultured brain cells. An attractive feature of the calcium hypothesis of Alzheimer's disease is that it helps to explain the heterogeneity of the disorder. In addition to functional abnormalities in excitatory amino acids, growth factors, amyloid protein, etc., calcium channels and binding proteins may also be involved. It is not without interest that various dietary and environmental factors (such as aluminium) may also contribute to the calcium defect, so leading to the disorder.

It should be emphasized, however, that not all investigators agree that the degenerative changes in cortical neurons are due to glutamate excitotoxicity. Thus, three groups of British and Swedish investigators have suggested that the glutaminergic system is hypoactive rather than hyperactive in Alzheimer's disease. Nevertheless, the development of drugs that block NMDA receptors may be of value in the treatment of multi-infarct dementia, in which there is evidence that excessive glutamate release, with the consequent neuron degeneration, follows the cerebral hypoxia.

It may be concluded that it is not possible at present to identify any one neurotransmitter system as being of primary importance in any of the dementias and that the recorded neurochemical changes are possibly secondary to more fundamental disturbances, the nature of which is unclear. Nevertheless, significant correlations have been shown to exist between neurotransmitter disturbances and behavioural symptoms which may be of value in formulating treatment strategies.

Excitotoxins

The concept of excitotoxicity

The amino acids glutamic and aspartic acids are known to be present in high concentrations in the mammalian brain, where they have been shown to act as excitatory neurotransmitters. Over 20 years ago, it was shown that the systemic administration of glutamic acid to newborn rodents resulted in a destruction of retinal cells and also some cells in the central nervous system. Later studies showed that high oral doses of this amino acid also caused brain damage in primates, such toxic effects being particularly apparent on the postsynaptic dendrosomal membranes where the excitatory amino acid receptors are located. Such findings led to the concept of excitotoxicity and, later, to the view that some neurological diseases such as epilepsy could be a consequence of nerve cell damage due to the excessive release of glutamate within the brain.

At least three types of excitatory amino acid receptors have been identified, termed the NMDA, alpha-amino-3-hydroxy-5-methyl-4-isoxazole proprionic acid (AMPA) and kainate receptors according to their affinity for specific excitatory amino acids (see p. 57). Antagonists of some of these receptor types, such as MK 801 and D-2-amino-5-phosphonopentanoate (AP 5), were then shown to protect neurons *in vivo* against the

Table 14.2. Potencies of some antagonists of NMDA receptors in chick embryo retina *in vitro*

	Potency
Competitive NMDA antagonists	
D-2-Amino-5-phosphonopentanoate (AP 5)	25 μM
D-2-Amino-5-phosphonoheptanoate (AP 7)	75 μM
Non-competitive NMDA antagonists	
MK 801	0.01 μM
Phencyclidine	0.5 μM
Ketamine	5 μM
(+/ −) Cyclazocine	5 μM
(+/ −) N-Allylnormetazocine (SKF 10047)	10 μM
Dextromethorphan	50 μM
Mixed excitatory amino acids	
Cyanonitroquinoxalinedione (CNQX)	50 μM
Kynurenic acid	300 μM
Barbiturates	
Amylobarbitone	50 μM
Thiopentone	200 μM

Potencies of compounds expressed as the minimal concentration (μM) required to provide total protection against the excitotoxic effects of NMDA.

neurotoxic effects of glutamate or NMDA. Table 14.2 lists some of the compounds that have been developed as antagonists of the most important of the excitatory amino acid receptors, the NMDA receptor.

So far, only the non-competitive antagonists of the NMDA receptors such as phencyclidine and MK 801 can readily penetrate the blood–brain barrier and therefore protect animals against the toxic effects of exogenous excitatory amino acids. The barbiturates (e.g. thiopentone) have an additional action in blocking both NMDA and non-NMDA (e.g. kainic acid) receptors and are therefore of some interest as broad-spectrum excitotoxin antagonists, while the quinoxalinedione derivative cyanonitroquinoxalinedione (CNQX) was the first compound to be synthesized that showed a greater potency in blocking non-NMDA excitatory amino acid receptors.

The essential features of the NMDA receptor are illustrated diagrammatically in Figure 14.8. The NMDA receptor controls the opening of the sodium/ calcium ion channel, which may be blocked by dissociation anaesthetics such as phencyclidine and ketamine or by magnesium ions. In addition to glutamate, glycine can also facilitate the opening of the ion channel by activating a strychnine-insensitive receptor site. It should be remembered that in the spinal cord glycine acts as an inhibitory transmitter by acting on a different type of glycine receptor; strychnine causes characteristic convulsions by blocking the action of glycine on these spinal cord receptors. Zinc ions can

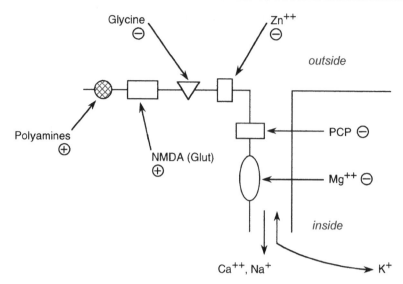

Figure 14.8. Sites of action of endogenous ligands and drugs that modulate the action of excitatory amino acids on the NMDA receptor. Recent evidence shows that glutamate (Glut) and possibly other excitatory amino acids released from presynaptic terminals activate the NMDA receptor site on postsynaptic membranes, resulting in the opening of the Na^+/Ca^{++} channels. Glycine acts on a strychnine-insensitive receptor while polyamines (e.g. spermine and spermidine) also have a modulatory role. Conversely Zn^{++} and Mg^{++} and drugs like phencyclidine (PCP) block the ion channel by acting at various sites on the NMDA receptor complex or the ion channel.

reduce the effects of glutamate and glycine on the NMDA receptor. In view of the complex inter-relationships between the various agonists that act on the NMDA receptor, it may be speculated that a pathological process affecting any of these factors might create an imbalance which leads to a malfunctioning of excitatory amino acid transmission in the brain.

Environmental excitotoxins

It is well established that *monosodium glutamate*, a widely used food additive and major component of soya sauce, can destroy nerve cells when administered orally to young animals. Those neurons lying immediately outside the blood–brain barrier, e.g. in the arcuate nucleus of the hypothalamus, are the most vulnerable. It is therefore possible that ingestion of a diet high in glutamate may contribute to degenerative changes in the brain later in life.

Neurolathyrism occurs in some tropical countries as a result of consuming large quantities of the legume *Lathyrus sativus*, which contains a potent excitatory amino acid analogue that can cause paralysis. In certain South Sea Islands, particularly the island of Guam, ingestion of the seeds of the cycad plant leads to the occurrence of a specific neurological disease with the combined features of amyotrophic lateral sclerosis, Parkinsonism and dementia. The analogue of alanine that causes this neurological disease has been identified.

Excitotoxins and neurodegenerative diseases

Epilepsy and related disorders may arise as a consequence of a dramatic release of glutamate from central nerve terminals. Sustained seizures of the limbic system in experimental animals result in brain damage that resembles that due to glutamate toxicity. Similar pathological changes are seen at autopsy in patients with intractable epilepsy. In animals, such seizure-related brain damage may be reduced by the administration of non-competitive NMDA antagonists (such as MK 801, phencyclidine or ketamine), but it would appear that not all seizure activity is suppressed by such drugs.

The precise mechanism whereby persistent seizure activity results in neuronal degeneration is incompletely understood. It seems possible that repetitive depolarization and repolarization of the nerve membrane eventually leads to an energy-deprived state within the cell, thereby preventing the restoration of the cell membrane potential. Each depolarization will also lead to an influx of calcium ions, and an efflux of potassium ions, which if prolonged can result in cell death. The reduced efficiency of glial cells to remove potassium ions and the ability of high extracellular concentrations of potassium ions to depolarize neurons and cause neurodegenerative changes also play a critical role in causing the degenerative changes that are a feature of status epilepticus and intractable epilepsy.

Hypoxia and ischaemia may also cause neurodegenerative changes in the mammalian brain. In animals, cerebral ischaemia has been shown to cause a marked elevation in the extracellular concentrations of glutamate and aspartate, particularly in the hippocampus. Such pathological changes can be prevented by the prior administration of NMDA receptor antagonists. The hypoxic state results in energy deficiency within the brain, so that the mechanism responsible for the maintenance of transmembrane potentials may become compromised. The net effect of the elevation in the extracellular concentrations of excitatory amino acids could be a failure of magnesium ions to reduce the functional activity of the NMDA receptor. This could result in persistent membrane depolarization, excessive intracellular accumulation of calcium ions and the extracellular accumulation of potassium ions. The movement of sodium ions, accompanied by water, into the cell further compromises cellular function and results in cell death. Somewhat similar pathological changes have been postulated to occur following *brain and spinal cord injury* and in *dementia pugilistica*, a concussive brain injury associated with boxing.

Other neurological diseases in which a disorder of central excitatory amino acid function has been implicated include *Huntington's disease*, *Alzheimer's disease* and *Parkinsonism*. Experimental studies have shown that the injection of excitatory neurotoxins such as kainic and ibotenic acids into the rat brain results in pathological changes that resemble those seen in Huntington's disease. More recently, an endogenous neurotoxin, quinolinic acid, has been found in human brain which, if present in excessive quantities, selectively destroys the striatum but leaves other regions largely unaffected. While it now seems unlikely that quinolinic acid is the endogenous excitotoxin responsible for the pathological changes found in Huntington's disease, it remains a possibility that some other excitotoxin with similar properties and selectivity of action on striatal function may be involved. The possible involvement of excitotoxins in the pathology of Alzheimer's disease and parkinsonism is considered in the appropriate chapters.

Figure 14.9 summarizes the various factors that contribute to cell death following the production of intracellular reactive oxygen species. The possible mechanism whereby β amyloid contributes to apoptosis is illustrated in Figure 14.10.

Inflammatory changes and the role of the immune system

There is increasing evidence that many of the changes in the brain of the patient with AD are the result of inflammatory mediators. The view is supported by the observation that anti-inflammatory drugs have a neuroprotective action. In patients with AD the acute phase inflammatory response is increased, as indicated by a rise in the pro-inflammatory cytokines interleukins-1 and 6 (IL-1, IL-6) and tumour necrosis factor (TNF) alpha, changes which are accompanied by an increase in the plasma of the acute phase proteins alpha-1 chymotrypsin and alpha-2 macroglobulin. The complement system has also been shown to be active in the brain of the AD patient, a change which is associated with the activation of lytic enzymes that damage the neuronal membranes and which may therefore contribute to premature neuronal death. TNF alpha has also been shown to act as a potent neurotoxin when present in excess in the brain. In addition to the inflammatory cytokines, the activity of cyclooxygenase 2, an enzyme which synthesizes the inflammatory mediator prostaglandin E_2 (PGE_2) in the brain, has been shown to be increased in the brain of the patient with AD, thereby adding to the cascade of inflammatory changes.

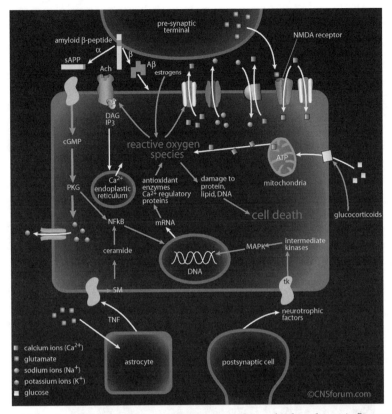

Figure 14.9. Summary of the role of glutamate, β-amyloid and pro-inflammatory cytokines such as tumour necrosis factor (TNF) in the production of reactive oxygen species leading to neuronal death.

Direct evidence for the role of inflammatory processes in the progression of AD has been provided by the study of IL-6 mRNA expression in the hippocampus. Thus a positive correlation has been found between the progression of the symptoms from the moderate to the severe form of the disease and the increase in IL-6 mRNA expression. From these observations it can be concluded that the increase in inflammatory mediators in the brain plays an important, but not the only, part in the development and progression of AD. Thus the deposition of Ab plaques in the cortex, an essential feature of the disease, may precede the changes in neurotransmitter function and the increase in inflammatory mediators. Whichever of these changes is eventually found to be of primary importance, it is now evident that AD is not due to a random failure of neuronal pathways but is the consequence of a systematic and progressive degeneration of different neuronal systems within the brain.

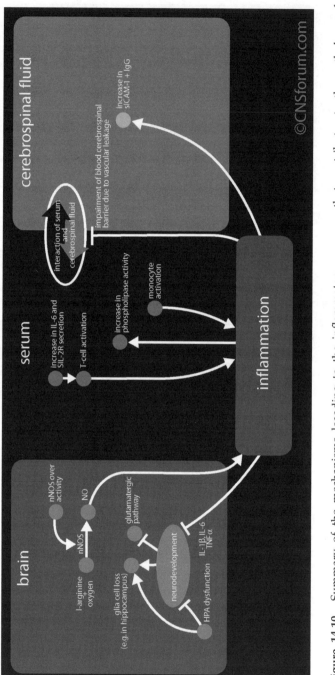

Figure 14.10. Summary of the mechanisms leading to the inflammatory response that contributes to the pathology of Alzheimer's disease.

Figure 14.10 summarizes the mechanisms involved in the inflammatory processes that contribute to Alzheimer's disease (see Chapter 18 for more detailed account of the role of inflammatory changes in diseases of brain function).

Treatment strategies based on correcting neurotransmitter defects

For the past 20 years, an increased understanding of the pathology of AD has led to the development of numerous drugs for the treatment of the disorder. At the present time, there are at least 60 drugs estimated to be in development for the symptomatic treatment of AD, some of which may ultimately be expected to affect the development of the disease. The drugs in current use can be broadly divided into those that are designed to enhance cholinergic function and those that reduce the synthesis of free radicals, the anti-inflammatory agents, the oestrogens and a miscellaneous group of natural products which include the *Ginkgo biloba* alkaloids. In addition, some drugs are in development which are aimed at counteracting the possible causes of neuronal cell loss by counteracting the neurotoxic effects of Ab. These include the inhibitors of gamma secretase and vaccines against Ab. Some of these drugs will now be considered.

Drugs enhancing cholinergic function

The cholinergic hypothesis of AD is based on the loss of histochemical markers of forebrain cholinergic neurons that correlate with diminished cognitive function and with the degree of accumulation of NPs and NFTs. Assuming that AD bore some resemblance to Parkinson's disease, in which dopaminergic agonists correct the endogenous deficiency of striatal dopamine, it was speculated that directly and indirectly acting cholinergic agonists should correct the symptoms of the disorder. In the past decade drug development has therefore largely focused on centrally acting anticholinesterases and, to a lesser extent, muscarinic agonists and acetylcholine releasing agents. Other approaches have included the administration of high doses of acetylcholine precursors (such as lecithin and choline), which have not been shown to be therapeutically effective, and more recently galanin receptor antagonists.

Because of the progressive neuronal loss that occurs in AD, drugs that enhance the endogenous cholinergic system are inevitably limited in their duration of action. However, at post-mortem the M_1 and M_4 type of cholinergic receptors appear to remain intact in patients with AD, which has strengthened an interest in drugs which have direct cholinomimetic effects. The loss of cholinergic tracts in the brain of a patient with Alzheimer's disease is illustrated in Figure 14.11.

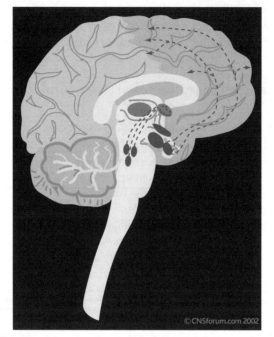

Figure 14.11.   Diagram showing loss of cholinergic tracts in a brain from a patient with Alzheimer's disease.

Anticholinesterases

Tacrine, donepezil, rivastigmine and galantamine are cholinesterase inhibitors which preserve endogenous acetylcholine following its synthesis. The inhibition of the cholinesterase may be either reversible, irreversible or pseudo-irreversible. In addition, the inhibitor may be either competitive or non-competitive for true (acetyl) cholinesterase, pseudo (butyryl) cholinesterase or for both types. Some anticholinesterases also have a weak affinity for the nicotinic cholinergic receptors. These drugs also differ in their pharmacokinetic properties (for example, protein binding, elimination half-life and in their drug interactions).

Tacrine is a non-competitive, irreversible inhibitor of both acetyl and butyryl cholinesterase, with a greater potency for the latter enzyme. Based on the outcome of placebo-controlled, double-blind studies, tacrine was the first anticholinesterase to be licensed for the symptomatic treatment of AD in the United States. The main disadvantage of tacrine lies in its hepatotoxicity (approximately 50% of patients were found to develop elevated liver transaminases which reversed on discontinuation of the drug). Because of such side effects and limited efficacy, tacrine is no longer widely prescribed.

Donepezil is primarily a reversible inhibitor of acetylcholinesterase with a long elimination half-life. It lacks the hepatotoxicity of tacrine but frequently causes nausea, vomiting and diarrhoea. These side effects, together with occasional bradycardia, sycope and changes in the sleep architecture, are directly associated with a central and peripheral enhancement of cholinergic function. At the present time, donepezil is the most widely prescribed anticholinesterase in the United States and Europe.

Rivastigmine is a pseudo-irreversible inhibitor of both acetyl and butyryl cholinesterases. Thus although the drug initially blocks the enzymes, it is metabolized by them thereby giving the drug a relatively short half-life. The top dose is often necessary to achieve therapeutic efficacy, at which dose the central and peripheral cholinergic side effects become apparent.

Galantamine, unlike the other anticholinesterases in clinical use, is derived from the alkaloids from the daffodil and snowdrop family. It is a reversible, competitive inhibitor of acetylcholinesterase with some inhibitory action on butyryl cholinesterase. It is also an agonist at nicotinic receptor sites. Although a clinically effective drug, galantamine frequently causes gastrointestinal side effects.

Other anticholinesterases recently licensed in Europe include metrifonate. This is an irreversible organophosphorus inhibitor of acetylcholinesterase and is a pro-drug for dichlorvos. The development of metrifonate was delayed because some patients developed muscle weakness and a delayed neurotoxicity has been described for compounds that are chemically related to the drug.

To complete the list of anticholinesterases, extended release physostigmine has been shown to have some therapeutic efficacy but has been restricted in its development because of the high frequency of nausea and vomiting.

In addition to their ability to increase the endogenous concentrations of acetylcholine, *in vitro* studies have demonstrated that the anticholinesterases can increase the synthesis of non-amyloidogenic APP and decrease the neurotoxicity of Ab. Regarding the effect of some anticholinesterases on nicotinic receptors, there is evidence that neurodegeneration is delayed, thereby suggesting that such drugs may be neuroprotective. This view has been supported by epidemiological studies in which the incidence of Parkinson's disease has been shown to be lower than expected in cigarette smokers.

Muscarinic receptor agonists

The first generation of cholinomimetics, such as arecoline, bethanecol and pilocarpine, were not designed for the treatment of AD and the results of the early clinical trials were consistently disappointing. In addition to their poor bioavailability and short duration of action, any therapeutic benefits were limited by their cholinergic side effects. The second generation of muscarinic agonists were therefore developed to specifically treat AD. These drugs, exemplified by milameline and xanomeline, have improved pharmaco-kinetic profiles relative to the first generation drugs. Thus in controlled clinical trials xanomeline has shown moderate clinical efficacy but, despite *in vitro* data showing that it was selective for M_1 and M_3 receptors, it still caused mild to moderate parasympathomimetic side effects. Milameline has equal affinity *in vitro* for all five muscarinic receptor subtypes; peripheral cholinergic side effects were clearly evident in the initial clinical trials. Neither of these cholinomimetics has been marketed at the present time.

Despite the theoretical interest in specific nicotinic agonists for the treatment of AD, to date none has reached clinical development.

Anti-inflammatory drugs

Inflammatory processes are well known to be associated with AD. Thus the elevation in circulating pro-inflammatory cytokines, acute phase proteins, complement and the presence of activated microglia have been described in patients with AD. It has also been shown that the complement cascade can be activated by Ab and result in neurotoxic changes. The seminal studies of McGeer and coworkers laid the basis for the preventative strategy for the treatment of AD. These investigators showed that the prolonged use of non-steroidal anti-inflammatory drugs for the treatment of arthritis and related conditions was associated with a significant decrease in the incidence of AD. Studies of siblings who had a differential exposure to anti-inflammatory drugs also showed that the incidence of AD was significantly reduced in those to whom such drugs were administered.

Despite the clinical evidence implicating the involvement of inflamma-tory processes in the pathology of AD, the mechanisms behind the accumulation of inflammatory mediators is complex. Nevertheless, it would appear that cyclooxygenase 2 (COX_2) plays a crucial role. It is known that COX_2 activity is elevated in the brain of the patient with AD and that there is an increased expression of COX_2 mRNA in the frontal cortex of such patients. Furthermore, the severity of the symptoms correlates with both the COX_2 activity and the increased expression of Ab.

A number of anti-inflammatory drugs have now been tested for their therapeutic efficacy in AD. For example, the steroid prednisolone, which is lipophilic, has been administered to patients with AD for up to a year but the results were disappointing. The potent non-steroidal anti-inflammatories diclofenac and indomethacin have also been tested but shown to have minimal benefit with a high frequency of side effects. Perhaps these results are not surprising as it seems likely that the inhibition of COX will have little beneficial effect on the symptoms of AD once neuronal death has occurred, as seems likely in the clinical studies in which the patients were in the advanced stage of AD. Another problem arising in the interpretation of the data concerns the effects of the selective COX_2 inhibitors such as celecoxib and rofecoxib which, in *in vitro* studies, have been shown to enhance the formation of the highly neurotoxic form of Ab, Ab 42. By contrast the non-selective COX inhibitors ibuprofen and suldinac were shown to reduce Ab to its less neurotoxic form of Ab 38. With regard to the mechanism of action of the non-steroidal drugs, it has been speculated that the beneficial effects might be linked to a reduction in the activity of gamma secretase, the enzyme assumed to be responsible for the cleavage of APP to its neurotoxic product. In addition, it is known that these drugs also act as free radical scavengers, which is unconnected with their inhibitory actions on COX.

The most positive result for the action of an anti-inflammatory has been obtained from the studies of propentofyline. This drug inhibits the action of microglia which act as macrophages within the brain and release inflammatory cytokines. However, while there was evidence of some therapeutic benefit, the results were modest and insufficient for the drug to be marketed either in Europe or North America. Thus the jury is still out regarding the potential therapeutic efficacy of the non-steroidal drugs, at least in the treatment of patients with established AD.

Antioxidants

Free radicals have been considered to play an important role in initiating neuronal death. Neurotoxic processes arising from an overactivity of the glutamatergic system, from ischaemia, and from the direct action of Ab lead to increased oxidative stress and free radical synthesis. It would therefore be anticipated that free radical scavengers and antioxidants could delay or prevent the progression of neuronal degeneration due to such causes. Of the compounds tested in a clinical situation, vitamin E has been the most extensively studied. The result of a 2-year placebo-controlled trial has shown that vitamin E, particularly when combined with the monoamine oxidase B inhibitor and free radical scavenger selegiline, had a significant beneficial effect but high doses of vitamin E which were necessary are also known to cause disorders of blood coagulation, so it seems unlikely that this will become a treatment of choice. Studies of the use of high daily doses of vitamin E alone in the treatment of AD have, at best, been inconclusive.

Chelating agents

It is known that metals such as zinc and copper become more concentrated in the brain with increasing age and that these metals can induce Ab aggregation, thereby enhancing the deposition of senile plaques. In addition, the presence of these metals with Ab initiates the formation of hydrogen peroxide which causes oxidative damage to neurons. By using metal chelating agents such as cliquinol, it has been possible to reduce the zinc and copper concentrations in the brains of patients with AD, leading to a small but significant improvement in cognitive function. The use of chelating agents may therefore be of some therapeutic benefit in the future.

Oestrogens

Like the potential usefulness of the non-steroidal anti-inflammatory drugs, the potential therapeutic value of the oestrogens came from their protective effect against AD in post-menopausal women. Experimental studies have shown that oestrogens protect hippocampal dendrites from damage and also augment the activity of choline acetyl transferase. Additional properties of oestrogens which may contribute to their neuroprotective effects include antioxidant properties and a facilitation of the processing of APP along a non-amyloidogenic pathway.

Despite the promising experimental and epidemiological studies, the clinical trials of the oestrogens in AD have been disappointing. There is some evidence that women who had taken oestrogens for the treatment of post-menopausal symptoms had a better response in terms of an improvement in cognitive symptoms than those who had not taken oestrogens. It seems possible that selective oestrogen receptor modulators (SERMs), which are drugs that act as selective agonists for central oestrogen receptors, may eventually be developed to replace the non-selective steroidal oestrogens which have been used to date.

Secretase inhibitors

Amyloid deposition is now regarded as one of the earliest changes that initiates AD. It would appear that, regardless of the position of the mutation, whether this is in the APP gene, presenilin-1 or 2, the final outcome is the increase in neurotoxic Ab 42 in the brain and plasma. A similar finding has been with the increased frequency of the apolipoprotein E_4 allele. This has led to the hypothesis that the aggregated form of Ab is primarily responsible for the symptoms of AD and therefore it might be possible to develop appropriate drugs to prevent the neurotoxic damage by blocking the synthesis of Ab.

It is known that beta and gamma secretases are responsible for cleaving APP to Ab so that by inhibiting these enzymes it might be possible to block the progression of the disease. Alternatively, enhancing the activity of alpha secretase, leading to the formation of a non-amyloidogenic end-product, might also be beneficial. Another approach could involve the increase in the breakdown of Ab once it has been formed. All these possibilities are actively under consideration, but so far no drugs have emerged.

Regarding the possibility of developing secretase inhibitors, it appears that the pancreas also contains beta secretase and it is presently unclear what the consequences could be if the pancreatic enzyme was inhibited in addition to the brain enzyme. With regard to gamma secretase, it is known to be closely associated with the presenilins, the enzymes that are critically involved in a number of metabolic pathways in addition to the formation of Ab. Thus there may be unexpected toxicity problems which arise by inhibiting gamma secretase.

Thus it would appear that despite some exciting experimental findings in mice that have been genetically programmed to develop the human form of Ab, so far there is no evidence to indicate that secretase inhibiting drugs have been developed that offer some prospects for treating AD.

There is evidence that cholesterol contributes to AD by enhancing Ab synthesis. This provides a theoretical basis for the use of statins to lower the blood cholesterol concentration. There is also recent evidence that the statins have unexpected anti-inflammatory properties by reducing the adhesion and activation of leucocytes which may contribute to the moderate improvement in the cognition scores which have been observed in a placebo-controlled trial.

Vaccines

Transgenic mice that overexpress Ab have been used to determine whether vaccines could be produced to reduce the concentration of the peptide in patients with AD. Experimental studies have shown that Ab peptide immunization reduces the cognitive impairments and the formation of plaques in rodent models of AD. This finding led to the development of vaccines for human use and while the phase 1 trials in the UK suggested that the vaccine was safe, more extensive studies in Europe led to the termination of the clinical trials because 5% of the patients develop meningioencephalitis. More studies are presently underway to induce an immune response against Ab without initiating T-cell activation which underlies the inflammatory process in the brain.

Conclusion

Major progress has been made in the past decade to develop drugs to treat the symptoms of AD. Some of the principal drugs that are available for clinical use are listed in Table 14.3. To date, important advances have been made regarding the reversal of the disease process. In particular with respect to preventing the accumulation of Ab and in defining strategies for preventing the central inflammatory response which appears to initiate the neurotoxic changes. Undoubtedly the following decade will see the development of vaccines, and other strategies, that will alter the course of the disease. Thus we can expect the therapeutic pessimism of the past to be replaced by therapeutic optimism in the future.

Table 14.3. Anti-dementia drugs currently available

Type	Possible efficacy
Noötropic agents, antihypoxic agents E.g. piracetam, amiracetam, pramiracetam, oxiracetam	No evidence for efficacy in AD
Cholinomimetics E.g. arecoline, levocarnitine, milameline, xanomeline	Limited efficacy in AD
Anticholinesterases E.g. physostigmine, tacrine, donepezil, metrifonate, huperzine A, eptastigmine, velnacrine, galantamine, rivastigmine	Efficacy in early stages of AD
Anti-inflammatory drugs E.g. prednisone, indomethacin, celecoxib, rofecoxib, propentofyline	May be preventative as evidenced by epidemiological studies; no evidence of efficacy in patients with AD
Antioxidants E.g. vitamin E+seligiline	Limited efficacy
Chelating agents E.g. desferroxamine, clioquinol	?Some improvements in cognitive function
Oestrogens	May have a preventative role but no efficacy in AD
Ginkgo biloba alkaloids	Slight effect on cognitive function but not sufficient for therapeutic use
Others E.g. memantine	Glutamate antagonist (AMPA receptors). Clinical trials show modest improvement in cognitive function

Other approaches

Benzodiazepine receptor agonists are known to cause amnesia, whereas those drugs which act as *inverse agonists on the benzodiazepine receptor* exert promnestic properties, at least under experimental conditions. Attempts are therefore being made to develop inverse agonists with cognitive-enhancing properties. ZK 93426 is a benzodiazepine inverse agonist which has similar cognitive-enhancing effects in human volunteers to drugs that facilitate central cholinergic transmission, and experimental evidence suggests that ZK 93426 facilitates acetylcholine release. In this respect this inverse agonist resembles some of the centrally acting *angiotensin-converting enzyme inhibitors*, such as captopril, which have been shown to exhibit cognitive-enhancing properties in experimental studies, possibly by stimulating acetylcholine release.

Despite the numerous animal studies in which *neuropeptides* (analogues of adrenocorticotrophic hormone, vasopressin, cholecystokinin, beta-endorphin) have been shown to have potent and reproducible effects in facilitating learning and memory, there is to date no convincing evidence to suggest that these drugs are of any therapeutic benefit to patients with Alzheimer's disease.

The ampakines are a group of compounds that facilitate transmission by stimulating the AMPA glutamate receptors (see p. 58). The AMPA receptor is believed to play a major role in long-term potentiation, a physiological process that is important in memory formation. Experimental studies in aged rats have already shown that the ampakines can reverse age-associated memory loss but their activity in Alzheimer's patients has yet to be determined.

Another approach has been based on the epidemiological finding that oestrogens, antioxidants and anti-inflammatory drugs might delay the onset of Alzheimer's disease. Of the drugs undergoing studies under the auspices of the Alzheimer's Disease Co-operative Study in the USA, particular attention is being given to the antioxidant vitamin E and the monoamine oxidase-B (MAO-B) inhibitor deprenyl (selegeline) which has been widely used as an adjunct to L-dopa therapy in the treatment of Parkinson's disease. In addition to its MAO-B inhibitory effects, deprenyl has also been shown to act as an antioxidant. The rationale for studying such drugs is based on the belief that reactive oxygen-free radicals are produced in excessive amounts in the ageing brain and that this process is particularly prominent in the brain of the Alzheimer's patient. Furthermore, there is evidence that excessive production of free radicals is linked to the neurotoxic effects of beta-amyloid which is predominantly found in degenerative nerve terminals in the brain of the Alzheimer's patient.

In cell culture, it has been found that beta-amyloid can increase the synthesis of hydrogen peroxide and free hydroxyl radicals which can act directly on neuronal membranes and thereby damage the integrity of the cell. The neurotoxicity of beta-amyloid can be prevented, at least *in vitro*, by the addition of antioxidants including vitamin E. Whether the prophylactic administration of such antioxidants will delay the degenerative changes that precede Alzheimer's disease in those patients who are predisposed to the disease is unknown but initial clinical findings are disappointing.

Finally, it may be possible to reduce the excessive influx of calcium into neurons which may be a contributing factor to cell death in Alzheimer's disease. It is known that the density of calcium channels is increased three-fold in the neurons of aged rats in comparison to younger animals. Such changes are correlated with memory and learning deficits in the animals. Thus the use of centrally acting calcium channel inhibitory drugs might have a neuroprotective role to play. Which, if any, of these approaches will lead to drugs that are both effective and safe in slowing the decline in neurodegeneration remains to be proven.

Table 14.4.   Treatment decisions for Alzheimer's disease

- Treatment of choice – a centrally acting cholinesterase inhibitor (e.g. donepezil, galantamine, rivastigmine)
- Switching – an alternative cholinesterase inhibitor
- Augmentation – a cholinesterase inhibitor plus vitamin E
- Other options – memantine, selegiline, *Ginkgo biloba* alkaloids

Note: There is no evidence that noötropics (e.g. piracetam, nimodepine) are beneficial but some (e.g. co-dergocrine) may cause a minor improvement in neuropsychological and behavioural parameters.

Treatment decisions for Alzheimer's disease are shown in Table 14.4.

In CONCLUSION, despite the very limited advances that have been made in developing drugs that are of real benefit to the patient with Alzheimer's disease, there have been some developments which may ultimately lead to this goal. The discovery of the defect in the forebrain cholinergic system has led to a treatment strategy which, although limited in its clinical value, raises the prospect of rational drug development.

Another important research strategy concerns the reasons why brain cells die prematurely in patients with Alzheimer's disease. Is this due to a genetically programmed change in the chemistry of the neurofibrillary tangles? One possible approach to this question would involve studying the nature of the cross-linking of the proteins that compose these filaments. It is not without interest that a dominant mutation has recently been described in a nematode worm (*C. elegans*) that results in a toxic gene product causing degeneration of specific neurons in the adult. Could such a toxic gene product also be responsible for selective neuronal degeneration in patients prone to Alzheimer's disease?

A third approach involves studies on the way neurotrophic factors affect the functioning and viability of brain cells. The finding that the synthesis of the neuropeptide somatostatin is defective in Alzheimer's disease lends added impetus to the assessment of the role of brain peptides which may have neuromodulatory and/or trophic functions.

Other strategies include detailed studies of the changes in brain carbohydrate metabolism in ageing and how this may differ in patients with Alzheimer's disease. Changes in the composition and biophysical properties of neuronal membranes may also be of crucial importance in regulating the cytosolic free calcium, which could affect cellular homeostasis.

Finally, there is an increasing need to evaluate the importance of environmental toxins in the pathology of Alzheimer's disease. There has been much interest lately in the role of aluminium as a causative factor, while the studies of dementia associated with the acquired immunodeficiency syndrome have focused attention on the effects of slow viruses in causing brain cell death.

The systematic study of Alzheimer's disease commenced only relatively recently, despite the fact that Alois Alzheimer described the disease over 90 years ago. In the last decade our knowledge of the disease and of its possible aetiology has advanced from almost total ignorance to the stage where it is possible to develop therapeutic strategies. Perhaps we should be optimistic that the next decade will enable early diagnosis of this devastating disease to be followed by effective symptomatic treatment and attenuation of the inevitable destruction of the brain.

Stroke

Brain injury from stroke is a major public health problem in most industrialized countries in the world. For example, in the United States over 0.5 million cases of stroke occur annually, the incidence of stroke doubles approximately each decade over the age of 45 and occurs in up to 2% in those over 75. Frequently, stroke causes major disability with the patient having difficulty in communication, ambulation and movement, or in reasoning. Fortunately, the incidence and severity of stroke has been reduced in many countries by the introduction of preventative measures aimed at controlling hypertension, hypercholesterolaemia, smoking and by the use of anticoagulants in high risk groups.

Ischaemic stroke commonly occurs due to the occlusion of blood vessels which perfuse the brain by the occurrence of a blood clot that originates from the heart or an atherosclerotic arterial plaque. To date, most therapeutic strategies have failed to prevent cerebral infarction but currently a number of experimental studies in animal models of stroke have led to the development of potential agents that can reduce infarct size. Some of these experimental approaches will now be considered.

Pathophysiology of brain infarction

The brain is uniquely vulnerable to the effects of energy deprivation. Metabolically the brain is largely dependent on oxygen and glucose to maintain normal physiological activity. Oxidative metabolism results in the formation of high energy phosphate compounds of which adenosine triphosphate (ATP) is the most important. A primary function of ATP is directed towards maintaining and restoring ionic gradients related to synaptic transmission and the action potential.

Excitatory transmitters such as glutamate utilize much of the energy demand of the brain and it is well established that excessive activation of central excitatory amino acid receptors may be neurotoxic even in the presence of normal glucose and oxygen. This type of neurotoxic damage is

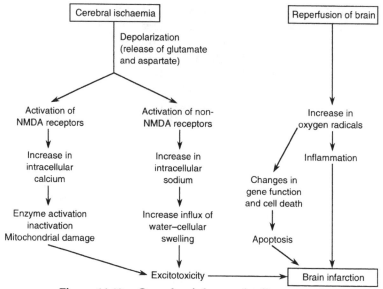

Figure 14.12.   Cascade of changes leading to stroke.

termed excitotoxicity and may also be involved in other neurodegenerative processes such as Alzheimer's and Huntington's disease.

In brain ischaemia, the excessive stimulation of glutamate receptors causes a marked increase in intracellular calcium activated enzymes (such as the proteases, kinases, phospholipases and endonucleases) which promote neuronal and glial cell death. In addition, free radicals are produced by the damaged mitochondria and by the reaction of molecular oxygen with iron released from protein binding sites by proteases, acidosis and oxygenases. The cascade of changes which occurs following cerebral ischaemia is illustrated in Figure 14.12.

Because it is necessary for the stroke patient to receive prompt treatment before brain cell death occurs, any useful drug must be effective even when there is considerable time lapse (often several hours) between the occurrence of the stroke and the onset of treatment. The term "therapeutic window" refers to the critical time of intervention between the onset of the ischaemia and occurrence of brain infarction. Some of the drugs that have been developed and shown to be effective in the treatment of various animal models of stroke are listed in Table 14.5. It should be emphasized that none of these drugs is currently marketed for the treatment of stroke. All have been developed on animal models and recent positron emission tomography and magnetic resonance imaging studies have shown that the therapeutic window may be much more variable and prolonged in man than in such models. Only extensive double-blind clinical trials (estimated

Table 14.5.   Neuroprotective agents of use in the treatment of cerebral ischaemia

1. Calcium channel antagonists – nimodipine, flunarizine
2. Free radical scavengers, antioxidants – ebselen, tirilazad
3. GABA agonists – chlormethiazole
4. Glutamate receptor antagonists – NMDA channel blocker: cerestat,
     dextromethorphan, dextrophan
     – Mg^{++} site: memantine, remacemide
     – polyamine site: eliprodil, ifenprodil
5. Opiate antagonists – naloxone, nalmefene
6. Sodium channel antagonists – fosphenytoin, lubeluzole

Note: Voltage-sensitive sodium and potassium channels are targets affecting depolarization whereas calcium channels control calcium influx which, following ischaemic stroke, enhances glutamate release which leads to cell death. GABA agonists attenuate excitotoxicity and free radical scavenger production, thereby acting as neuroprotectants.

to require 600–2000 patients to demonstrate statistical reliability) will demonstrate which, if any, of these drugs is therapeutically useful.

Pharmacological strategies for the treatment of stroke

Drugs blocking glutamate receptors

NMDA receptor antagonists or channel blockers such as phencyclidine or dizocilpine reduce the size of focal ischaemia in many animal models of stroke but are less effective in models of global ischaemia that simulate the conditions following cardiac arrest. Theoretically the NMDA receptor ion channel antagonists may be advantageous in the treatment of acute stroke when the high glutamate concentration in the synapse is more likely to stimulate ion channel openings. Those drugs that modulate the NMDA receptors via an action on the polyamine or glycine sites (for example eliprodil) promote the NMDA ion channel opening and may be useful as neuroprotective agents in those patients liable to suffer from stroke. Some non-NMDA receptor antagonists have also been found to be neuroprotective in animal models of focal and global ischaemia. For example, compounds such as CNQX have been shown to be effective in animal models of global ischaemia.

Free radical scavengers

Oxygen free radicals are highly reactive molecules that damage lipids, nucleic acids, carbohydrates and proteins, thereby contributing to excitotoxic-induced neuronal death. In addition, free radicals can contribute to increased permeability of the blood–brain barrier, to brain oedema and to the movement of macrophages into the ischaemic zone. The gaseous neurotransmitter nitric oxide contributes to cell death by combining with superoxide to form the highly reactive peroxynitrite anion. Two drugs are undergoing clinical trial at present, tiriliazad and pergorgotein, for the treatment of head trauma.

Thrombolysis and anticoagulants

Heparin-like anticoagulants such as nadroparin have been found to be useful in some clinical trials in stroke patients as have streptokinase-like drugs which dissolve the fibrin matrix of blood clots.

Anti-inflammatory agents

White blood cells readily traverse the blood–brain barrier 12–24 hours after ischaemia and contribute to the excessive production of oxygen free radicals. Eventually the infarcted zone becomes infiltrated with lympho-cytes, polymorphs and macrophages. The cytokines released from the macrophages contribute to the injury of the vessel walls and to the consequent oedema, haemorrhage and necrosis. Thus the function of the anti-inflammatory agents is to reduce the initial adhesion of the white blood cells and thereby limit the extent of the inflammatory response.

Voltage-dependent channel blockers

The release of neurotransmitters is triggered by the opening of the calcium channels in the neuronal membrane which results from the depolarization of the neuron. The conventional calcium channel blockers (e.g. nimodipine) block the L-channels only and therefore do not affect those calcium channels necessary for neurotransmitter release. Nevertheless, the L-channel blockers may prevent excess calcium influx into the cytoplasmic and mitochrondrial compartments which may assist in preventing stroke in those patients at risk from vasospasm following subarachnoid haemorrhage. In addition to a variety of N-channel blocking compounds which are still largely experi-mental, drugs such as lamotrigine (an anti-epileptic drug which also modulates NMDA receptors), lubeluzole, rolizole and fosphenytoin have been shown to be effective in reducing ion flux through the sodium channel in the neuron and thereby attenuating neurotransmitter release.

In CONCLUSION, the future drug treatment of stroke will probably depend on a combination of both neuroprotection (e.g. hypothermia, glutamate receptor antagonists, free radical scavengers, etc.) with thrombolysis which attempts to re-establish normal blood flow. Such treatments may help to expand the window between the initial ischaemic episode and brain damage. Whether any of the drugs mentioned here will ultimately be of any value in the prevention and/or treatment of stroke is still a matter of conjecture.

15 Psychopharmacology of Drugs of Abuse

Mankind has always shown a surprising ingenuity for finding drugs which have a pleasurable effect. Alcohol in its various forms is perhaps the oldest drug to be used for its effects on the brain, closely followed by various naturally occurring hallucinogens; for example fungi have long been known to be an important component of religious ritual in many societies. Other drugs, some of which have had therapeutic uses, include the opioid analgesics such as morphine and codeine, cannabis, cocaine (until recently in a relatively crude form extracted from the leaf of the Andean coca plant) and the milder stimulants, caffeine and nicotine. The use of extracts of opium, coca leaves and khat, a plant growing in some Middle Eastern countries that contains several stimulant components, has had social importance in some non-industrialized societies, where such substances are commonly used as social alternatives to alcohol and also have a role in counteracting hunger and fatigue. Most societies in which these drugs are used recognize their potential dangers to health should they be consumed to excess. Thus both the non-medical use of drugs and the related problem of drug abuse have been widely recognized since antiquity. This chapter concentrates on the psychopharmacological properties of drugs of abuse (Table 15.1).

Definitions

The term "drug abuse" refers to the use of any drug in a manner which is at variance with the approved use in that particular culture. Thus the term refers to socially disapproved use and is not descriptive of a particular pattern of abuse. For example, chewing the leaves of *Catha edulis*, or khat, is socially acceptable in the Yemen and other Middle Eastern countries, where there is little evidence that, within the confines of that culture, it is abused or that it causes major health problems. In most European countries, however, its use is illegal and it is treated as a criminal offence to be in possession of this substance. Conversely, alcohol is a major health hazard in most

Fundamentals of Psychopharmacology. Third Edition. By Brian E. Leonard
2003 John Wiley & Sons, Ltd. ISBN 0 471 52178 7

Table 15.1. Drugs of abuse and how their effects may be treated

Mechanism involved	Main neuro-transmitter affected	Potential treatment
Action on endogenous receptors for endogenous ligands		
Opioids	Endorphins, enkephalins	Partial agonists (e.g. buprenorphine) Antagonists (e.g. naltrexone)
Alcohol	GABA, endorphins	Partial agonists (e.g. bretazenil) Opiate antagonists (e.g. naltrexone)
Benzodiazepines	GABA	Partial agonists (e.g. bretazenil) Antagonists (e.g. flumazenil)
Nicotine	Acetylcholine	Antagonists (? mecamylamine)
Cannabinoids	? Anandamide	Antagonists (e.g. SR 141716A)
LSD and related hallucinogens	5-HT	$5-HT_2$ receptor antagonists (e.g. ritanserin)
Increasing the release of endogenous neurotransmitters		
Cocaine	Dopamine	D_2 receptor antagonist* Antagonist of the uptake site (e.g. SSRI)
Solvents	? Noradrenaline	? Receptor antagonists
Antagonizing the action of natural transmitters		
Alcohol	Glutamate	NMDA antagonists (e.g. dizocilpine)
Barbiturates	Glutamate	AMPA antagonists (e.g. 2,3-benzodiazepines such as GYKI 52466) and some dihydro-quirioxalines such as CNQX)

*Most typical (e.g. haloperidol) and atypical (e.g. sulpiride, tiapride, risperidone) neuroleptics have a high affinity for D_2 receptors.

industrialized countries where it is socially accepted, but is banned in many Muslim countries, with dire consequences for those transgressing the ban.

"Non-medical drug use" covers, for example, the occasional use of alcohol and the regular use of the opioid analgesics. This term includes the occasional recreational use of licit and illicit drugs for their pleasurable effects (e.g. the use of amphetamines or cannabis) and outside their approved medical indications.

"Drug dependence" is defined as a syndrome in which someone continues to take the drug because of the reinforcing effect which is derived from it. This behaviour occurs despite the adverse social or medical consequences which it may have; the dependent person is motivated to continue taking the drug for his/her continued well-being. Often the dose of the drug must be increased to maintain its desired effect. This leads to a change in the behaviour of the dependent person, which varies from a mild desire to obtain the drug to a craving or compulsion. With some drugs of abuse, for example the opioids, physical and psychological dependence on the drug may occur so that lifestyle becomes dominated by the need to secure further supplies of the drug.

The term "addiction" is so non-specific that it should no longer be used. When used, it suggests that the person is severely dependent on a drug of abuse.

Drug dependence

Three factors are generally involved in drug dependence: tolerance, physical dependence and psychological dependence.

Tolerance

Tolerance often occurs, whereby an increasing amount of the drug must be administered to obtain the required pharmacological effect; tolerance may occur as a result of the drug being more rapidly metabolized, so-called *metabolic tolerance*, or through a drug-induced insensitivity of the receptors or target sites upon which it acts within the brain, termed *tissue tolerance*. Thus tolerance should be considered a general phenomenon that is not restricted to drugs of abuse. For example, tolerance is known to develop to anticholinergic agents.

Regarding drugs of abuse, tissue tolerance commonly occurs to the opioids, ethanol, and the sedatives of the benzodiazepine type. Tolerance does not develop to all drugs of abuse, however. Thus cocaine and the amphetamines maintain their stimulant and euphoriant effects for a prolonged period of administration without any need to increase the dose appreciably.

Psychological tolerance is the term used to describe the reduction in the desired psychological effects of the drug; this may not be paralleled by an increase in the metabolic tolerance.

Physical dependence

This term is used to describe the phenomenon in which abnormal behavioural and autonomic symptoms occur when the drug is abruptly withdrawn or its effects are terminated by the administration of a specific antagonist. Most drugs of abuse (e.g. the opioids, sedatives, alcohol) produce some physical dependence, although withdrawal symptoms are relatively mild following the abrupt withdrawal of cannabis, the stimulants, and cocaine.

The nature of the withdrawal symptoms depends upon the neurotransmitter systems which are the target of the drug. Thus cocaine and the amphetamines alleviate fatigue, cause anorexia and elevate mood; withdrawal therefore results in feelings of fatigue, hyperphagia and depression. Abrupt withdrawal from the sedatives, such as barbiturates or following high doses of benzodiazepines, can be associated with anxiety, insomnia and spontaneous seizures.

It must be emphasized that the relationship between tolerance, physical dependence and compulsive drug use is complex and depends both on the category of drug and the personality of the abuser. For example, it appears that the majority of patients prescribed benzodiazepines for periods of many months experience relatively minor withdrawal symptoms when the drugs are abruptly stopped. Others, however, experience severe anxiety states and have extreme difficulty in stopping the drug.

Psychological dependence

Psychological dependence occurs with most drugs of abuse. Such drugs produce an immediate pleasurable effect and, following their continuous administration, the individual experiences dysphoria and intense craving should the drug be abruptly stopped. Many drugs of abuse cause both physical and psychological dependence.

Cross-dependence

Cross-dependence arises when a drug can suppress the symptoms of withdrawal due to another drug. For example, the effects of alcohol withdrawal can be suppressed by the administration of a benzodiazepine. As both drugs enhance gamma-aminobutyric acid-ergic (GABAergic) transmission, albeit by different mechanisms, a benzodiazepine can prevent the withdrawal symptoms that arise following the abrupt cessation of alcohol. However, cross-tolerance and cross-dependence can only occur between drugs with a similar mechanism of action at the cellular level. For example, benzodiazepines cannot directly suppress the effects of morphine withdrawal.

Withdrawal syndrome

The occurrence of the withdrawal syndrome following the abrupt termination of administration of the drug is the only objective evidence of physical dependence. The symptoms of withdrawal have at least two origins: (a) the abrupt removal of the drug of dependence and (b) the hyperarousal of the brain due to re-adaptation following the absence of the drug. The pharmacokinetic properties of the drug are of major importance in determining the amplitude and duration of the withdrawal syndrome. The symptoms of drug withdrawal are characteristic for the specific category of the drug and are usually the opposite of those produced when the drug is first administered. For example, an opioid agonist such as morphine produces constricted pupils and bradycardia but on abrupt withdrawal dilated pupils and tachycardia occur.

Tolerance, physical dependence and withdrawal are a natural consequence of the properties of drugs of dependence. They can be produced in experimental animals as readily as they can in man but the symptoms do not always imply that the individual is dependent on a drug of abuse. For example, a patient with hypertension who is receiving a beta-adrenoceptor antagonist such as propranolol will probably exhibit a withdrawal syndrome consisting of a rebound hypertension when the drug is abruptly withdrawn.

Are there some basic neuronal mechanisms which are affected by all drugs of abuse?

In recent years, many of the molecular targets for drugs of abuse have been identified and cloned. In addition, it has been possible to integrate this information into a system that extends from the neuron to the behavioural consequences that follow prolonged drug abuse.

Some years ago, converging evidence suggested that all drugs of abuse affected the dopaminergic system in the brain. It was suggested that although the different classes of drugs of abuse (e.g. stimulants, depressants, hallucinogens, opiates, cannabinoids) influence many different neurotransmitter systems within the brain, all drugs of abuse appear to directly or indirectly enhance dopaminergic function in the limbic system. For example, it is known that opiates act as agonists at opioid receptors but that these receptors also increase the activity of the mesolimbic dopaminergic system. This pathway projects to the prefrontal cortex and also to the striatum. The nucleus accumbens, located near the striatum, is of primary importance in mediating the rewarding effects of stimulants such as cocaine and the amphetamines; this is associated with an increase in the concentration of dopamine in this region of the brain. The relevance of such changes is suggested by results of experimental studies in which rats self-administer amphetamine to the nucleus accumbens and increase the amount of drug administered when the dopamine receptors are partially blocked by a neuroleptic. Such positive reinforcement is evidence that dopamine is the neurotransmitter involved in the behaviour of reward and is supported by the observation that lesions of the dopaminergic system completely block the self-administration of amphetamine. Other experimental studies have shown that other types of abused drugs, such as nicotine, the opiates and alcohol, also induce positive behavioural reinforcement by enhancing dopamine release in the mesolimbic pathway while abrupt withdrawal of such drugs leads to a dramatic reduction in the concentration of dopamine in the nucleus accumbens. Thus it appears that the reinforcing effects of drugs of abuse partly depend on the functioning mesolimbic dopaminergic system which normally mediates the motivational properties of food and sex.

Other aspects of the dopaminergic system have also been implicated in drug dependence. For example, different allelic forms of the dopamine D_2 receptor gene have been implicated in predisposing some individuals to drug abuse. In addition, the dopamine transporter is undoubtedly involved in the stimulant action of cocaine and the amphetamines. The importance of the dopaminergic system is further suggested by the use of "knock-out" mice which lack the D_2 receptor. These mice show a reduction in the amount of cocaine which they self-administer. Interestingly, in brain imaging studies, it has been shown that the subjective responses to cocaine do not correlate with its action on the dopamine transporter. Thus the simplistic view that enhanced mesolimbic dopaminergic function explains all aspects of drug dependence must be treated with caution.

Of the other transmitters believed to be involved in drug abuse, serotonin has achieved some prominence. There is physiological evidence to suggest that serotonergic and dopaminergic systems are mutually inhibitory. Cocaine, like the SSRI antidepressants such as fluoxetine and citalopram, blocks the serotonin transporter. Again, it seems improbable that the serotonergic system provides the common neurochemical pathway. Thus mice lacking the 5-HT_{1B} receptor self-administer cocaine more readily than normal mice but paradoxically 5-HT_{1B} receptor agonists have the same effect.

Other approaches that have been used to find a common pathway which accounts for all drugs of abuse include the effects of such drugs on gene expression. Experimental intercellular second messenger systems increase the activity of adenylate cyclase and cyclic AMP dependent kinase, factors which increase gene transcriptase. Thus the cyclic AMP response element binding protein (CREB) increases the expression of the immediate early genes c-fos and c-jun. Chronic morphine administration reduces CREB while fos-like proteins are induced by stimulants, morphine and nicotine. It has been speculated that the genetic composition could affect neurodevelopment which then leads to adaptive changes to the presence of the drugs, thereby leading to an increase in the reinforcing properties of the drugs of abuse.

Attempts to develop novel drugs to treat dependence usually focus on the reward region of the brain, namely the dopamine-rich median forebrain bundle. However, it is now apparent that at least in the rat the reward region functions independently of the area concerned with craving. Experimentally it has been shown that when rats become dependent on cocaine and are then withdrawn from the drug, they will increase their electrical self-stimulation of the median forebrain bundle to a greater extent than they do when cocaine is administered. By contrast, stimulation of the ventral subiculum, a glutamate-rich region of the hippocampus, has been shown to produce behaviour associated with craving for cocaine. Thus while it would appear that stimulation of either the median forebrain bundle or ventral subiculum leads to dopamine release, it is only when the stimulus originates in the hippocampus that the stimulus triggers the memory that is integral to craving. It therefore appears that drug dependence entails two separate processes, one that involves neuroadaptive changes that are a direct result of the drug and another that involves the establishment of memory traces that are located in the hippocampus.

It is well known that, despite the widespread availability of drugs of dependence, particularly alcohol and nicotine, the majority of individuals do not become drug abusers. The neurophysiological explanation is that inhibitory mechanisms within the brain normally hold potentially maladaptive behaviour in check. Such a mechanism is usually attributed to the neural networks involving the prefrontal cortex and striatum. In fact, some of the behavioural and cognitive characteristics of drug abuse, such as impulsivity, risk-taking and poor-decision making abilities, resemble those changes which follow damage to the ventromedial prefrontal cortex. For example, in decision-making tasks, chronic amphetamine abusers perform similarly to patients with damage to the prefrontal cortex. However, opiate abusers show only part of this deficit. These differences appear to be related to the fact that chronically administered amphetamine causes a reduction in the serotonin content of the orbitofrontal cortex; similar changes have been reported to occur in those abusing methenedioxymethamphetamine (MDMA, "ecstasy").

These general comments on the cellular basis of drug abuse and dependence, while emphasizing the common features that may be ascribed to all drugs of abuse, also indicate that there are differences which may be of primary importance in predisposing the individual to prolonged drug abuse.

Sedative drugs of abuse

Alcohol, the barbiturates and the benzodiazepines are included in this group, all of which facilitate GABAergic activity.

Alcohol

The use of alcohol (ethanol) prepared from the fermentation of sugars, starches and other carbohydrates dates back to the beginning of recorded history. Alcohol is the most important drug of dependence in all industrialized countries, and the clinical and social problems that arise from its widespread abuse are legion. In the US, the total annual economic cost of alcoholism and its related disorders has been estimated to be approximately $80 billion, and this does not take into account the human cost, which is impossible to quantify. It has been calculated that the lifetime prevalence of alcohol abuse and alcohol dependence (alcoholism) in the United States is 5–10% for men and 3–5% for women.

The American Psychiatric Association (1994) defines "alcohol abuse" as a condition whereby social life is impaired for at least one month as a result of alcohol. "Alcoholism" is defined as the occurrence of tolerance and physical dependence that results from prolonged alcohol abuse.

It has been calculated that alcoholism now rivals heart disease and cancer as the major health problem in industrialized countries, with 9% of men and 5% of women currently at risk. In lifetime prevalence rates, alcoholism now ranks first of all psychiatric disorders. However, it is not yet possible to identify any biological, psychological, social or cultural variable which is predictive of alcohol abuse or alcoholism.

There is some epidemiological evidence to show that there is a family predisposition to alcoholism. The incidence of the illness is four times greater in the offspring of alcoholics, and the rate among identical twins is greater than among non-identical twins. There are many animal studies which also show that some inbred strains have an increased sensitivity to the effects of alcohol and have a greater alcohol intake when given a free choice. From the numerous animal and human studies it has been concluded that alcoholism is a polygenic and multifactorial problem in which genetic factors contribute to the risk of developing the illness.

Recent epidemiological evidence shows that very moderate alcohol consumption, amounting to under three units per day for men and two units for women (one unit being equivalent to about 0.25 litres of beer, one glass of wine or spirits), may protect against myocardial infarction. However, regular consumption of alcohol above 21 units per week for men and 14 units for women predisposes to brain, liver, heart and gastrointestinal tract malfunction. Additional health problems arise as a consequence of the multiple drug abuse which many alcoholics exhibit, particularly of tobacco, minor tranquillizers, sedatives and caffeine.

Criteria for the diagnosis of drug or alcohol dependence are shown in Table 15.2.

Pharmacokinetics

Alcohol is readily absorbed from an empty gastrointestinal tract; the rate of absorption is impeded by food. It is widely distributed throughout the body according to the water content of the tissue, easily penetrating both the blood–brain and placental barriers. More than 90% of the drug is oxidized in the liver to carbon dioxide and water by dehydrogenases, while the remainder is excreted unchanged through the lungs, skin and kidneys. The rate of oxidation is dependent on the degree of tolerance of the individual, the non-tolerant person oxidizing approximately 10–15 ml of absolute

Table 15.2. Criteria for diagnosis of drug or alcohol dependence

---

Any three of the following are sufficient for the diagnosis.
1. The substance is often taken in larger amounts or over a longer period than the person intended.
2. Persistent desire or one or more unsuccessful efforts to cut down or control substance use.
3. A great deal of time spent in activities necessary to get the substance, taking the substance, or recovering from its effects.
4. Frequent intoxication or withdrawal symptoms when expected to fulfil major role obligations at work, school, or home, or when substance use is physically hazardous.
5. Important social, occupational, or recreational activities given up or reduced because of substance use.
6. Continued substance use despite knowledge of having a persistent or recurrent social, psychological, or physical problem that is caused or exacerbated by the use of the substance.
7. Marked tolerance, i.e. the need for markedly increased amounts of the substance to achieve intoxication or a desired effect, or markedly diminished effect with continued use of the same amount of substance.
8. Characteristic withdrawal symptoms, depending on the individual drug, upon stopping its use.
9. Substance often taken to relieve or avoid withdrawal symptoms.

---

alcohol per hour. The alcohol metabolizing system is thus easily saturated, and its elimination is governed by "zero-order" kinetics (see Chapter 2).

The daily intake of one or two units of alcohol rapidly leads to tissue tolerance, which is not as extensive as that observed after the administration of any of the opiates and is readily lost after a few days of abstinence.

Psychological tolerance to alcohol develops at a faster rate than metabolic tolerance. Thus death from alcohol overdose can occur in a psychologically tolerant person following only a moderate increase in alcohol intake above that normally consumed.

A "reverse tolerance" has also been described, whereby an alcoholic taking a small quantity of alcohol may become intoxicated, aggressive, and antisocial. This occurs in those who have brain or liver damage and therefore show an enhanced sensitivity to the disinhibiting actions of the drug or a decreased metabolism.

Cross-tolerance also readily occurs between alcohol and other central depressants, for example the benzodiazepines and the barbiturates.

Mode of action

Meyer, in 1901, was the first to suggest that alcohol acted like general anaesthetics by dissolving into cell membranes and thereby disrupting the lipid network that comprises the cell wall. It is now known that, at pharmacologically relevant concentrations (in the range 25–100 mmol/L), alcohol increases the fluidity of cell membranes following its acute administration, these changes correlating with the sedative effects of the drug. This suggests that alcohol produces its effects in a relatively non-specific manner, but it is now known that the nerve membrane is structurally and functionally heterogeneous and that specific regions of the membrane are more sensitive to the disordering effects of the drug than other regions. Thus alcohol may affect the calcium flux across the nerve membrane or, by disrupting the phosphatidyl inositol system intracellularly, affect the intraneuronal availability of calcium. This could have a profound effect upon neurotransmitter release.

While there is little evidence to suggest that alcohol produces its pharmacological effect via a specific "alcohol receptor", some lipids do show a particular vulnerability to the disorganizing effects of the drug. For example, alcohol selectively inhibits monoamine oxidase-B, and not the A form, in human platelets and brain; similarly, it inhibits sodium/potassium-dependent adenosine triphosphatase in the neuronal membrane but not in the glial membrane.

With regard to its effect on neurotransmitter function, alcohol increases adenylate cyclase activity, possibly via the membrane-bound G protein complex. The effect of alcohol on the secondary messenger system appears to depend on its location; the noradrenaline-linked cyclase in the cortex seems to be directly affected by the drug, whereas the dopamine-linked enzyme in the basal ganglia appears to be altered by a combination of changes in the membrane fluidity, together with those in the G protein–cyclase complex.

As alcohol has pronounced sedative properties, it is not surprising to find that it facilitates central inhibitory transmission. It has been shown that alcohol has a direct effect on a portion of the GABA–benzodiazepine complex that controls the chloride ion channel. In clinical studies it has been shown that such inhibitory effects may be reversed by some partial inverse benzodiazepine receptor agonists, but their development as therapeutic agents has been discontinued because they do not reverse other detrimental effects of alcohol on brain function (see Figure 15.1).

Alcohol tolerance has been explained in terms of the adaptational changes in lipids in the nerve membranes. Thus acute alcohol administration is associated with enhanced membrane fluidity due to the disordering effects of the drug, whereas after chronic administration the membranes become more rigid owing to an increased replacement of the unsaturated by saturated fatty acids. Nevertheless, it seems unlikely that such changes are due to a single type of lipid and more likely that different populations of lipids within the nerve membrane show adaptational changes at different rates.

Another approach that has been used to elucidate the biochemical mechanisms associated with tolerance in animals has been to use specific

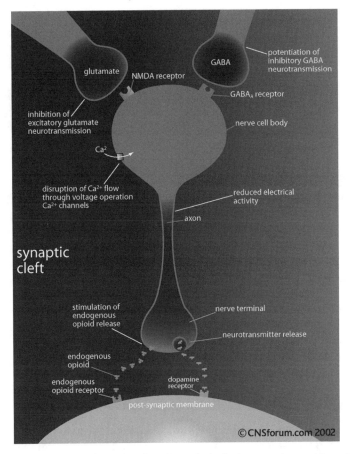

Figure 15.1. Summary of mode of action of alcohol on amino acid, opioid and dopamine dependent neurotransmission in the brain.

neurotoxins to lesion the noradrenergic and serotonergic systems. Thus lesions of the central noradrenergic system block the development of both environmentally dependent and independent tolerance. (Environmentally dependent tolerance is the situation in which tolerance to alcohol develops more rapidly when the drug is consumed or administered in the same environment.) Lesions of the serotonergic system are associated only with a block of the environmentally linked tolerance. The results of such studies suggest that tolerance is a phenomenon which can be separated from the development of physical dependence, and may not therefore be a part of a unitary mechanism for all drugs of abuse.

With regard to the neurotransmitter correlates of alcohol withdrawal and dependence, there is evidence of decreased GABA–benzodiazepine receptor function following chronic alcohol administration, which may be causally related to dependence. Changes in the number of cholinergic muscarinic receptors in the cortex and hippocampus have been reported to occur in alcohol-dependent animals, which return to control levels following withdrawal, but the precise significance of this is unknown.

Experimental studies have also suggested that alcohol may reduce N-methyl-D-aspartate (NMDA) receptor function following acute administration, and following withdrawal of alcohol the functioning of these receptors is enhanced.

Drugs interacting with alcohol

Disulfiram (Antabuse) and calcium carbide are sometimes used to assist the detoxified alcoholic to remain abstinent. The rationale behind the use of disulfiram is that it inhibits liver aldehyde dehydrogenase. Any alcohol consumed will lead to an elevation in blood acetaldehyde levels and the aversive toxic effects of acetaldehyde will become apparent. These include facial flushing, nausea, vomiting, gastrointestinal distress and potentially hazardous hypotension and tachycardia. It should be noted that other drugs which may be given for other medical conditions can also inhibit liver aldehyde dehydrogenase and can cause the disulfiram reaction. These include the sulphonylurea antihyperglycaemics, metronidazole and furazolidone (both antimicrobial agents). It must also be emphasized that alcohol will potentiate the action of any drug that has a sedative effect.

Activating drugs and the treatment of alcohol dependence

The aversive effects of alcohol withdrawal are associated with decreased mesolimbic dopaminergic activity and increased extracellular glutamate in the nucleus accumbens. The recently introduced anti-craving drug *acamprosate* has been shown to reduce the enhanced glutamate release that occurs following abrupt alcohol withdrawal. In addition, the neuronal hyperexcitability which occurs during alcohol withdrawal is accompanied by an increased expression of the immediate–early gene *c-fos* in several regions of the rat brain; acamprosate has been shown to suppress the elevated *c-fos* expression in these structures. Unlike the sedative drugs, such as the benzodiazepines, which by enhancing GABAergic function are cross-tolerant with alcohol, acamprosate has no effect on the GABAergic system but acts primarily by modulating the activity of the glutamatergic system. In neocortical neurons for example, it has been shown that acamprosate reduces the activation of excitatory glutamatergic synapses and the depolarizing responses evoked by the iontophoretic application of glutamate and NMDA without changing the membrane potential or the input resistance of the cells. In the hippocampus, the NMDA-initiated changes following the block of transmission have been shown to be enhanced by acamprosate. These effects suggest that acamprosate may act postsynaptically to modulate excitatory transmission in both the neocortex and hippocampus. In addition to the specific changes in the glutamatergic–NMDA system, acamprosate interacts with voltage-gated calcium channels and inhibits the up-regulation of calcium channels in alcohol withdrawn rats.

Clinically it has been shown that acamprosate can prevent relapse in alcoholics. In a large double-blind, placebo-controlled European study, acamprosate was shown to be effective in the treatment of alcoholism. Thus at the end of a 1-year period of treatment followed by a 1-year period without medication, 39% of the patients were still abstinent compared with 17% of the placebo-treated patients. Its main clinical effect would appear to be due to its anti-craving properties as it does not interfere with the pharmacokinetics or pharmacodynamics of alcohol. Furthermore, it does not have any reinforcing effects or discriminative stimulus properties of its own. Acamprosate has now been registered for the treatment of alcoholism in most European countries.

Numerous pharmacological and behavioural studies suggest that alcohol interacts with endogenous opioids. Earlier studies had suggested that condensation products of alcohol-derived acetaldehyde and dopamine, tetrahydroisoquinoline, may stimulate opioid receptors but *in vivo* evidence is lacking. However, experimental studies have shown that transgenic mice lacking beta-endorphin showed a reduction in voluntary consumption when compared to their wild-type, suggesting that a high alcohol intake is associated with an enhancement of endogenous opioid activity. These findings support the hypothesis that drugs blocking the opioid receptors will decrease alcohol intake. Numerous experimental and clinical studies have now indicated that the opiate antagonist naltrexone reduces alcohol intake and the drug has been registered in many countries as an adjunct for the treatment of alcoholism. However, there is evidence that its ability to facilitate abstinence when compared to placebo diminishes over time.

The mechanism of action of *naltrexone* in reducing alcohol consumption is complex but experimental studies show that opiate antagonists have direct effects on alcohol-seeking behaviour. A possible site for this action could be the mesolimbic dopaminergic reward circuit in which opioid receptors are located. The activity of endogenous opioids in the ventral tegmental area, the site of origin of the A_{10} mesolimbic dopaminergic neurons, blocks the activity of the GABAergic interneurons that impinge on the A_{10} neurons which leads to disinhibition. Thus an increase in the endogenous opioid system induced by alcohol would indirectly enhance dopamine release in the mesolimbic system and thereby induce the reward-enhancing effects of the drug. Naltrexone and other antagonists have been shown to antagonize these effects. As naltrexone and other antagonists such as naloxone block the opiate receptors and have been shown in both experimental and clinical studies to suppress alcohol-induced reinforcement, it can be assumed that the activation of the endogenous opioid system is crucially involved in the mediation of alcohol reinforcement.

In summary, naltrexone and acamprosate act via different mechanisms. Naltrexone interferes with the positive reinforcement effects of alcohol and attenuates the effects of conditioned stimuli that had been previously paired with the positive reinforcing effects of alcohol. Acamprosate appears to act by reducing neuronal hyperexcitability and probably inhibits reactivity induced by stimuli that are paired with alcohol withdrawal, an action which may explain the anti-craving action of the drug. While both drugs have been shown to prevent relapse after long abstinence periods, there is no evidence that these drugs also reverse the lasting changes in sensitivity to alcohol that is induced by their long-term use. Other compounds that act on NMDA receptors, such as the non-competitive antagonist memantine, appear to hold promise for the treatment of alcoholism in the future.

Anxiolytics and sedatives

The pharmacological properties of these drugs are dealt with in Chapter 5, and therefore only their propensity to cause physical and psychological dependence is considered here. Because of their lack of efficacy, and particularly because of their toxicity, barbiturates should never be used now as anxiolytic or sedative drugs. For this reason, emphasis is placed here on the benzodiazepines, which are not only effective but also relatively safe. Nevertheless, problems have arisen regarding their ability to cause dependence, and so this aspect of their pharmacology must be considered.

Considering their widespread use, intentional abuse of prescribed benzodiazepines is relatively rare. Normally, following the administration of a benzodiazepine for several weeks, there is little tolerance or difficulty in stopping the drug when the condition no longer warrants its use. Following prolonged treatment however (several months for example) tolerance often develops and the abrupt cessation of treatment results in withdrawal symptoms. These consist of: anxiety; agitation; increased sensitivity to light and sound; paraesthesiae; muscle cramps, myoclonic jerks; sleep disturbance and dizziness. These effects are usually short lived and their onset following withdrawal of the benzodiazepine depends on the half-life of the drug. Following the administration of a high dose of a benzodiazepine however, seizures and delirium can also occur.

It is often difficult to distinguish withdrawal symptoms from the reappearance of the underlying anxiety state for which the benzodiazepine was originally prescribed. Furthermore, some patients may increase the dose of the drug over time, particularly if they are taking the drugs for the treatment of insomnia as tolerance often develops to their sedative effects. However, there is little evidence to suggest that tolerance develops as quickly to the anxiolytic effects of the benzodiazepines and most patients continue to take their medication for years without increasing the dose. The American Psychiatric Association (1990) formed a task force that reviewed these issues and published guidelines for the correct medical use of the benzodiazepines. They recommend intermittent use of these drugs when possible to reduce the occurrence of tolerance and dependence. Patients with a history of alcohol or drug abuse have an increased risk to develop benzodiazepine abuse and therefore their use in such patients should be avoided.

The benzodiazepines are the most widely used drugs for the management of insomnia, anxiety, muscle spasticity and seizures. About 12% of the adult population in the US have used such drugs on more than one occasion during the past year for the treatment of insomnia, while approximately 2.4% of adults have taken such drugs continuously for 4 months or longer. Figures from European countries vary, some being higher and some lower than those reported in the US, but in all cases detailed studies of the prescribing of benzodiazepines show that they are being used appropriately both in the US and in most European countries. Nevertheless, despite this there has been concern over the dependence potential of these drugs following their therapeutic use, and this has led to restrictions on their prescribing and the recognition of the need to limit administration to less than 6 weeks in most cases.

Opioid analgesics as drugs of abuse

The medical use of opium as a pain-relieving drug dates back to the third century. Arab physicians used extracts of the oriental poppy to treat diarrhoea and probably introduced it to the Far East. However, because of its erratic absorption from the gastrointestinal tract, its use as an effective analgesic only became possible with the introduction of the hypodermic syringe in the middle of the last century.

Opium is obtained from the dried juice from the seed capsule of the oriental poppy, *Papaver somniferum*. The dried juice contains up to 17% morphine and 4% codeine by weight, as well as other, non-additive alkaloids that lack analgesic activity such as noscapine, papaverine, and thebaine. Papaveretum is a standardized preparation of opium containing 50% morphine.

The term "opioid" is used to designate a group of drugs that have opium-like or morphine-like properties. The term "opiate analgesic" is often used as an alternative. The term "narcotic analgesic" is now obsolete; it was formerly used to describe potent opiate analgesics which had sedative properties.

The opioids produce their pharmacological effects by interacting with a closely related group of peptide receptors, thereby suggesting that endogenous opioid-like polypeptides exist, which presumably have a physiological function.

In recent years there has been a major research effort, so far without success, to produce potent, centrally acting analgesics that do not have an abuse potential. The discovery of various types of opioid receptor, which may have different effects on central neurotransmitter function, may ultimately lead to the development of such a drug. In the meantime, the most widely used opioids, for example morphine, heroin (also called diacetylmorphine) and codeine are therapeutically effective but are liable to be abused and produce dependence. The structure of some of the morphine-like analgesics and their antagonists are shown in Figure 15.2.

Substitution of an allyl group on the nitrogen atom of morphine produces drugs which act as antagonists, such substances thereby reversing the analgesia, euphoria and respiratory depressant effects of such agonists as morphine and heroin. The structurally related antagonist naltrexone is frequently used as an antagonist of morphine and related opioid agonists. Other structural analogues of morphine, such as nalorphine, act as partial agonists. When nalorphine, for example, is injected into an animal, it will produce analgesia, but will also counteract such an effect of morphine should this pure agonist be given concurrently. All the opioids exert their pharmacological effects by binding to specific receptors located in the brain and on peripheral organs. The seminal studies of Kosterlitz and Hughes in the 1970s clearly demonstrated the relationship between opioid receptor occupancy and the ability of a drug to inhibit electrically stimulated contractions of the guinea pig ileum *in vitro*.

Later studies showed that the opiates have a high affinity for specific building sites in the brain and gastrointestinal tract which is both saturable and stereospecific. However, there does not appear to be a direct relationship between the affinity of an agonist for the central opioid receptors and its analgesic potency. This can be partly explained by the relative lack of accessibility of many opiates to the brain owing to their low lipophilicity, but other factors, such as the differences in their affinity for the various types of opioid receptors, must also be considered. Ligand-binding studies, subcellular fractionation to determine the location of the receptors at the cellular level, and the application of histochemical and immunocytochemical techniques to map the distribution of the receptors in the brain have now enabled a detailed assessment to be made of their distribution, and possible function, in man and other mammals.

The highest concentration of opioid receptors appears to be in the sensory, limbic and hypothalamic regions of the brain, with particularly high concentrations being found in the amygdala and the periaqueductal grey

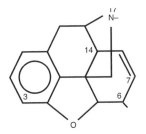

Drug	Chemical groups inserted in positions:		
	3	6	17
Morphine	–OH	–OH	–CH₃
Heroin	–OCOCH₃	–OCOCH₃	–CH₃
Levorphanol*	–OH	–H	–CH₃
Levallorphan*	–OH	–H	–CH₂CH=CH₂
Codeine	–OCH₃	–OH	–CH₃
Hydrocodone**	–OCH₃	=O	–CH₃
Nalorphine	–OH	–OH	–CHCH=CH₂
Naloxone**	–OH	=O	–CHCH=CH₂
Naltrexone**	–OH	=O	–CH₂ —◁
Buprenorphine***	–OH	–OCH₃	–CH₂ —◁
Butorphanol* **	–OH	–H	–CH₂ —◇

*–OH group added to position 14.
**Oxygen bridge missing.
***Etheno bridge inserted between positions 6 and 14 rings, plus hydroxy, trimethyl propyl substitution on position 7.

Figure 15.2. Structures of opiate analgesics and their antagonists (last five listed).

matter. The importance of receptors in these regions was evaluated by applying morphine to these sites using microinjection. Injection of morphine into the periaqueductal grey matter was found to be associated with analgesia, while retrograde amnesia resulted when the drug was applied to the amygdala, and hyperactivity when injected into the basal ganglia. The high density of opioid receptors in the spinal cord, particularly the substantia gelatinosa, which is an area that is highly innervated by peripheral type C fibres, accounts for the spinal analgesia which many opiates possess.

Actions of opioids on opioid receptors

The first endogenous ligands for the opioid receptors were isolated by Kosterlitz and Hughes and were found to be the pentapeptides methionine and leucine enkephalin (meta- and leu-enkephalin). The structures of these,

Table 15.3. Structures of some opioid peptides

Leucine enkephalin
Tyr–Gly–Gly–Phe–Leu–OH

Methionine enkepahlin
Tyr–Gly–Gly–Phe–Met–OH

Gamma-endorphin
Tyr–Gly–Gly–Phe–Met–Thr–Ser–Glu–Lys–Ser–Gin–Thr–Pro–Leu–Val–Thr–Leu–Phe

Alpha-endorphin
Tyr–Gly–Gly–Phe–Met–Thr–Ser–Glu–Lys–Ser–Gin–Thr–Pro–Leu–Val–Thr

Beta-endorphin
Tyr–Gly–Gly–Phe–Met–Thr–Ser–Glu–Lys–Ser–Gin–Thr–Pro–Leu–Val–Thr–Leu–
    Phe–Lys–Asn–Ala–Ile–Ile–Lys–Asn–Ala–Tyr–Lys–Lys–Gly–Glu–OH

---

and related peptides which also act as endogenous ligands for these receptors, are shown in Table 15.3.

Two further families of opioid peptides have since been isolated, namely the endorphins and the dynorphins. Each family of peptides is derived from a distinct precursor polypeptide, which has been identified as pro-enkephalin (from which both met- and leu-enkephalin are derived), pro-opiomelanocortin (which gives rise to alpha and gamma melanocyte-stimulating hormone (MSH), adrenocorticotrophin hormone (ACTH), beta-lipotropin and met-enkephalin) and pro-dynorphin, which produces alpha- and beta-neoendorphins and leu-enkephalin. Detailed binding studies in the brain and peripheral tissues have now established that these various opioids interact with different categories of receptors, which have been designated mu, kappa and delta receptors. The synthetic opioid compound N-allylnormetazocine (SKF 10047) has been shown to bind preferentially to another class of receptor, termed the sigma receptor, but it is now recognized that this category of opioid receptor is not directly associated with the pharmacological activity of the opioid analgesics.

In addition to the opioid peptides which occur in the mammalian brain, it is now evident that morphine, codeine and related benzomorphans occur naturally, in trace amounts, in the brain, where they exist in a conjugated form usually bound to brain proteins. The significance of these substances to brain function is unclear.

All opioids produce their effect by activating one or more of the three types of receptors. Thus analgesia involves the activation of the mu receptors that are located mainly at supraspinal sites and kappa receptors in the spinal cord; delta receptors may also be involved but their relative contribution is unclear. Nevertheless, the actions of the opioids on these receptors is complex, as there is evidence that the same substance may act as a full agonist, or as an antagonist at different sites within the brain.

Table 15.4. Effects of some opiate agonists and antagonists on opioid receptors in mammalian brain

Opiate agonist or antagonist	Receptor type		
	Mu	Delta	Kappa
Morphine	++	+	+
Butorphanol	−	0	++
Pentazocine	−	0	++
Buprenorphine	±	0	−
Naloxone	−	−	−
Nalorphine	−	0	+

Potency of agonist or antagonist shown as + and − respectively.
0 = inadequate data available; ± = partial agonist.

In man, the changes that result from the activation of different receptors have been inferred from clinical observation and from extrapolation from studies on animals. A summary of the interaction of morphine and a number of synthetic opioids on the three main receptor types is shown in Table 15.4.

To add a further complication to the understanding of ways in which the opioids act, it now appears that the mu receptors may be further subdivided into μ_1 and μ_2 subtypes, the former being high-affinity receptors that mediate supraspinal analgesia, while the latter are of relatively low affinity and are involved in respiratory depression and in the gastrointestinal effects of the agonists.

Certain benzomorphan analgesics related to pentazocine selectively bind to kappa receptors in the spinal cord, thereby producing analgesia. This analgesia is still present in animals that have been made to tolerate the analgesic effects of morphine, suggesting that there is a distinct separation of the functional effects of these receptor subtypes. The kappa agonists produce dysphoria, rather than the euphoria caused by morphine-like drugs, and occasionally such psychomimetic effects as disorientation and depersonalization.

The precise role of the delta receptors in man is uncertain, as specific agonists have not yet been developed which cross the blood–brain barrier. The structures of pentazocine and some other opiates are shown in Figure 15.3.

Mechanism of action

Of all the drugs of abuse which have been investigated, the mechanisms responsible for opioid-induced physical dependence have been the most thoroughly studied. There does not appear to be a significant change in the opioid receptor number following chronic drug administration, but there is evidence of a decrease in the functional activity of these receptors, as shown by a decrease in adenylate cyclase activity. This action is mediated by the inhibitory guanine nucleotide binding regulatory protein (Gi). Following abrupt withdrawal of the opioid, the cyclase activity returns to normal. This may be the explanation for the excessive sympathetic activity associated with the abrupt withdrawal of these drugs, particularly as some opiate receptors are located in the local coeruleus. This relationship between the opioid and adrenergic system in the brain may help to explain why the α_2-adrenoceptor agonist clonidine can attenuate some of the symptoms of opiate withdrawal. Nevertheless, the fact that opiates act on at least two different types of opioid receptors in the brain, the *mu* and *delta* receptors, which are widely distributed in the central and peripheral nervous systems, means that the pharmacological effects of these drugs and the symptoms seen on withdrawal cannot be entirely ascribed to changes in central noradrenergic transmission.

The mechanism of action of opioids at their receptor sites is complex and incompletely understood. However, they all share a number of characteristics. Thus they all facilitate inhibitory transmission in the brain and gastrointestinal tract, and appear to be located on presynaptic receptor sites, where they function as heteroreceptors. Furthermore, they all appear to be coupled to guanine nucleotide-binding regulatory proteins (G proteins), and thereby regulate the transmembrane signalling systems. In this way, the opioid receptors can regulate adenylate cyclase, the phosphatidyl inositol system, ion channels, and so on. There is evidence that the mu and delta receptors appear to operate via potassium channels and the adenylate cyclase system, while kappa receptors inhibit voltage-dependent calcium channels.

Pharmacological properties

Drugs in this therapeutic group include morphine, heroin, pethidine, methadone, codeine, dihydrocodeine, dextropropoxyphene, pentazocine, phenazocine, levorphanol and buprenorphine. The principal antagonists in clinical use are naloxone and naltrexone (see Figure 15.3).

All agonists in this therapeutic group decrease the sensation of painful stimuli, which is their main clinical application. They tend to subdue dull, persistent pain rather than sharp pain, but this difference is to some extent dose dependent. The major difference between the non-opioid analgesics such as aspirin and the opiates is that the former reduce the perception of peripherally mediated pain, by reducing the synthesis of local hormones that activate the pain fibres, whereas the latter attenuate the affective reaction to pain without affecting the perception of pain. This clearly suggests that the site of action of the opiate analgesics is in the central nervous system.

Euphoria is a common side effect of most opiates after chronic use, and undoubtedly this effect contributes to their dependence-producing

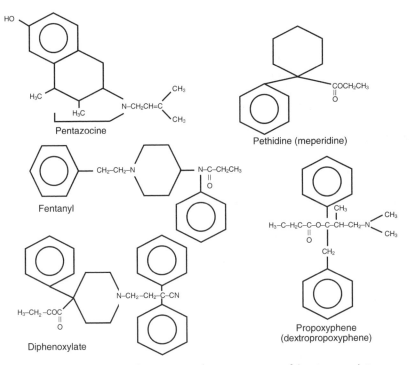

Figure 15.3.   Chemical structure of some non-morphine-type opiates.

tendency. This may play an important part in modifying the response of the patient to chronic pain. Many opiates also produce sedation, particularly after acute administration.

The opiates reduce anxiety, possibly through their sedative effects, and induce nausea and vomiting. These effects are more marked after acute administration. The emetic effect is due to their stimulant effects on the chemoreceptor trigger zone in the area postrema on the floor of the fourth ventricle, an effect that has been ascribed to an activation of dopamine receptors. The emetic effect is particularly pronounced in the case of the non-analgesic analogue of morphine, apomorphine, which has been used experimentally in the treatment of parkinsonism and in inducing emesis following a drug overdose.

The opiates cause constipation by inducing spasm of the stomach and intestines, presumably by the stimulation of opioid receptors in the myenteric plexus and reducing the release of acetylcholine. This property can be used therapeutically for the symptomatic relief of diarrhoea. Biliary colic and severe epigastric pain can occur because of the contraction of the sphincter of Oddi and the resulting increase in pressure in the biliary ducts.

One of the serious complications of the use of the opiate analgesics, even at therapeutic doses, is respiratory depression, an effect which is further complicated by the ability of these drugs to decrease the sensitivity of the respiratory centre to carbon dioxide. The administration of oxygen to a patient whose respiration has been depressed by the opiates is therefore counterproductive and may lead to total respiratory paralysis.

Many opiate analgesics are effective cough suppressants (also called anti-tussives), although only codeine and dihydrocodeine are generally used for this purpose. As there is a dissociation between the anti-tussive and analgesic action of the opiates, dextromethorphan and noscapine are now commonly used as cough suppressants because of their efficacy and lack of dependence-producing properties.

Miosis is a characteristic symptom of opiate administration, and while tolerance develops to many of the pharmacological effects of this class of drugs, tolerance to the miotic effects occurs at a much slower rate. Miosis is due to an excitatory action of the autonomic segment of the nucleus of the oculomotor nerve, an effect attributed to the stimulation of the mu receptors. In general, it would appear that the actions of morphine and its analogues on the brain, spinal cord and gastrointestinal tract are due to stimulation of the mu receptors.

Tolerance and dependence

An acute dose of 100–200 mg morphine, or its equivalent, in the non-tolerant adult can lead to respiratory depression, coma and death. In the tolerant individual, single doses or more than 10 times this amount are tolerated and have little visible effect. The development of tolerance to the opiates does not appear to be due to enhanced metabolism (metabolic tolerance) but is probably due to opioid receptor insensitivity (tissue tolerance). The dependent person therefore ultimately requires high doses of the opiate to prevent withdrawal effects.

Cross-tolerance occurs between all opiates that act primarily via the mu receptors. This is the basis of the methadone substitution therapy which is commonly used to withdraw people who are dependent on heroin or morphine; methadone is used because of its relatively long half-life (about 12 hours) and its ease of administration in an oral form. Cross-tolerance does not occur between the opiates and other classes of dependence-producing drugs such as the barbiturates, alcohol or the amphetamines, which act through different mechanisms.

The sudden reduction in plasma opiate levels, or the administration of an opiate antagonist such as naloxone, leads to withdrawal symptoms. These include restlessness, craving, lacrimation, perspiration, fever, chills, vomiting, joint pain, piloerection and mydriasis. These effects are maximal

2 or 3 days after the abrupt withdrawal of heroin, morphine or related drugs, but are slower in onset and less severe in the case of drugs like methadone which have a longer half-life and whose tissue concentration therefore decreases more slowly.

Endogenous opioids and the pain response

It has long been known that stress can elevate the pain threshold. In rodents this may be quantified by measuring the increase in the pain threshold following prolonged unavoidable foot shock. Under conditions of environmental stress, the pain threshold has also been shown to increase in man. Such effects have been attributed to a rise in opioid peptides in the cerebrospinal fluid (CSF). Conversely, in chronic pain syndromes, the CSF concentration of the endorphins decreases.

While the physiological basis of acupuncture is incompletely understood, it is now apparent that the endogenous opioid systems are activated by such techniques. Furthermore, when acupuncture is simulated in animals there is a decrease in the pain response to noxious peripheral stimuli, which can be reversed by naloxone.

From such studies, it may be concluded that physical stress leads to an activation of endogenous opioid systems, which raises the pain threshold. The euphoriant effect of physical exercise may also be attributed to the effects of these opioids acting on limbic regions of the brain.

The discovery that the opioid peptides cause analgesia and have anti-tussive and antidiarrhoeal effects led to the widespread search for synthetic peptides that could be administered orally but that would not have the dependence-producing effects of morphine and related drugs. Synthetic peptides modelled on the endogenous opioids have been synthesized which have longer half-lives than the endogenous substance and which are resistant to the enkephalinases which rapidly degrade the endogenous opioids. Unfortunately, to date, all of the experimental and clinical studies have been disappointing, as it has been found that morphine-dependent animals show cross-tolerance with all such compounds.

The endogenous opioid peptides have a range of affinities for the different types of opioid receptor. Some met-enkephalin derivatives, for example, show affinity for mu and delta receptors, whereas other peptides, derived from pro-enkephalin, show a preference for the delta sites. All peptides from prodynorphin act predominantly on kappa sites, while beta-endorphin behaves like the enkephalins and shows selectivity for the mu and delta sites.

Perhaps it may be possible to use this diversity and selectivity of action to develop new synthetic opiates that will have therapeutic advantages over morphine and its analogues which, in one form or another, have been used by mankind for nearly 2000 years.

Nicotine as a drug of abuse

Nicotine is an alkaloid derived from the leaves of the *Nicotiana* species. It originated in South America where it has been smoked by the native population for hundreds of years. It was introduced into Western Europe in the 16th century but shortly after its introduction into Great Britain it was condemned as a habit "injurious to the lung" by King James I.

Nicotine has both stimulant and depressant actions on the brain. The stimulant and rewarding action is attributed to the action of the drug on the nicotinic cholinergic receptors that indirectly increase the release of dopamine from the nucleus accumbens reward system; an increase in dopamine release has been detected in this brain region following the administration of the drug to rats. This action is a common property of most drugs of abuse and has already been covered in detail at the beginning of this section. In addition, nicotine indirectly increases the release of endogenous opioids and glucocorticoids which add to the complexity of action of the drug.

Because nicotine provides the reinforcement for the smoking of cigarettes in particular, it is arguably the most influential dependence-producing drug available. The dependence, both psychological and to a lesser extent physical, is extremely durable as exemplified by the failure rate among smokers who try to stop the habit. For example, it has been calculated that although over 80% of smokers wish to stop the habit, only 35% succeed each year. It has been estimated that dependence can occur in individuals who smoke more than 5 cigarettes per day; most smokers consume about 20 cigarettes per day.

Nicotine is readily absorbed through the skin, mucous membranes and lungs but smoking is the preferred route because of the rapid absorption of the drug across the mucosa of the lung leading to an effect on the brain within about 7 seconds. Thus each puff of a cigarette produces a discrete reinforcement and it has been calculated that with an average of 10 puffs per cigarette, 20 cigarettes per day will reinforce the habit 200 times daily. In dependent smokers, there is evidence that the urge to smoke correlates with a low blood nicotine concentration and it has been concluded that those who are dependent smoke not only in order to obtain the reinforcing effect of the drug but also to avoid the symptoms of nicotine withdrawal. The symptoms of nicotine withdrawal include: irritability; impatience; hostility; anxiety; dysphoria; difficulty in concentrating; restlessness; bradycardia, increase in appetite; and weight gain.

Smokers who have been abstinent for several weeks, or those who smoke for the first time, often experience nausea even at low blood nicotine concentrations. This aversive effect is due to the action of the drug on the chemoreceptor trigger zone whereby it indirectly activates the release of dopamine. Apomorphine and related dopamine agonists also cause nausea by activating the dopaminergic system in this brain region.

The nicotine withdrawal syndrome can be alleviated by nicotine replacement therapy. There are several forms of nicotine replacement products which are widely available. These are nicotine gum, transdermally delivered nicotine (nicotine patch) and nasal nicotine spray. Both the nicotine gum and the patch have shown efficacy in increasing short term abstinence rates, reducing the symptoms of nicotine withdrawal and relieving the craving for cigarettes. Nasal nicotine spray appears to be efficacious in sustaining abstinence from smoking and has the advantage over the other nicotine formulations in that the venous pharmacokinetic profile of nicotine administration closely follows that of smoking a cigarette. Unlike the patch or gum, nicotine spray can cause nasal and throat irritation.

Of the more recently introduced methods for smoking cessation, bupropion (an antidepressant with dopaminomimetic properties) has recently been introduced. Clinical trial data, in which the nicotine patch, bupropion at 300 mg, and a combination of the two drugs were compared with placebo treatment, have shown cessation of smoking rates of 36% for the patch, 49% for bupropion and 58% for the combined treatments following 7 weeks of treatment. The placebo response rate was 23%. All subjects received relapse prevention therapy. Thus bupropion appears to be a reasonably safe and effective treatment for nicotine dependence. It is however contraindicated in those subject to epilepsy; its main side effects are dry mouth and insomnia.

The psychostimulants: cocaine and the amphetamines

Cocaine is a major alkaloidal component from the Andean bush *Erythroxylon coca*. Leaves of this plant are chewed by Andean Indians to decrease the feeling of hunger and fatigue; there is little evidence that dependence is caused by this means of administration. A major health problem arises, however, when cocaine is used in industrialized countries. Thus in the US over 20 million people are estimated to use the drug, by nasal administration ("snorting"), injection of the salts, or smoking the free alkaloid ("crack").

The subjective effects of all the psychostimulants depend on personality, the environment in which it is administered, the dose of the drug, and the route of administration. For example, moderate doses of D-amphetamine (10–20 mg) in a normal person will produce euphoria, a sense of increased energy and alertness, anorexia, insomnia, and an improvement in the conduct of repetitive tasks. Some people become anxious, irritable and talkative. As the dose of amphetamine is increased, the symptoms become more marked and the influence of the environment less pronounced.

Most psychostimulants produce qualitatively similar effects, and include such drugs as methylamphetamine, phenmetrazine, methylphenidate and diethylpropion. The shrub khat, from Yemen and other Middle Eastern countries, contains the stimulant ($-$)cathinone, which has properties similar to those of the synthetic psychostimulants.

The main difference between cocaine and the amphetamine-like drugs lies in its shorter duration of action, the half-life for cocaine being about 50 minutes while that of amphetamine is 10 hours.

Because of its widespread abuse, particularly in the US, detailed studies have recently been undertaken on the pattern of abuse of cocaine. Some 20% of those experimenting with the drug go on to become regular users (i.e. psychologically dependent). Once dependent, the individual may administer the drug as frequently as every 15 minutes for up to 12 hours at a time. The initial positive social effects, such as increased energy and motivation, eventually give rise to the individual becoming asocial and preoccupied with the drug-induced euphoria. Severe psychological and social impairment finally intervenes. The consequence of long-term abuse is unclear, but it does seem that people taking cocaine by the intranasal route may recover without progressing to other forms of drug abuse.

Mechanisms of action

The reinforcing (i.e. dependence-producing) effects of cocaine are thought to result from its ability to inhibit the reuptake of dopamine and thereby to increase dopaminergic activity, particularly in the ventral tegmental area and the nucleus accumbens, so enhancing the activity of the dopaminergic system in the mesolimbic area (the reward area) of the brain.

By contrast, the stimulant amphetamines, such as D-amphetamine and methylamphetamine, release dopamine from most brain regions. These drugs also inhibit the reuptake of all biogenic amines, but the effects on the noradrenergic and serotonergic systems do not appear to be directly associated with the dependence potential of the drugs.

Fenfluramine is an amphetamine that selectively stimulates the release of 5-HT and lacks dependence and stimulant properties. This drug is used as an anorexiant, a property which it shares with the stimulant amphetamines.

The structures of some of these stimulants are shown in Figure 15.4.

Toxicity

Cocaine

The most serious toxic effects of cocaine involve changes in the cardiovascular system. These include cardiac arrhythmias, myocardial ischaemia and infarction, and cerebrovascular spasm, all of which can be largely explained by the facilitation of the action of catecholamines on the cardiovascular system. Another explanation of the cardiotoxicity of cocaine lies in the direct vasoconstrictive properties of its major metabolite, norcocaine. It seems likely

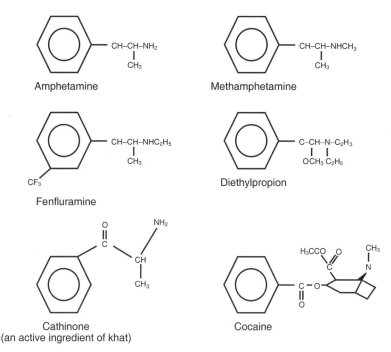

Figure 15.4. Chemical structure of some centrally acting stimulants.

that the vasoconstrictor effects of cocaine are due to a reduction in sodium flux across the cardiac cell wall, as all local anaesthetics block sodium channels but only cocaine causes vasoconstriction. It has been estimated that about 20% of those dying of cocaine overdose show myocarditis at autopsy. Nevertheless, it has also been established that cocaine increases the release of adrenal catecholamines (adrenaline and noradrenaline) and sensitizes the cardiac adrenoceptors of their action.

Seizures, possibly due to the local anaesthetic effects of the drug at toxic doses, can occur particularly in those predisposed to epilepsy. Although such toxic and often fatal effects occur more frequently after intravenous and inhalational administration, nasal administration has also been reported to result in such toxicity even in young, apparently healthy people. There is a poor correlation between the euphoriant effects of cocaine and its cardiotoxicity, so that someone who uses the euphoriant effects of the drug to regulate the dose may be unaware of the cardiovascular toxicity. Thus one of the main reasons why the cocaine user may die suddenly is the differential psychological and cardiovascular tolerance. This occurs more rapidly in the brain than the heart, and therefore a slight overdose with the drug can lead to heart failure.

Anxiety and panic attacks may be associated with high doses of cocaine. These effects may be associated with paranoid ideation, visual and tactile hallucinations (called formication) and visual pseudohallucinations (seeing snow lights). Ideas of reference, characteristic of stimulant psychosis, also occur.

Similar effects have been reported after abuse of the amphetamines which, in addition, may be associated with increasing stereotyped behaviour and a full psychotic episode (auditory, visual and tactile hallucinations often unassociated with cardiovascular symptoms) which may be difficult to differentiate from paranoid schizophrenia. This is the basis for using amphetamine as a model for schizophrenia, in both animals and human volunteers. The central effects of high doses of cocaine and the amphetamines may be suppressed by the administration of neuroleptics.

Amphetamines

The toxicity following the administration of high doses of amphetamines arises as a consequence of the release of catecholamines from peripheral and central sympathetic neurons, combined with their reduced metabolism owing to the reduction in their reuptake. The cardiotoxicity is similar to that described for cocaine, in which sympathetic drive to the heart is increased. There is now evidence that high, chronic doses of the amphetamines can cause a degeneration of dopaminergic neurons, possibly because of the formation of an endogenous neurotoxin, 6-hydroxydopamine.

The amphetamines are weak MAO-B inhibitors, and this may limit the oxidative deamination of such a metabolite and thereby lead to its accumulation. The pronounced anhedonia seen after chronic amphetamine abuse may be ascribed to a degeneration of dopaminergic neurons in the mesolimbic region of the brain.

Acute intoxication with amphetamine is associated with tremor, confusion, irritability, hallucinations and paranoid behaviour, hypertension, sweating and occasionally cardiac arrhythmias; convulsions and death may occur. The cardiovascular effects of the stimulants may be treated by beta-blockers, or by the combined alpha- and beta-blocker labetalol; calcium channel antagonists such as nifedipine may correct the arrhythmias, while intravenous diazepam is of value in attenuating seizures.

Tolerance

This only develops to some of the effects of cocaine, for example the euphoric "rush" following intravenous administration and some of the cardiovascular effects, but the degree of tolerance is limited. However, most long-term users do require increasing amounts of the drug to produce the same subjective effects to those experienced initially when taking the drug.

Amphetamine users also develop a tolerance to some of the central effects, such as the euphoria and anorexia, which may lead to the escalation of the dose; this may be partly ascribed to enhanced excretion of the drug. Cross-tolerance occurs between the psychostimulants.

Reverse tolerance, or sensation, can occur with all the psychostimulants, and may be partly related to enhanced mesolimbic forebrain dopaminergic function. Such increased sensitivity to the effects of these drugs need not depend on the drugs being given daily. The stereotyped behaviour seen in amphetamine abusers may be attributed to the increased activity of the striatal dopaminergic system.

Kindling may account for the lowered seizure threshold following chronic cocaine abuse. This phenomenon has been described elsewhere (e.g. in the use of carbamazepine in the treatment of mania), and occurs when small, subconvulsive doses eventually give rise to spontaneous seizures.

Withdrawal effects following the abrupt termination of the administration of psychostimulants comprise depression, anxiety and craving, followed by a general fatigue and disturbed sleep pattern. Hyperphagia and anhedonia are common. In general, the mood returns to normal after several days. There are no grossly observable signs of physical dependence following prolonged psychostimulant abuse. In the US, desipramine has been found to be beneficial in treating the withdrawal effects from cocaine (so-called "cocaine crash"). The precise mechanism whereby this tricyclic antidepressant produces such an antagonistic effect is uncertain.

The abuse potential of "designer" drugs

The term "designer drug" was first used in the US to describe a synthetic opioid analogue that was sold to heroin addicts in California in 1980 as a very potent form of heroin (called "China white", and reputed to be 200 times more potent than morphine). Subsequently the compound was identified as alpha-methyl fentanyl, an analogue of the dissociative analgesic fentanyl. It has been estimated that this compound has caused several hundred deaths through overdose in California alone, the main danger being the narrow margin between the dose producing euphoria and that leading to respiratory depression. People using these fentanyl derivatives show all the features of opiate abuse.

Another synthetic heroin-like compound was sold to heroin-dependent individuals in California in 1982 as "new heroin", which was soon recognized to cause severe Parkinsonian symptoms in young people. Eventually it was discovered that "new heroin" contained pethidine together with an N-methyl-phenyl-tetrahydropyridine (MPTP) contaminant. It is now established that MPTP is converted to a neurotoxic metabolite, MPP+, by the action of MAO-B in the substantia nigra, where it acts as a neurotoxin and destroys the dopamine cell bodies. MPTP thus acts as a pro-toxin. Its neurotoxicity can be prevented by inhibiting the action of MAO-B by deprenyl, for example, or by the administration of mazindol, which inhibits the dopamine carrier mechanism whereby MPP+ is transported into the dopaminergic neurons. Should MPP+ enter the dopaminergic neurons, irreversible parkinsonism occurs which is amenable to treatment with L-dopa. Treatment of rodents and monkeys with MPTP is now used to produce a model of the disease.

The Health Authorities in many countries are concerned over the widespread use of methylenedioxymethamphetamine, *MDMA* ("Ecstasy") as a recreational drug. This has been a reflection of the increase in reports in both the medical and popular press of MDMA related fatalities and severe adverse effects. MDMA is structurally related to methylenedioxyamphetamine (MDA), known amongst recreational drug users as "Eve". Both drugs cause euphoria and are drugs of abuse which are similar to methamphetamine. The acute effects of these drugs in volunteers who have had previous experience of MDMA include symptoms commonly seen after use of stimulants, for example, tachycardia, hypertension, dry mouth, mood elevation and a subjective sense of increased energy. Impaired judgement has also been frequently noticed. Other psychiatric symptoms which have been reported in weekend users of MDMA include a significantly reduced mood during the week following the use of the drug and an impairment of memory which may reflect the temporary depletion of brain serotonin. Reduced non-REM sleep and a disturbed sleep pattern have also been described in these users. In a study of individuals with a history of MDMA abuse, a PET imaging study showed that there was a decreased global and regional binding of a specific ligand for the serotonin transporter which suggests that, in man as in primates and rodents, regular use of MDMA is neurotoxic to serotonergic neurons. The mechanism of this neurotoxicity is unclear but there is experimental evidence to suggest that free radicals, produced by the oxidation of metabolites of MDMA, are implicated. In contrast to these chronic effects of MDMA, the acute effects include both the sympathomimetic effects and those symptoms such as hyperthermia, hyperreflexia and myoclonus which are attributed to the enhanced release of serotonin. Both the acute and chronic effects of MDMA seen in rodents and primates occur at doses commonly taken by recreational drug users (75–150 mg).

MDMA and MDA abuse has been associated with panic disorder, depression and chronic paranoid psychosis. As these conditions may also occur independently of these drugs, it is difficult to prove causality but it seems reasonable to conclude that some individuals are more vulnerable to such psychiatric disorders which are exacerbated by these drugs. In

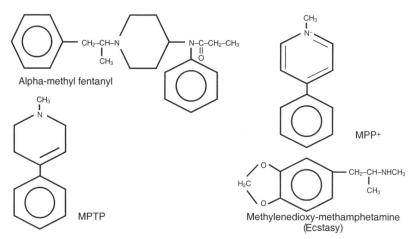

Figure 15.5. Structures of some "designer drugs" of abuse. Compare the structure of alpha-methyl fentanyl with that of fentanyl, MMP⁺ with that of pethidine, and ecstasy with that of methamphetamine.

addition to the neurological and psychiatric effects that are elicited by these amphetamines, recent evidence suggests that some aspects of cellular immunity are suppressed for several hours even after a single dose of MDMA. It is currently unclear what impact this might have, particularly after regular recreational use, on the resistance of the immune system to infections but clearly these drugs have effects which far exceed those anticipated from the pharmacology of amphetamine.

In conclusion, recent evidence suggests that MDMA and related compounds do not deserve the widespread belief that they are harmless substances which should be legally available. They constituted a potentially serious risk for acute toxic reactions that cannot be predicted by the dose taken. The acute reactions carry with them significant mortality and morbidity while the neurotoxicity shown to occur in rodents, primates and now in man suggests that they have a potential to cause permanent brain damage.

The structures of some of these "designer drugs" are shown in Figure 15.5. Their relationship to the amphetamines and opiates is apparent.

Hallucinogens

Clinical effects

Many different classes of drugs can produce hallucinations when given in toxic doses (e.g. the anticholinergics, such as atropine and scopolamine), but such symptoms are generally associated with confusion and lack of sensory clarity. As such, hallucinations are a component of a toxic psychosis.

True hallucinogens, also called psychedelics or psychotomimetics, produce their effects without causing changes in the level of consciousness. Such effects are usually associated with a heightened sensory awareness but a diminished control of the incoming sensory impressions. Thus the individual frequently finds it impossible to differentiate between one sensory impression and another, thereby leading to a feeling of being "in union with mankind or the universe", a chemically induced equivalent of a religious experience.

The drugs usually included among the hallucinogens are of the indolealkylamine type (like lysergic acid diethylamide, LSD), the phenylethylamine (mescaline-like) or phenylisopropranolamine (amphetamine-like) types. Figure 15.6 gives the structures of some of the more common hallucinogens.

Another method of classification has been based on such criteria as their subjective effects, the neurophysiological changes they produce, and their ability to cause cross-tolerance with members of the same or different chemical series. This has led to the classification into:

1. LSD-like (e.g. LSD, psilocybin and psilocin).
2. Dimethoxyamphetamine (DMA), dimethoxymethylamphetamine (DOM), dimethyltryptamine (DMT) and related drugs.
3. Drugs which lack the effects of LSD but which are hallucinogenic, such as the cannabinoids (e.g. delta-9-tetrahydrocannabinol from cannabis), bufotenin and phencyclidine.

LSD was discovered accidentally by the Swiss chemist Hofmann in 1943 while he was trying to prepare oxytocin derivatives related to the ergot alkaloids. The profound visual hallucinations which LSD produced suggested that an understanding of the mechanism of action of such drugs may give some insight into the basis of psychotic disorders. Although drugs like LSD have had no lasting clinical application, they have been used illicitly for over two decades. However, while the illicit use of LSD has declined, particularly in the US, a resurgence of its use has occurred in the UK recently with the arrival of the "acid house" culture.

Mechanism of action

Research into the action of the hallucinogens has largely concentrated on the serotonergic system, following the seminal hypothesis of Woolley and Shaw (1954) that LSD blocked 5-HT receptors in the brain. It was subsequently found that the firing rate of dorsal raphé neurons was specifically attenuated by low doses of LSD applied systemically or micro-iontophoretically. It is now known that such drugs stimulate the presynaptic 5-HT receptors, thereby inhibiting the firing of the raphé neurons; similar effects can be produced by applying 5-HT. The net result is a decreased activity of 5-HT terminals in the forebrain. It would appear that the hallucinogens produce their effects by activating 5-HT_2-

type receptors, effects which can be selectively blocked by the specific antagonist ritanserin. Most hallucinogens can also affect the activity of the locus coeruleus, again via the 5-HT$_2$ receptors located on the noradrenergic cell bodies. These receptors are linked to the phosphatidyl inositol second messenger system, and it has been observed that drugs like LSD have an effect on this system more like a partial than a full agonist. The rapid development of tolerance to the hallucinogenic effects of LSD-like drugs has been related to the rapid desensitization of these receptors.

Pharmacological effects

Doses of 20–50 µg LSD in the normal adult can produce pronounced effects on the brain, with negligible changes in peripheral organs. Higher doses produce such peripheral sympathomimetic effects as pupillary dilatation, tachycardia, hypertension, hyper-reflexia, tremor, nausea, piloerection and hyperthermia. With slightly higher doses, the euphoriant effects tend to predominate initially, closely followed by visual hallucinations and peripheral changes after two or three hours; auditory hallucinations are rare.

The term "synaesthesia" refers to the phenomenon whereby sensory modalities overlap, so that music is "seen" and colours "heard". This loss of sensory boundaries can be highly disturbing, and can lead to severe anxiety and even panic. At this stage, mood is often labile. After 4 or 5 hours, should the effects of a "bad trip" not occur, the individual may become detached in thinking and behaviour. Doses of LSD in the range 1–16 µg/kg are associated with an accentuation of all these effects, which may last for 12 hours; the half-life of the drug is 3 hours. There is no evidence of long-term personality changes.

The pattern of effects of other hallucinogens is somewhat similar to that of LSD, but most of these drugs are less potent and often must be inhaled or injected because of their poor oral absorption. With the hallucinogenic amphetamines, such as DOM, low doses produce mild euphoria with hallucinations and enhanced self-awareness, while higher doses have LSD-like effects. These changes can be effectively blocked by selective 5-HT antagonists, suggesting that all hallucinogens act via a common serotonergic pathway.

Tolerance and dependence

Tolerance to the effects of LSD can occur after only three or four daily doses, presumably because of desensitization of the 5-HT$_2$ receptors; the cardiovascular system shows a much slower development of tolerance.

Cross-tolerance occurs between LSD, mescaline and psilocybin, but not between this group and the amphetamine type of hallucinogens. This

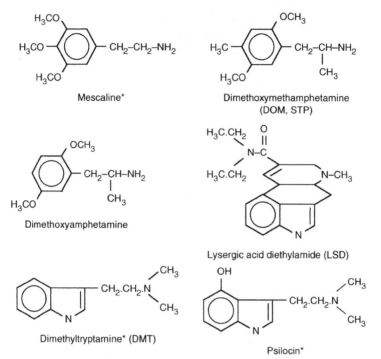

Figure 15.6. Structures of some naturally occurring (*) and synthetic hallucinogens.

suggests that the latter must produce their effects by acting on other transmitter processes in addition to the 5-HT system.

Unlike other drugs of abuse, the hallucinogens do not produce a pattern of regular use and they appear to be confined only to occasional use. Abrupt withdrawal is not associated with any noticeable physical or psychological effects. The primary adverse effect of these drugs (a "bad trip") is associated with severe anxiety and panic, which usually respond to anxiolytics. A recurrence of hallucinations when the user is not taking the drug, termed a "flash-back", can occur in about 15% of former hallucinogen users. It is often precipitated by anxiety and may occur several years after the last administration of a hallucinogen.

In some people, the use of hallucinogens can precipitate a severe psychiatric disorder, such as depression or a schizophrenic-like psychosis.

Phencyclidine and related compounds

Historical background

Phencyclidine (PCP) was first developed as a dissociative anaesthetic in the 1950s, but its use was mainly confined to veterinary anaesthesia after it had been established that it caused delirium and hallucinations in patients undergoing anaesthesia. A closely related congener, ketamine, is however still used clinically, especially in children, as a dissociative anaesthetic, as such psychotomimetic effects are minimal. Both drugs produce intense analgesia, amnesia and finally anaesthesia after intravenous administration. Recovery from ketamine-induced anaesthesia is nevertheless often accompanied by nightmares and occasionally hallucinations, many patients also experiencing delirium and excitement.

Phencyclidine has been favoured as an illicit drug of abuse for some 20 years, but such a use appears to have declined recently owing to the availability of relatively inexpensive cocaine. The drug has the street names of "PCP", "angel dust' and "crystal". The structures of phencyclidine and ketamine are shown in Figure 15.7.

Both phencyclidine and ketamine are arylcyclohexylamines with stimulant, depressant, hallucinogenic and analgesic properties. In man, small doses produce signs of intoxication, as shown by staggering gait, slurred speech and nystagmus. Higher doses also cause sweating, a catatonic rigidity and disorientation; drowsiness and apathy may also be apparent. Such a state is sometimes accompanied by physical aggression. As such drugs are potent amnestic agents, the individual may be unaware of violent acts on recovering from the effects of the drug. Increasing doses lead to anaesthesia and eventually coma. Heart rate and blood pressure are elevated and the individual shows hypersalivation, fever and muscular rigidity. Convulsions may occur at high doses. The effects of a single dose may last 4 to 6 hours; perceptual disturbances, disorientation and intense anxiety commonly occur.

Mode of action

Both phencyclidine and ketamine bind with high affinity to a number of receptors in the brain, but it is now accepted that the primary target is the sigma-PCP receptor site located in the ion channel of the NMDA excitatory amino acid receptor complex. The precise function of this receptor in the brain is still the subject of debate. It is now known that there are two distinct sigma receptor sites in the mammalian brain (σ_1 and σ_2) which are not associated with the NMDA receptor complex. Haloperidol and the atypical neuroleptic remoxipride bind with high affinity to such sites, and it has been postulated that some typical and atypical neuroleptics may owe some of their pharmacological effects to their action on such receptors.

Considerable attention is now being paid to the way in which phencyclidine and ketamine block the ion channel controlled by the NMDA receptor. This prevents the movement of calcium ions in particular into the cell which, in the case of the NMDA receptors situated in the hippocampus, inhibits long-term potentiation and thereby blocks memory

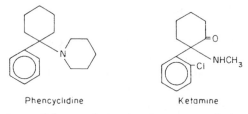

Figure 15.7.   Structures of the psychotomimetic compound phencyclidine and the
structurally related dissociative anaesthetic ketamine.

formation. These drugs can also exhibit a neuroprotective effect against
nerve cell damage arising from cerebral hypoxia. Such an action is of
potential importance in the future development of drugs to prevent brain
damage that arises as a consequence of stroke.

The pronounced effects of phencyclidine on locomotor activity in both
animals and man, and the psychotomimetic effects in man, may be a
consequence of its facilitatory effects on dopaminergic transmission,
particularly in mesolimbic regions of the brain. This is unlikely to be due to a
direct effect of the drug on dopamine receptors, but is probably due to its action
on NMDA heteroceptors on dopaminergic terminals in these brain regions.

After chronic use, the drug appears to have an extended half-life of up to
3 days. This is due to the extensive enterohepatic circulation combined with
the increased concentration of its metabolites, some of which are
pharmacologically active.

Tolerance and dependence

Tolerance to the effects of phencyclidine develops in both animals and man.
A slight physical dependence has been reported in man, characterized by a
craving for the drug, persistent amnesia, slurred speech and difficulty in
thinking, which may last up to 1 year after discontinuing the drug. Severe
personality changes have also been reported.

Cannabis and the cannabinoids

Principal sources

The hemp plant, *Cannabis sativa*, has been known for its commercial use as a
source of hemp for the manufacture of rope, sacking and so on for well over
2000 years. The hemp seeds have also been used as a source of oil, as an
animal feed and as a form of soap, while the leaves were first used in China
because of the psychoactive ingredients they contained. From China, the

use of hemp spread first to India and then to Europe via the Middle East in the 16th century.

All parts of the hemp plant contain psychoactive substances; some 60 active ingredients, the cannabinoids, have been isolated from the plant to date. In addition, over 300 non-cannabinoid compounds have been identified which do not appear to contribute to the psychoactive properties of the plant. The highest cannabinoid concentrations are found in the flowering heads.

There are three main types of cannabis preparation in use. *Herbal cannabis*, known variously as "grass", "pot", "joint" or "marijuana", is prepared by collecting the flowering heads or the upper leaves of the plant, allowing them to dry, and then removing the stems and stalks by rubbing the dried material. The resultant material is then rolled into cigarettes, or placed in a pipe, and smoked. The cannabinoid content of herbal cannabis varies according to the climate and growing conditions, but it comprises up to 8% cannabinoids.

Cannabis resin, an exudate secreted from the hairs on the leaves of the plant, is also collected from the upper leaves, and comprises up to 14% cannabinoids. The resinous material is powdered and usually compressed into a hard, brownish mass, which darkens in the air as a result of oxidation. This form of the drug is known as "hash", "resin" or "charas".

The purest form of the drug produced for illicit use is *cannabis oil*. This is prepared by solvent extraction of the resin followed by further purification to produce an oil that comprises up to 60% cannabinoids. Cannabis oil is generally added in small quantities to tobacco and smoked.

Cannabis in its various forms is still the most commonly used illicit drug in most countries. In the US, more than 50% of young adults report the use of this drug on some occasion, but it would appear that its casual use has declined among young people in that country from 37% in 1978 to about 18% 10 years later. Despite statements from the advocates for its decriminalization, there is evidence that the smoke from the dried leaves contains potential carcinogens, together with carbon monoxide, and is therefore liable to affect the respiratory and cardiovascular systems adversely, in a similar manner to tobacco.

The main active ingredients of cannabis are cannabinol, cannabidiol and several isomers of tetrahydrocannabinol, of which delta-9-tetrahydro-cannabinol (THC) is probably responsible for most of the psychoactive effects of the various preparations. It is of interest to note that THC does not contain nitrogen in its three-membered ring system. The structure of THC is shown in Figure 15.8.

Tetrahydrocannabinol and related compounds are very lipophilic and therefore readily absorbed from the lung and gastrointestinal tract. The bioavailability of oral THC varies from 4% to 12%, depending on the way in which it is delivered, whereas the availability of THC when smoked can be

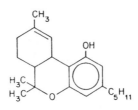

Figure 15.8. Structure of tetrahydrocannabinol (delta-9-THC), the main psychoactive ingredient of the cannabis plant.

as high as 50%. Under optimal conditions, this could mean that a cigarette
containing 1 g could lead to the delivery of up to 10 mg of THC to the
circulation. The plasma concentration peaks after about 10 minutes, and the
psychoactive effects reach a maximum after 20–30 minutes and last for
about 2–3 hours. The time of peak effect and the duration of the
pharmacological response is slower after oral administration.

Tetrahydrocannabinol is metabolized in the liver to form active
metabolites which are further metabolized to inactive polar compounds;
these are excreted in the urine. Some metabolites are excreted into the bile
and then recycled via the enterohepatic circulation. Because of their high
lipophilicity, most active metabolites are widely distributed in fat deposits
and the brain, from which sources they are only slowly eliminated. The
half-life of elimination for many of the active metabolites has been
calculated to be approximately 30 hours. Accordingly, accumulation occurs
with regular, chronic dosing. Traces of the cannabinoids can be detected in
the blood and urine of users for many days after the last administration.
There is some evidence of metabolic tolerance occurring after chronic use of
the drug. THC and related cannabinoids readily penetrate the placental
barrier and may possibly detrimentally affect foetal development.

Mechanisms of action

The high lipophilicity of THC and related compounds implies that these
drugs are widely distributed throughout the brain, particularly in the grey
matter; they appear to be taken up into neurons rather than the glia.

Understanding the pharmacological properties of the cannabinoids has
been greatly increased by the recent discovery and cloning of specific
cannabinoid receptors in the mammalian brain, spleen and macrophages. In
addition, possible endogenous candidates which act on these receptors have
also been identified. In the brain, the cannabinoids act on the CB1 type of
receptor. These are distributed in regions of the brain concerned with motor
activity and postural control, such as the basal ganglia and cerebellum, with
emotion (for example the amygdala and hippocampus), sensory perception

(thalamus) and autonomic and endocrine functions (hypothalamus, pons and medulla). The distribution of the CB1 receptors in the brain is similar to the distribution of tetrahydrocannabinol and other cannabinoids so it is not unreasonable to assume that they exert their pharmacological effects by activating the CB1 receptors. A second type of cannabinoid receptor, the CB2 receptor, has been detected on the surface of immune cells in the spleen and probably mediates the immunological effects of these drugs. Both types of receptor are present in peripheral tissues.

The first endogenous substance which was shown to interact with cannabinoid receptors was anandamide (from the Sanskrit word for bliss, ananda). This is a derivative of the polyunsaturated fatty acid arachidonic acid, namely arachidonyl ethanolamide. It appears that several other endogenous ligands also exist which include 2-arachidonylglycol. Stimulation of neurotransmitter receptors appears to play a determinant role in initiating the synthesis of these ligands. Thus it has been shown that anandamide release in the striatum is strongly enhanced by activation of dopamine D_2 receptors. Once released, anandamide activates CB1 or 2 receptors or is accumulated in the adjacent cells by an energy and sodium-dependent transport mechanism. Thus anandamide and 2-arachidonylglycerol can be released from neuronal and non-neuronal cells when the need arises, utilizing distinct receptor-mediated pathways from those used by conventional neurotransmitters. The non-synaptic release mechanisms and short half-lives of these endogenous cannabinoids suggests that they act near the sites of their synthesis to regulate the effects of primary neurotransmitters and hormones. A major implication of the discovery of the cannabinoid receptors is that it should be possible to develop selective cannabinoid agonists and antagonists for use either as therapeutic agents or as tools to unravel the precise physiological function of the cannabinoid system.

As the endogenous cannabinoids might serve important regulatory functions, it is not unreasonable to assume that they may have important therapeutic applications. The following account summarizes such possibilities.

Modulation of pain. Cannabinoids strongly reduce pain responses by interacting with CB1 receptors in the brain, spinal cord and peripheral sensory neurons. In the case of neuropathic pain, these drugs have been shown to be potent inhibitors of allodynia (pain from non-noxious stimuli) and hyperalgesia (increased sensitivity to noxious stimuli). In a rat model of neuropathic pain, the CB1 receptor agonist WIN 552122 has been shown to attenuate such responses at doses that do not cause overt side effects. These beneficial effects were antagonized by the CB1 antagonist SR 141716A. In addition, CB1 receptor agonists have been shown to alleviate peripherally mediated pain, possibly by affecting the gating mechanism by enhancing the opioid peptides. The clinical impact of these advances is still modest but the development of novel cannabinoid receptor agonists may lead to the discovery of novel drugs to treat these often intractable conditions.

Neuroprotection. CB1 receptor agonists inhibit both glutamatergic transmission and long-term potentiation which suggests that the endogenous cannabinoids may play an important role in the regulation of excitatory transmission. In cultures of rat hippocampal neurons, the stimulation of glutamate release causes neuronal death. CB1 receptor agonists prevent this response but do not protect the neurons against the effects of exogenous glutamate. Similar protective effects of CB1 agonists have been shown to occur in *in vivo* models of cerebral ischaemia, these effects being blocked by CB1 receptor antagonists. Thus it seems possible that cannabinoids may be of potential value as neuroprotective agents.

Dopamine transmission, movement disorders and psychosis. CB1 receptors are densely expressed in the basal ganglia and cortex, a distribution which provides an anatomical substrate for the functional interaction between the cannabinoid system and ascending dopaminergic pathways. There is experimental evidence to show that anandamide modulates the dopamine-induced facilitation of psychomotor activity. In support of this hypothesis, "knock-out" mice lacking the CB1 receptor show a profound decrease in locomotor activity. The therapeutic implications of this discovery have been shown by the discovery that CB1 receptor agonists alleviate the spasticity in various conditions, and tics in Tourette's syndrome. With regard to psychosis, there is consensus that heavy cannabis abuse can precipitate psychotic episodes in those with an underlying schizophrenic condition. It is possible that CB1 antagonists may therefore be of some therapeutic value in the treatment of psychotic disorders. CB1 agonists such as tetrahydrocannabinol have however been shown to inhibit amphetamine-induced stereotypy, a drug used in rodent models of psychosis. However, it has been shown that the chronic administration of cannabinoids causes an increase in the stimulant effects of amphetamine which suggests that CB1 receptor desensitization can exacerbate psychosis. Thus there is a need to investigate a wide variety of drugs which modulate the cannabinoid system.

In CONCLUSION, it would be surprising if the cannabinoid system which appears to serve such an important function in the brain and peripheral system, did not facilitate the development of novel drugs in the near future.

Tolerance and dependence

Regular use of cannabis can lead to an intake of THC which would be toxic to the naïve user. This suggests that tolerance develops. While there is some evidence that metabolic tolerance may arise, it would appear that tissue tolerance is the most likely explanation for the effects observed. Tolerance develops to the drug-induced changes in mood, tachycardia, hyperthermia and decrease in intraocular pressure. Tolerance also develops to the effects of THC on psychomotor performance and changes on electroencephalography.

Cross-tolerance occurs between THC and alcohol, at least in animal studies, but this does not appear to occur between the cannabinoids and the psychotomimetics.

The abrupt withdrawal of very high doses of THC from volunteers has been associated with some withdrawal effects (irritability, insomnia, weight loss, tremor, changed sleep profile, anorexia), suggesting that both physical and psychological dependence may occasionally arise.

Pharmacological effects

Smoking a cigarette comprising 2% THC causes changes in memory, motor coordination, cognition and sense of time, all of which are adversely affected. There is an enhanced sense of well-being and euphoria, accompanied by a feeling of relaxation and sleepiness. The intensity of these effects depends to some extent upon the environment in which the drug is taken. The effect upon short-term memory and the impairment of the ability to undertake memory-dependent, goal-directed behaviour is called *temporal disintegration*. This process is correlated with a tendency to confuse the past, present and future, and to feel depersonalized. Such effects may last for several hours and may be intensified should the subject also consume alcohol.

Higher doses of THC are associated with hallucinations, delusions and paranoid ideas; the sense of depersonalization also becomes more intense. The possibility that high doses of THC can trigger a schizophrenic episode in predisposed people is well recognized. "Flashbacks" have been reported in those who have been exposed to high doses of the drug.

Chronic cannabis users frequently exhibit the *"amotivational syndrome"*, characterized by apathy, impaired judgement, memory defects and loss of interest in normal social pursuits. Whether chronic cannabis abuse leads to more permanent changes in brain function is uncertain, but it is known that chronic administration to animals results in permanent damage to the hippocampus. Regular use of cannabis by adolescents frequently predisposes them to other types of drug abuse later. This may reflect the social pressures placed upon them rather than the pharmacological consequences of abusing cannabis.

The most consistent effects of THC upon the cardiovascular system are tachycardia, increased systolic blood pressure and a reddening of the conjunctivae. As myocardial oxygen demand is increased, the chances of angina are enhanced in those who may be predisposed to this condition.

Pulmonary function is impaired in chronic cannabis smokers, despite the clear evidence that the acute use of the drug results in a significant and long-lasting bronchodilatation. However, it should be noted that the tar produced by cannabis cigarettes is more carcinogenic than that obtained from normal cigarettes, so that the risks of lung cancer and heart disease are increased in chronic cannabis smokers.

There are conflicting reports on the effects of chronic high doses of THC on human sexual function, but there is some evidence that spermatogenesis and testosterone levels are decreased. In women, a single cannabis cigarette can suppress release of luteinizing hormone, so that lack of ovulation frequently occurs in women who abuse this drug. Lowered birth weight and increased chances of malformations have also been reported in the offspring of women who abuse THC during pregnancy. It is also possible that *in utero* exposure to this drug causes behavioural abnormalities in childhood.

There are two features of the cannabinoids which may ultimately be of therapeutic importance. THC lowers intraocular pressure, which may be of benefit in the treatment of glaucoma. There is also evidence that THC is a moderately effective antiemetic agent. Such a discovery has led to the development of nabilone, a synthetic cannabinoid, as an antiemetic agent, but its use is limited because of the dysphoria, depersonalization, memory disturbance and other effects which are associated with the cannabinoids. Whether the bronchodilator action of THC will ever find therapeutic application in the treatment of asthma remains an open question.

Conclusions

Whether a person will self-administer a drug depends on a number of factors in addition to the pharmacological properties of the drug, the dose administered and its route of administration. These factors include the environment in which the drug is taken and the nature of the previous experience following administration of another drug with similar proper- ties. With some exceptions, any mammal given continuous access to a drug of dependence will show a pattern of self-administration which is similar to that found in man. This suggests that a pre-existing psychopathology is not a prerequisite for the initial, or even continual, drug use, and that drugs of dependence have powerful reinforcing properties whether or not they cause physical dependence.

16 Paediatric Psychopharmacology

Introduction

When any psychotropic drug is to be given to either a very young or an elderly patient, the general rule is to start with the lowest dose that is therapeutically beneficial in contrast to the standard dose that would be given to a young adult. There are a number of reasons for this practice. The rates of drug absorption, metabolism and distribution differ. In the case of the young child and aged person, hepatic microsomal enzyme metabolism, which is largely responsible for the metabolism of psychotropic drugs, is suboptimal. In the elderly patient, the cardiac output and renal perfusion rates are substantially decreased, even in the physically healthy person. There is also evidence that tissue sensitivity to many psychotropic drugs is altered at the extremes of age. Thus the general rule is to start at the lowest possible dose and, if necessary, increase the dose slowly until optimal therapeutic benefit is achieved.

In the treatment of psychiatric disorders of children, the clinician is faced with a problem which is less apparent in the adult patient. In adult psychiatry, the diagnosis of the condition assists in ensuring optimal treatment. For example, the treatment of the symptoms of anxiety will depend on the underlying condition with which the anxiety is associated. Thus the type of drug used will depend, for example, on whether the patient is an anxious schizophrenic, an anxious depressive or a patient with panic disorder. As psychiatric diagnosis of childhood disorders is at a more elementary stage than it is in adult psychiatry, the diagnostic approach to treatment still leaves much to be desired. This chapter will therefore be confined to a discussion of those disorders of childhood for which there seems to be reasonable agreement over diagnosis and treatment.

Despite the success in the use of psychotropic drugs for the treatment of psychiatric disorders in adults, and to some extent in adolescents, the application of psychotropic drugs for the treatment of children has been less encouraging. This has been due to the use of invalid diagnostic

Fundamentals of Psychopharmacology. Third Edition. By Brian E. Leonard
© 2003 John Wiley & Sons, Ltd. ISBN 0 471 52178 7

classifications, limitation of the methods for measuring response to treatment and the utilization of concepts drawn from adult psychiatry being inappropriately applied to children. These difficulties are reflected in the greater variability in the use of psychotropic drugs in children. This unfortunate situation is reflected in the fact that methylphenidate, imipramine and chlorpromazine still form the bulk of the prescriptions of child psychiatrists.

There are four main areas where psychotropic drugs are useful in children:

1. To provide relief from symptoms until the child matures, for example, in enuresis.
2. As an adjunct to other treatments as, for example, when a child refuses to attend school.
3. To suppress symptoms and thereby prevent the negative effects on other psychogical parameters. An example of this would be a child who suffers from tic disorders which causes embarrassment.
4. In severe conduct disorders when other non-drug-based methods have been unsuccessful.

It must be emphasized that the use of psychotropic drugs is only part of the treatment process, particularly when considering children.

Short-term side effects of psychotropic drugs

As with all types of medication, the side effects of psychotropic drugs should be weighed against their benefits. Symptoms such as dizziness, appetite suppression and sleep disturbance occur quite commonly but often diminish following continual use. Other more serious side effects may involve changes in endocrine and cardiac function, effects which can sometimes be controlled by reducing the drug dose. Finally there are idiosyncratic and allergic reactions such as agranulocytosis which are difficult to predict and which can be fatal in some cases.

Other side effects may only be manifest in the behaviour of individual patients. For example, benzodiazepines have a calming effect in most cases but can occasionally be associated with behavioural dysinhibition and lead to aggressiveness in a disturbed child. Similarly, neuroleptics can suppress aggression but also cause emotional flattening and cognitive dysfunction. Such side effects are particularly important in the younger child. Longer-term side effects such as growth retardation as a result of stimulants and tardive dyskinesia following the prolonged use of typical neuroleptics are particularly important. It is presently unclear whether the long-term use of stimulants leads to dependence, although there would appear to be little evidence that this is the case.

Use of psychotropic drugs in specific childhood disorders

Attention deficit hyperactivity disorder (ADHD)

This is a heterogeneous disorder of inattention, hyperactivity and impulsivity that starts in childhood and may persist into adulthood. Children with the disorder can be identified by their inattention which leads to daydreaming, distractability and difficulty in sustaining an effort to complete a task. Their impulsivity makes them accident prone and disruptive while their hyperactivity, combined with excessive talking, is poorly tolerated particularly in schools. As teenagers, the hyperactivity and impulsivity tend to diminish but other symptoms persist. The adolescent with ADHD often has low self-esteem, poor relationships with peers and often becomes subject to drug abuse. To what extent ADHD persists into adulthood is open to debate, but some longitudinal, family and genetic studies would favour this view. ADHD is often co-morbid with conduct, depressive, bipolar and anxiety disorders.

Psychopathology of ADHD

Evidence of fronto-limbic dysfunction with poor inhibitory control of the cortex over the limbic system would appear to account for many of the physical and psychological symptoms. Neuroimaging studies have implicated a disorder of the right frontal cortex while PET imaging studies have shown that there is an approximate increase of 70% in the dopamine transporter in this brain region. Genetic and twin studies have shown that the heritability of the hyperactivity of ADHD is greater than 65%, while that of the attention deficit is greater than 70%. In molecular genetic studies there is evidence of an association between ADHD and a defect in the D_4 receptor gene, but it must be emphasized that not all studies have replicated this. D_4 receptor "knock-out" mice show supersensitivity to cocaine and methamphetamine that may have some bearing on the pathology of ADHD in children. ADHD is also associated with an abnormal allelic form of the dopamine transporter protein.

The catecholamine hypothesis of ADHD is the most widely supported hypothesis at the present time. This is largely based on the efficacy of the drugs used to treat the disorder and which act on the noradrenergic and dopaminergic systems. The drugs would appear to be most effective during the initial phase of the daily treatment when the plasma drug concentration is rising. This parallels the acute release of noradrenaline and dopamine and it has been argued that these changes in the catecholamines increase the inhibitory effect of the pre-frontal cortex on the subcortical regions of the brain. There is less convincing evidence regarding the involvement of 5-HT in ADHD; SSRIs have little benefit in treating the disorder. Recently, evidence has emerged that the nicotinic cholinergic receptors are defective, a view which is supported by the finding that nicotine applied as transdermal patches can improve some of the symptoms of the disorder. Nicotinic receptors can act as heteroceptors on dopaminergic terminals in the frontal cortex, which again serves to emphasize the importance of the dopaminergic system in the pathology of this disorder.

Pharmacological treatment of ADHD

The stimulants methamphetamine, dexamphetamine, methylphenidate and pemoline have been shown to improve the main symptoms of the disorder in up to 70% of children; they may be of some benefit in adults also.

Conduct disorders

The symptoms consist of a collection of symptoms such as defiance, disobedience, temper tantrums, fighting, destructiveness, stealing and lying. These disorders frequently lead to the child being brought to the child psychiatric clinic and requiring treatment as they predict potentially serious outcomes in terms of later psychiatric disorders.

While there has been an emphasis on the use of different psychotherapeutic techniques for treating these disorders, there is increasing evidence that psychotropic drugs have an important role to play.

Neuroleptics such as chlorpromazine and haloperidol have been used to treat aggressive behaviour in mentally handicapped children, but there is always a risk that such drugs have a negative impact on the cognitive, social, emotional and developmental aspects. Such side effects necessitate the use of such drugs for a very short period only. Whether the atypical antipsychotics such as risperidone could be used as safer alternatives to the first-generation neuroleptics is unknown but because of their better side effects, are worthy of consideration.

Anticonvulsants have sedative side effects and therefore drugs such as carbamazepine have occasionally been used to treat conduct disorders. There is no evidence that such drugs are useful in the control of aggressive symptoms.

Lithium may be of some value in the treatment of difficult, impulsive and aggressive adolescents and children but the results from the studies in which lithium was used are few and the outcome uncertain.

Thus, at present, there is little evidence that psychotropic drugs have a major role to play in the treatment of conduct disorders.

Emotional disorders

These disorders in children are considered to be particularly amenable to psychological treatment and therefore there has been a reluctance to use psychotropic drugs to treat them. In addition, problems of diagnostic classification have confounded research into drug treatment. Nevertheless the benzodiazepines and tricyclic antidepressants have been used. Thus the benzodiazepines have been used for childhood emotional disorders but there are no satisfactory controlled studies regarding their efficacy. Clearly only the short-term use, using short half-life drugs such as temazepam, is acceptable. So far there is no evidence of benzodiazepine dependence occurring in children.

Of the tricyclic antidepressants used, clomipramine has been shown to be effective in the treatment of children with obsessional symptoms, effects which have been shown to be independent of the antidepressant action of the drug. More recent studies have provided evidence that the SSRI antidepressants such as fluoxetine are as effective, with fewer side effects.

Tic disorders

These range from transient disorders lasting a few weeks or months to chronic conditions lasting more than a year. The most severe form of a tic disorder is Tourette's syndrome.

Neuroleptics are the drugs of choice in the treatment of tic disorders but they should only be considered in situations where the life of the child is seriously affected and when behavioural treatments have failed. Of the classical neuroleptics which have been used, haloperidol and pimozide have shown success but so far there have been no adequately controlled trials of any neuroleptic to objectively validate their efficacy. It would appear that only low doses of haloperidol are necessary (2–3 mg/day) to obtain a significant reduction in tic frequency. It would seem reasonable to consider the use of the atypical antipsychotics for these disorders but, to date, there is no evidence of their efficacy in children. Recently there have been studies in which clonidine was used in the effective treatment of motor tics. The side effects are similar to those seen in the adult and include sedation, headache, irritability and sinus bradycardia.

Nocturnal enuresis

This is quite a common condition affecting some 7% of 7 year olds who continue to wet the bed at least once a week. The cause of nocturnal enuresis is complex and beyond the scope of this volume. It is evident, however, that various treatments are available including retention control, dry-bed training, enuretic night alarms and waking the child to urinate during the night. The most effective treatment (estimated at 80%) is the use of the enuretic night alarm.

Drug treatments include sympathomimetic stimulants, anticholinergics, tricyclic antidepressants and synthetic antidiuretics. Of these, imipramine and desmopressin have been found to be the most effective.

The efficacy of imipramine has been repeatedly demonstrated in controlled trials; about 85% of children treated within a week of the start of medication, but tolerance frequently develops after a number of weeks and relapse is high after discontinuation of the treatment. Relatively low doses of imipramine only are needed, but the typical side effects of tricyclic antidepressants limit the prolonged use of the drug. The mechanism of action of imipramine in the treatment of nocturnal enuresis is unclear but one possible action is through a direct anticholinergic action on the bladder wall.

The synthetic vasopressin peptide, desmopressin, has been extensively investigated and shown to be effective as tricyclic antidepressants in the control of nocturnal enuresis and to enhace the enuretic night alarm treatment. The side effects are relatively few (nasal pain, conjunctivitis) when given by nasal spray. The precise mechanism of action of this peptide is unknown.

Affective disorders of childhood and adolescence

There is much controversy regarding the occurrence of major depressive disorder in prepubertal children. However, several studies in both the United States and Britain have suggested that depressive disorder does exist, although the frequency appears to be lower than in adolescents. There is endocrinological evidence, based on the hypersecretion of cortisol and an abnormal growth hormone response to insulin-induced hypoglycaemia, to suggest that children with major depressive disorder show similar endocrine abnormalities to those of adolescents and adults. However, the number of patients in these studies is small and clearly more thorough investigations must be undertaken before any conclusion may be reached.

Regarding the drug treatment of depression in children, there is so far a paucity of good clinical trials to show that antidepressants are effective. Several small studies suggest that daily doses of up to 5 mg/kg of imipramine may be beneficial, but there is no data to show whether other types of antidepressant medication are effective. The side effects and toxicity of tricyclic antidepressants are legion and have been discussed in detail elsewhere. Undoubtedly the SSRIs should now be the drugs of first choice in the treatment of depression in children.

Manic disorders would appear to be extremely rare in young children and only single case reports have appeared in the clinical literature. They are more common in adolescence but not as frequent as among adults. Some authorities have argued that the extent of mania among adolescents is underestimated and that many patients have been misdiagnosed as schizophrenics. Regarding treatment, lithium would appear to be the drug of choice. Since children and adolescents appear to have a higher lithium renal clearance than adults, it is occasionally necessary to give the drug in a higher oral dose than would be usual for the adult. Apart from the possible detrimental effect of lithium on bone growth in children, the monitoring of the young patient should follow the same procedures as outlined for the adult.

Anxiety disorders

The DSM–IV classifies anxiety disorders in children into four categories, namely social anxiety, over-anxious disorder, phobias and separation anxiety. Only separation anxiety, a fear of losing a loved one or a close attachment, has been reasonably well studied from the point of view of drug treatment. School phobia is perhaps the most severe form of separation anxiety and there are several trials to show that imipramine, in daily doses of up to 5 mg/kg, is effective. Many patients require drug treatment for at least 6 to 8 weeks before an optimal response is achieved. Frequently, children remain symptom free after a 3–4 month course of treatment. In addition to the usual anticholinergic effects of imipramine, it should be noted that children are often susceptible to withdrawal symptoms such as nausea and gastrointestinal spasm. This may be reduced if the drug is slowly withdrawn over a 2-week period.

Obsessive–compulsive disorders

These occur only rarely in children but more frequently in adolescents. There have been no extensive studies of drug treatments of this condition in young patients, but anecdotal reports suggest that tricyclic antidepressants such as clomipramine may be as effective as they are in adults but the SSRI antidepressants should be considered as first line treatments.

In SUMMARY, the relatively small number of psychotropic drugs which have been used for the treatment of psychiatric diseases in children and adolescents reflects the diagnostic uncertainty regarding the clinical status of the patients, the lower frequency of established psychiatric disorders in these groups of patients and, as a consequence, the paucity of good clinical trials in which the efficacy of drug treatments may be established. Nevertheless, there is good evidence that psychostimulants, particularly methylphenidate, are of value in the treatment of hyperkinetic disorders, while conventional neuroleptics and tricyclic antidepressants may have an application in the treatment of a diverse group of disorders ranging from depression to separation anxiety and aggression. In view of the well-established side effects and toxicity of such drugs, it is to be hoped that they will soon be superseded by safer drugs whose efficacy has already been established in adult patients.

It is apparent from the discussion of the drugs used in the treatments of childhood psychiatric disorders that the role of psychotropic drugs is far from clear. Many of the drugs in use were developed long before the strict guidelines of the regulatory authorities became mandatory and therefore the few drug treatments which are available have not always been subjected to the rigorous assessments which all other drugs are subject to. Clearly there is a need for more extensive research not only into the psychiatric disorders and their possible aetiologies but also into the efficacy of the drugs used to treat the disorders. There is very little evidence concerning the potential value of the second generation of antipsychotics and antidepressants that are increasingly replacing the older drugs at least in the industrialized countries. Hopefully not only will more research into the nature of childhood disorders be undertaken but also more attention given to the new psychotropic drugs that have an improved safety profile, at least in adult patients.

17 Geriatric Psychopharmacology

Introduction

The elderly person is likely to experience many socioeconomic, emotional and physiological changes which will have a major bearing on psychotropic drug treatment. Such a population is therefore more likely to be exposed to more types of drug treatment than younger age groups.

It has been found that the vast majority of elderly patients being treated for a psychiatric disorder also have at least one physical disorder that requires medication; 80% of all elderly patients in the United States have at least one chronic physical illness. Thus the elderly are the most likely group to experience adverse drug reactions and interactions. Studies show that patients over the age of 70 years have approximately twice as many adverse drug reactions as those under 50 years.

Another problem which particularly affects the elderly population concerns compliance with prescribed medication. Factors such as impaired vision, making it difficult for the patient to recognize the various medications, hearing, manual dexterity and cognition all contribute to the non-compliance. Perhaps one of the most important factors that governs non-compliance is the increased frequency and severity of the side effects that occur with most types of medication in the elderly. This may be illustrated by the tricyclic antidepressants and phenothiazine neuroleptics, both these classes of drugs having pronounced antimuscarinic activity even in the physically healthy young patient. In the elderly there is evidence of excessive sensitivity to the anticholinergic effects of drugs. This is compounded by the decline in cognitive function which accompanies ageing. Thus one must anticipate that patient compliance for any psychotropic drug with pronounced anticholinergic and sedative side effects will be low.

Another problem which can compromise compliance concerns the hypotensive actions of many psychotropic drugs (e.g. tricyclic antidepressants, phenothiazine neuroleptics). Due to the alpha$_1$ receptor antagonistic action of these drugs, they are likely to cause severe orthostatic

Fundamentals of Psychopharmacology. Third Edition. By Brian E. Leonard
© 2003 John Wiley & Sons, Ltd. ISBN 0 471 52178 7

hypotension in some elderly patients. This can cause patients to fall and damage themselves. The increased sensitivity of the elderly to the sedative effects of drugs is also well known. As hypnotics and anxiolytics are frequently administered to the elderly, the sedative effects of these drugs can be minimized by using drugs that have a short to medium half-life. There seems little justification for using the long half-life sedative hypnotics in the elderly patient.

Dementia

The pathological and clinical features of the various types of dementia have been the subject of detailed discussion elsewhere in this book (see Chapter 14). A variety of conditions that occur in the elderly must be differentiated from true dementia. Delirium, for example, is associated with an alteration in the level of consciousness, disordered thinking and fluctuating cognitive impairment. Such a delirious state can occur for a variety of reasons, including inadequately treated diabetes, hyperparathyroidism or hepatic encephalopathy. Dementia must also be distinguished from psychosis, in which the patient shows impairment of thinking but not impairment of memory. The term "pseudo-dementia" is often used to describe a depressive episode in which the patient presents with abnormalities of mood, appetite and sleep disturbance with cognitive dysfunction which is directly caused by the depression. The cognitive deficits usually resolve with treatment of the underlying condition. Finally cerebrovascular disease (as exemplified by multi-infarct dementia, which is the second most common cause of dementia) or carotid occlusion may be associated with episodic memory loss. It is therefore important to diagnose correctly the cause of the memory and cognitive impairment so that appropriate treatment may be given. Should the results of clinical and neurological investigation clearly establish the existence of Alzheimer's disease, then the appropriate symptomatic therapy (e.g. a cholinesterase inhibitor) may be considered (see Chapter 14).

Pseudodementia

This is defined as any condition which mimics dementia. The commonest psychiatric disorder which mimics dementia is depression in which the retardation can be confused with the apathy of dementia. The guiding principle is careful clinical assessment and, if in doubt, a trial of an appropriate antidepressant.

Depression

A disturbance in the sleep pattern is a common symptom of depression but changes in the sleep pattern also occur as a consequence of ageing. Once depression has been diagnosed, there are several types of antidepressants which may be given. Because of their potent anticholinergic side effects, there seems little merit in prescribing the older tricyclic antidepressants (e.g. amitriptyline, imipramine) to such patients. There is now sufficient evidence to suggest that sedative antidepressants such as mianserin or trazodone given at night reduce the likelihood that the patient will require a sedative hypnotic. For the more retarded elderly patient, a non-sedative antidepressant such as lofepramine or one of the SSRIs (e.g. fluoxetine, fluvoxamine or sertraline) may be used.

The side effects and cardiotoxicity of the tricyclic antidepressants have been discussed in detail elsewhere in this volume and, while there is ample evidence of their therapeutic efficacy, it seems difficult to justify their use, particularly in a group of patients who are most vulnerable to their detrimental side effects. Of the newer antidepressants, the reversible inhibitors of monoamine oxidase type A such as moclobemide may also be of value in the elderly depressed patient, particularly in those patients who fail to respond to the amine uptake inhibitor type of antidepressant.

The safety of antidepressants should be the first priority for the elderly. For this reason, the second-generation antidepressants, or the atypical tricyclic antidepressant lofepramine, should be the drugs of choice. Undoubtedly the SSRI antidepressants have a major role to play and of these, citalopram and fluvoxamine have been extensively studied in the elderly depressed patient.

The pharmacological properties of the antidepressants has been extensively covered in Chapter 7. It should also be remembered that electroconvulsive therapy (ECT) can be potentially life-saving in the elderly, particularly if the patient is suffering from delusions or is retarded and depressed. ECT should also be considered when antidepressant drug treatment has failed.

Psychosis

A variety of psychotic conditions occur in the elderly, but it is important to remember that an elderly person who develops agitation, paranoid ideation or delusions may be suffering from a drug-induced delirium. The most common causes of such a condition are drugs that have potent central muscarinic-blocking properties, such as the antiparkinsonian agents, antihistamines, tricyclic antidepressants and antipsychotics. Withholding all psychotropic drug medication for a few days may be the most judicious management for this type of toxic psychosis.

Agitation and aggression are often symptoms of advanced Alzheimer's disease and high potency atypical antipsychotics such as risperidone or olanzapine may be of value in demented patients. Drugs such as chlorpromazine and thioridazine are more likely to produce hypotension, cardiac abnormalities and excessive sedation in the elderly patient, and side effects are, of course, a problem with the high potency neuroleptics in the elderly; centrally acting anticholinergic agents that are used to reverse some of the symptoms of parkinsonism in such patients should be used as little as possible and in the lowest possible doses.

Mania can occur in any age group. Acute manic episodes in the elderly may best be managed with high potency neuroleptics. The use of *lithium* is not contraindicated in the elderly provided renal clearance is reasonably normal. The dose administered should be carefully monitored, as the half-life of the drug is increased in the elderly to 36–48 hours in comparison to about 24 hours in the young adult. The serum lithium concentration in the elderly should be maintained at about 0.5 mEq/litre. It is essential to ensure that the elderly patient is not on a salt-restricted diet before starting lithium therapy. The side effects and toxicity of lithium have been discussed in detail elsewhere (see p. 198 *et seq.*), and, apart from an increase in the frequency of confusional states in the elderly patient, the same adverse effects can be expected as in the younger patient.

Paranoid disorders

DSM–IV has abandoned the terms paranoia and paraphrenia and replaced them with the term delusional disorder to describe non-affective and non-bizarre delusional states.

Neuroleptics have been the group of drugs most widely recommended for delusional states. Of the first-generation neuroleptics, the sedative, cognitive impairing and extrapyramidal side effects are likely to be particularly prominent in the elderly. The introduction of the atypical neuroleptics should improve the treatment of these disorders as they are generally better tolerated due to their improved side-effect profile.

TCAs, together with neuroleptics should be avoided as they may aggravate psychotic symptoms and potentiate any anticholinergic side effects. In the case of the very aggressive patient, parenteral administration of lorazepam or diazepam will usually be sufficient to enable the patient to be managed.

Anxiety and insomnia

Anxiety states are often expressed somatically in the elderly and therefore it is important to exclude any physical disorder, such as cerebrovascular disease and thyroid dysfunction, which can be associated with apprehension and agitation.

Most psychotropic drugs are highly lipophilic, and the increased fat to lean body mass ratio and the decreased metabolism and excretion in the elderly patient mean that the half-lives of most psychotropic drugs are increased. The benzodiazepine anxiolytics and hypnotics are no exception. Following a single dose of chlordiazepoxide, diazepam or flurazepam, the time for elimination of the parent compounds and their active metabolites can be as long as 72 hours. For this reason, it is now general practice to administer a short-acting benzodiazepine (e.g. oxazepam, alprazolam or temazepam) only as needed and for as short a period as possible. Such drugs should only be used for a period not exceeding 6 weeks. Supportive psychotherapy, either as an adjunct to drug therapy or as an alternative, has an important role to play in treating mild anxiety states in the elderly.

Insomnia is a common complaint in the elderly. As people age they require less sleep, and a variety of physical ailments to which the elderly are subject can cause a change in the sleep pattern (e.g. cerebral atherosclerosis, heart disease, decreased pulmonary function), as can depression. Providing sedative hypnotics are warranted, the judicious use of short half-life benzodiazepines such as temazepam, triazolam, oxazepam and alprazolam for a period not exceeding 1–2 months may be appropriate. Because of their side effects, there would appear to be little merit in using chloral hydrate or related drugs in the treatment of insomnia in the elderly. It should be noted that even benzodiazepines which have a relatively short half-life are likely to cause excessive day-time sedation. The side effects and dependence potential of the anxiolytics and sedative hypnotics have been covered elsewhere in this volume (Chapter 9).

In addition to the benzodiazepines, there may be a role for the non-benzodiazepine drugs such as zalaplon, zolpidem or zopiclone in the treatment of anxiety and insomnia in the elderly. These drugs appear to be well tolerated in younger populations of patients, but it is essential to await the outcome of properly conducted trials of these drugs on a substantial number of elderly patients before any conclusions may be drawn regarding their value as alternatives to the benzodiazepines.

In SUMMARY, it can be seen that the types of psychotropic drug medication that may be used in the elderly are essentially similar to those used in the younger adult patient. The main difference lies in the reduction in distribution, metabolism and elimination of the drugs, which necessitates their administration in lower doses initially followed by a slower escalation of the dose until optimal benefit is obtained. Side effects, particularly anticholinergic effects, are more pronounced in the elderly and can contribute to poor compliance. Clearly the use of the older psychotropic medications, such as the tricyclic antidepressants and typical neuroleptics, should be avoided in elderly patients whenever possible and due consideration given to the second-generation antidepressants and antipsychotics. It is essential to emphasize that the side effects of psychotropic drugs, particularly the sedative and anticholinergic effects, are usually more pronounced in the elderly than in the younger patient.

18 The Inter-relationship Between Psychopharmacology and Psychoneuroimmunology

The background

The adverse effects of stress and depression, the effects of bereavement, unemployment and social isolation on mental and physical health have been known since antiquity. Aristotle advised physicians, "Just as you ought not to attempt to cure eyes without head or head without body, so you should not treat body without soul." One of the fathers of modern medicine put it more scientifically in the 19th century when he recommended that when attempting to predict health outcomes from tuberculosis in patients, it is just as important to know what is going on in a man's head as it is in his chest.

These are two of the numerous examples, largely anecdotal, that document the complex and intimate connection between the mind and the body. In the past 20 years this has given rise to a new science of psychoneuroimmunology that is devoted to the study of the inter-relationship between the brain, behaviour and the immune system. Interest in this area of neuroscience has undoubtedly been due to the impact of acquired immune deficiency syndrome (AIDS) in which it has been estimated that at least 10% of these patients will develop mood, behavioural, cognitive and memory changes before they develop somatic signs of the illness. Similarly, studies have shown that 6 months before patients with pancreatic cancer develop clinical signs of the disease, a significant proportion develop depression. Such observations suggest that not only does the brain influence the immune system by way of the endocrine and efferent neuronal pathways but also that products of immune cell activity, such as the cytokines, play a role in modifying human behaviour by directly modulating central neurotransmitter pathways.

Fundamentals of Psychopharmacology. Third Edition. By Brian E. Leonard
2003 John Wiley & Sons, Ltd. ISBN 0 471 52178 7

Basic structure of the immune system

It is not the purpose of this short introduction to psychoneuroimmunology to give a comprehensive view of the immune system, and readers are referred to the key references cited at the end of the book.

Most of the cells comprising the immune system can be divided into one of two categories depending on the targets of their action. Thus the immune cells are either primed to eliminate specific pathogens or to respond to any type of cell that is not recognized as being a normal body component. The first category of cells comprises the different types of lymphocytes which are divided into the B-lymphocytes (B cells) that are responsible for antibody production, and the T-lymphocytes (T cells) that directly phagocytose pathogens or release specific biologically active proteins, the cytokines, that regulate the activity of other cells in the immune system. Both T and B cells respond in a highly specific manner when attacking pathogens. In addition to these specific immune cells, there are phagocytic cells, such as the monocytes and neutrophils, that respond to any cell type or foreign molecule that is not recognized as being a normal constituent of the body.

The phagocytic cells such as the monocytes and neutrophils are basically scavenger white blood cells that ingest invading bacteria or viruses. Some of the monocytes also enter the tissues where they become macrophages. They can also provide signals enabling T cells to respond more efficiently to the pathogen. In this situation the antigen becomes attached to the monocyte membrane which is then presented to a T-lymphocyte together with the cytokine interleukin-1 (IL-1). This initiates a further activation of T-lymphocytes. Monocytes also produce mediators of inflammation, the complement proteins, which help to create a hostile environment for foreign organisms. In addition to complement proteins other mediators of the immune response include histamine (which acts as a local hormone to cause capillary dilatation), the prostaglandins and leukotrienes which act to initiate and terminate the activities of the macrophages and T cells.

Lymphocytes are derived from bone marrow but, whereas some of the cells remain in the bone marrow until they reach maturity (the B cells), others migrate early in their development to the thymus gland to become T cells. Thus B (from bursa) and T (from thymus) cells learn to distinguish between the normal constituent cells of the body and foreign objects, due to the presence of specific memory cells which are under genetic control. B and T cells circulate throughout the vascular system before concentrating in lymphoid tissue (spleen and lymph nodes) where they remain inactive until stimulated by specific antigens. Because of the specificity of function imparted on the T and B cells by the memory cells, the lymphocytes are highly selective in responding to relatively few antigens. The main

Table 18.1. The main properties of the immune cells that are altered in psychiatric illnesses

Natural killer cells (NKCs)	Recognize changes on cell-membrane virus-infected and cancer cells and destroy the cells. NKCs bind to surfaces of target cells and inject cytotoxic molecules into the cell membrane, destroying the cells. There are several types of cells that have NKC activity
Phagocytes	Two major classes of WBCs are involved in removing invading microorganisms by a process of phagocytosis. These are polymorphonuclear leukocytes and mononuclear phagocytes, or monocytes. In tissues, monocytes differentiate into macrophages and, in the brain, into microglia
T and B lymphocytes	Produced by lymphoid tissue. Lymphocytes represent about 20% of the WBCs in adults; they have a long life span (sometimes several years). They probably serve as memory cells for the immune system. These mononuclear cells may be small, agranular structures (T and B cells) or large, granular cells (NKCs). Different types of T cells may only be differentiated by their cell-surface markers (CD markers – clusters of differentiation). CD markers are identified using labelling antibodies

properties of the immune cells that are altered in psychiatric illnesses are summarized in Table 18.1.

T cells exist in several different forms. Thus the T-helper cells (Th cells) play a regulatory role by facilitating the antibody production by B cells and also activate the macrophages. Other types of T cells can directly attack pathogens or normal cells that have been infected with a virus or bacterium for example. These are the cytotoxic T cells, or natural killer cells (NKCs). Not only can such cells destroy pathogens but they also secrete such cytokines as IL-1 which have a key role to play in orchestrating the immune system both peripherally and in the brain. The immunoglobulins (the most important in man being IgM, IgG, IgE, IgD and IgA) are produced following the activation of B cells by specific antigens.

Fever and sleep are important events which assist recovery following an infection by helping to destroy heat-sensitive foreign microorganisms. One of the key promoters of sleep and fever following an infection is IL-1. This cytokine can penetrate some areas of the blood–brain barrier and raise the temperature "set point" in the hypothalamus thereby producing a fever. Similarly IL-1 promotes slow-wave sleep and thereby facilitates tissue repair due to the secretion of growth hormone during that sleep phase. In addition to facilitating tissue repair, growth hormone can also boost the immune system. Whereas the precise mechanism whereby the cytokines can enter the brain and initiate subtle changes in brain function is uncertain, CNS changes initiated by peripherally produced IL-1 (and also by the microglial cells within the brain) provides convincing evidence that the immune system directly impacts upon the brain.

The endocrine immune relationship

One of the major pathways whereby the central nervous system regulates the immune system is via the hypothalamic–pituitary–adrenal (HPA) axis. Various neurotransmitters (e.g. serotonin, noradrenaline, acetylcholine) regulate the secretion of corticotrophin releasing factor (CRF) which controls the release of adrenocorticotrophic hormone (ACTH) from the anterior pituitary. ACTH directly activates the adrenal cortex to produce glucocorticoids (e.g. cortisol). Following the rise in the plasma concentration of the glucocorticoids, a negative feedback mechanism normally operates to block the further release of ACTH from the pituitary. In depression, however, there would appear to be an insensitivity of the central glucocorticoid receptors to this feedback regulation. As a consequence, the plasma concentration remains elevated and cannot be easily suppressed by a potent synthetic glucocorticoid such as dexamethasone. This forms the basis of the dexamethasone suppression test (DST) which is often used as a biological marker of depression.

T cells are particularly sensitive to the inhibitory effects of the glucocorticoids. In particular, the nascent T cells, which represent about 90% of all T cells in the thymus gland, are very sensitive to the inhibitory effects of these steroids; high steroid concentrations can also prematurely induce the migration of T cells from the thymus to other immune tissues. This leads to a decrease in the size of the thymus gland. It should be emphasized that the effects of the glucocorticoids on the immune system are biphasic; in high concentrations they suppress major components of the immune system whereas in low concentration they activate it. In addition to glucocorticoid receptors, T cells also contain receptors for prolactin and growth hormones which suggests ways in which the endocrine system can directly affect the immune system.

The adrenal gland secretes glucocorticoids in a pulsatile rhythmical way with the highest plasma concentrations being reached during the day. It has been shown that the lowest plasma concentration of the glucocorticoids coincides with the time at which the lymphocytes respond most actively to antigens. As the hypersecretion of cortisol is a characteristic feature of depression and other psychiatric conditions, it is perhaps not surprising to find that components of the immune system are also abnormal in this condition.

Anatomical links between the brain and the immune system

What is the mechanism whereby the nervous system can influence the immune system? Two major routes serve to link the brain with the immune system. The first is via the HPA axis, already referred to. The second is via the autonomic nervous system.

It has been known for over 20 years that there were adrenoceptors on T cells, B cells and macrophages. In addition, noradrenergic fibres directly innervate the bone marrow, thymus, spleen, lymph nodes and virtually all other immune organs. These sympathetic nerve terminals not only release noradrenaline but also possibly neuropeptides as well. There is evidence that many sympathetic nerve terminals innervating the immune organs make direct contact with the parenchyma, ending adjacent to the cells of the immune system. In the spleen for example, the sympathetic terminals penetrate the areas that contain a high density of helper T cells and also cytotoxic and suppressor T cells. Electron microscopic evidence suggests that the sympathetic nerve terminals can form direct physical contact with T-lymphocytes and macrophages.

The functional connection between the peripheral sympathetic system and the immune system can be illustrated by the changes which take place in ageing. It is known that in the aged animal the sympathetic innervation of the spleen is dramatically reduced. This appears to be associated with deficiencies in T cell function and in cellular immunity. At the cellular level, immunosenescence is associated with a change in responsiveness of the immune cells and in their ability to regulate the beta adrenoceptors on their cell surfaces. Such changes appear to shift the metabolism of the sympathetic nervous system to a state that encourages apoptosis (or programmed cell death) possibly by inducing an increase in the production of cytotoxic metabolites. Experimental evidence suggests that the mono-amine oxidase-B (MAO-B) inhibitor deprenyl (selegiline) can reduce these neurodegenerative changes in the peripheral sympathetic system and lead to the restoration of sympathetic innervation of the spleen.

Figure 18.1 summarizes the inter-relationship between the nervous system and the immune system.

Stress and the immune system

All forms of stress result in the activation of the pituitary–adrenal axis, with a consequent rise in circulating catecholamines and glucocorticoid hormones from the adrenal gland. The secretion of ACTH from the pituitary gland, which is controlled by hypothalamic CRF, triggers the secretion of adrenal glucocorticoids, while stress-induced activation of

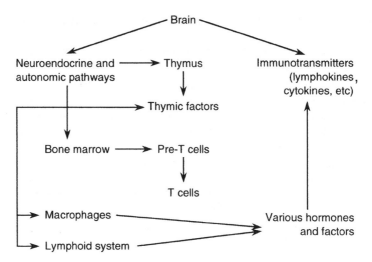

Figure 18.1.   Summary of the pathways postulated to be involved in the interaction
between the nervous and immune systems.

the sympathetic system is responsible for the catecholamine secretion. It is
now apparent that ACTH secretion can also be increased by thymic
peptides (such as thymopoietin), while interleukin-1 (IL-alpha), a product
of macrophage activity, has been shown to enhance ACTH secretion.

Such events show how the immune, endocrine and central nervous
systems are integrated in their responses to any form of stress. It is well
established that physical or psychosocial stress causes increased secretions
of prolactin, growth hormones, thyroid, and gonadal hormones, in addition
to ACTH. Endogenous opioids are secreted under such conditions and
function as immunomodulators, while also elevating the pain threshold.
Receptors for such hormones exist on immunocompetent cells, along with
receptors for catecholamines, serotonin and acetylcholine.

In addition to the regulatory effects of the nervous system on the immune
system, there is now convincing evidence that the immune system can
influence brain function. Thus changes in the activity of specific nuclei in
the hypothalamus of the rat have been described following the formation of
antibodies to specific antigen challenges. Alterations in electrical activity
appear to be linked to specific decreases in noradrenaline concentrations in
these nuclei. Changes in the activity of the serotonergic neurons in the
hippocampus also occur shortly after the occurrence of the immune
response. These findings illustrate how the immune system, presumably via
the release of immunoregulatory peptides (also called immunotransmitters)
such as interleukins from macrophages, can influence the activity of the

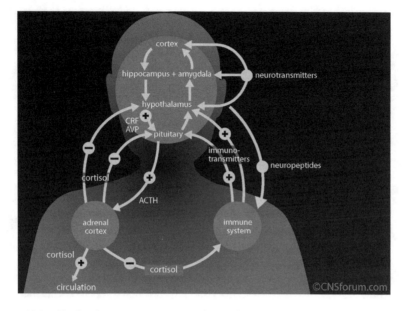

Figure 18.2. Endocrine–immune inter-relationship in normal subject. The hypotha-lamic–pituitary–adrenal (HPA) axis is a feedback loop that includes the hypothalamus, the pituitary and the adrenal glands. The main hormones that activate the HPA axis are corticotrophin releasing factor (CRF), arginine vasopressin (AVP) and adrenocorticotrophic hormone (ACTH). The loop is completed by the negative feedback of cortisol on the hypothalamus and pituitary. The simultaneous release of cortisol into the circulation has a number of effects, including elevation of blood glucose for increased metabolic demand. Cortisol also negatively affects the immune system and prevents the release of immunotransmitters. Interference from other brain regions (e.g. hippocampus and amygdala) can also modify the HPA axis, as can neuropeptides and neurotransmitters.

hypothalamic–pituitary axis and also higher centres of the brain (such as the hippocampus), which are involved in short-term memory processing. The triad of inter-relationships between the brain, endocrine and immune systems is illustrated in Figures 18.2, 18.3, 18.4 and 18.5.

The effect of stress on the endocrine and immune systems depends upon its duration and severity. Following acute stress, the rise in ACTH in response to the release of corticotrophin releasing factor (CRF) from the hypothalamus results in a rise in the synthesis and release of cortisol from the adrenals. The increase in the plasma cortisol concentration results in a temporary suppression of many aspects of cellular immunity. Due to the operation of an inhibitory feedback mechanism, stimulation of the central glucocorticoid receptors in the hypothalamus and pituitary causes a decrease in the further release of CRF, thereby decreasing the further

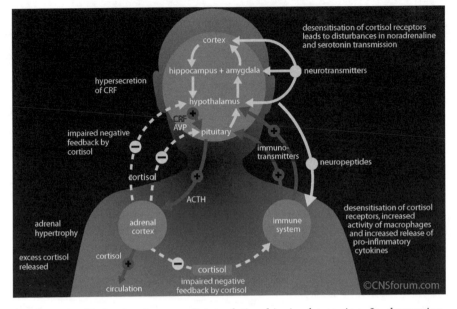

Figure 18.3. Endocrine–immune inter-relationship in depression. In depression, the hypothalamic–pituitary–adrenal (HPA) axis is up-regulated with a down-regulation of its negative feedback controls. Corticotrophin releasing factor (CRF) is hypersecreted from the hypothalamus and induces the release of adrenocortico-trophic hormone (ACTH) from the pituitary. ACTH interacts with receptors on adrenocortical cells and cortisol is released from the adrenal glands; adrenal hypertrophy can also occur. Release of cortisol into the circulation has a number of effects, including elevation of blood glucose. The negative feedback of cortisol to the hypothalamus, pituitary and immune system is impaired. This leads to continual activation of the HPA axis and excess cortisol release. Cortisol receptors become desensitized leading to increased activity of the pro-inflammatory immune mediators and disturbances in neurotransmitter transmission.

synthesis and release of cortisol. Arginine vasopressin (AVP) also plays a role in activating the release of ACTH from the anterior pituitary gland.

Following chronic stress, however, the regulatory feedback inhibitory mechanism is dysfunctional due to the desensitization of the central and peripheral glucocorticoid receptors. Thus cortisol continues to be secreted primarily due to the activation of the hypothalamic–pituitary axis by AVP and the elevated pro-inflammatory cytokines such as interleukin-1. Due to the desensitization of the glucocorticoid receptors on the immune cells and in the brain, and a lack of inhibition by glucocorticoids of central macrophage activity (the astrocytes and glial cells), glucocorticoids continue to be secreted.

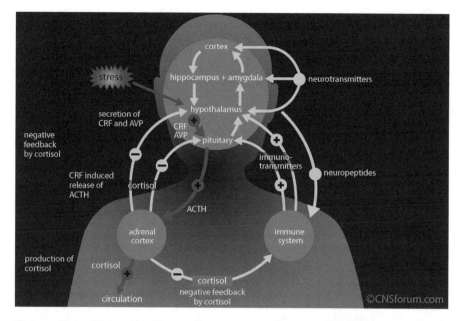

Figure 18.4. Endocrine–immune inter-relationship following acute stress. In response to stress, corticotrophin releasing factor (CRF) and arginine vasopressin (AVP) are secreted from the hypothalamus causing the release of adrenocortico-trophic hormone (ACTH) from the pituitary. ACTH interacts with receptors on adrenocortical cells and cortisol is released from the adrenal glands. Release of cortisol into the circulation has a number of effects, including elevation of blood glucose. The negative feedback of cortisol on the hypothalamus, pituitary and immune system remains unaffected in acute stress – the release of CRF, AVP and immunotransmitters is still inhibited, preventing the continual activation of the HPA axis.

Immune system in affective disorders

Susceptibility to bacterial and viral infections, and to the establishment of tumours, is reported to arise more frequently in those who are depressed than in those who are not. An analysis of the immune systems of those suffering the severe psychological stress of bereavement has shown that the activity of those immune cells that are fundamentally involved in the host defence against infections (e.g. NKCs and T-lymphocytes) is dramatically reduced. Such an effect can occur following chronic and subchronic stress.

The past 20 years have witnessed a broad interest in the role of the hypothalamic–pituitary–adrenal axis in the psychobiology of affective disorders. In depressed patients, increases in serum cortisol are frequently reported in addition to disruptions of circadian patterns of cortisol secretion

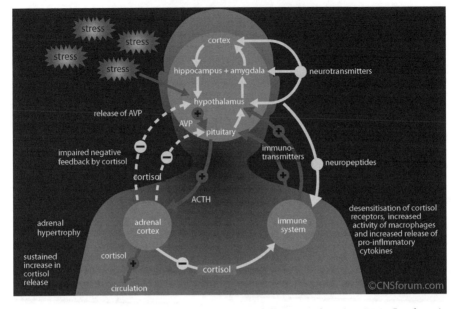

Figure 18.5. Endocrine–immune relationship following chronic stress. In chronic stress, the hypothalamic–pituitary–adrenal (HPA) axis is up-regulated with a down-regulation of its negative feedback control. Arginine vasopressin (AVP) is secreted from the hypothalamus and induces the release of adrenocorticotrophic hormone (ACTH) from the pituitary. ACTH interacts with receptors on adrenocortical cells and cortisol is released from the adrenal glands; adrenal hypertrophy can also occur. Release of cortisol into the circulation has a number of effects, including elevation of blood glucose. Unlike in acute stress, the negative feedback of cortisol to the hypothalamus and pituitary is impaired. This leads to continual activation of the HPA axis and excess cortisol release. Cortisol receptors become desensitized leading to increased activity of the pro-inflammatory immune mediators.

and an insensitivity of cortisol secretion to suppression by glucocorticoids such as dexamethasone.

The potential association between the immune system and mood disorders has become a major topic of interest in biological psychiatry in the past decade. In general, three immune measures have been examined, namely white blood cell counts, functional measures of cellular immunity such as natural killer cell activity and immune cell markers as exemplified by human lymphoctye antigen (HLA). The cumulative data from these studies suggests that depressed patients have a decreased number of lymphocytes, reduced mitogen-induced lymphocyte proliferation and a reduction in the number of natural killer cells. However, this does not apply to all depressed patients. Furthermore, not all aspects of immune function are decreased despite the presence of hypercortisolaemia. Thus the activity of macrophages (that include the microglia and astrocytes in the brain which are part of the immune system) has been shown to increase in depression. These immune cells release cytokines that not only act as immunoregulators but also as neuromodulators of central neurotransmitters. In general, the cytokines are either of the pro-inflammatory type (called Th-1 type, and largely stimulatory in their action) or anti-inflammatory type (called Th-2 type and largely inhibitory in their action). The pro-inflammatory cytokines are exemplified by interleukins (IL-) 1, 6 and tumour necrosis factor (TNF-) alpha while the anti-inflammatory cytokines are IL-4, 10 and 13. The presence of elevated blood concentrations of the pro-inflammatory cytokines, and in the concentration of IL-1 in the CSF, has led to the macrophage hypothesis of depression which suggests that the changes in brain neurotransmitter function are a consequence of the increase in inflammatory changes (involving the inflammatory mediators prostaglandin E_2 and nitric oxide which are increased in response to IL-1). The neural damage occurring in cortical and subcortical regions of the brain of depressed patients has been ascribed to the shift in the balance to pro-inflammatory cytokines from anti-inflammatory cytokines. These changes occur both in the brain and in the periphery and, in chronic depression, the brain damage is accentuated by the elevation of glucocorticoids which are hypersecreted due to the desensitization of the glucocorticoid receptors on neurons and on immune cells.

If a malfunctional immune system plays a role in the pathogenesis of depression, it would be anticipated that antidepressants have an immunoregulatory action. Because immune cells express neurotransmitter receptors, mediators such as noradrenaline and serotonin, as well as various neuropeptides, are able to modulate the immune response. Moreover, neurons and glial cells express cytokine receptors and the release and action of neurotransmitters are modulated by cytokines. Antidepressants appear to affect cytokine release from macrophages, monocytes and glial cells in addition to their well-known effects on monoamine synthesis. Antidepressants can also modulate intracellular signals such as cyclic AMP and neurotrophic factors (such as brain derived neurotrophic factor, BDNF) and in this way alter the synthesis of the pro-inflammatory cytokines. The beneficial long-term effects of antidepressant treatments in depression may therefore result from a shift in the balance of the pro-inflammatory to the anti-inflammatory cytokines in addition to improving the brain repair mechanisms (by increasing neurotrophic factor synthesis and reducing the brain concentration of the neurotoxic glucocorticoids).

Clearly, more detailed studies must be undertaken to validate this hypothesis, but these preliminary findings link proven neurotransmitter

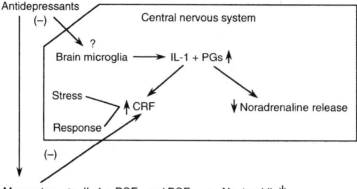

Figure 18.6. Possible changes in immune function and the brain in depression.

changes in depressed patients with the delays in onset of action of antidepressants and the changes in cellular immunity. Figure 18.6 summarizes the possible links between depression and changes in some aspects of the immune system.

It now seems probable that specific disturbances occur in the immune system in psychiatric illness that are not artefacts of non-specific stress factor, institutionalization or medication. The known effects of the neuroendocrine system on the immune response, and the recent evidence that receptor sites for neurotransmitters and neuroendocrine factors occur on lymphocytes and macrophages, support the hypothesis that immunological abnormalities may assist in precipitating the symptoms of anxiety and depression, commonly symptoms of major affective disorders.

Changes in the immune system in schizophrenia

Evidence suggesting an abnormality in immune function in those subject to severe stress or suffering from depression largely relates to an abnormality in function. Such abnormalities do not appear to occur in schizophrenia. Possibly because of its well-established genetic component, many aspects of the immune system would appear to be deranged in schizophrenic patients. Thus abnormalities in the concentration of serum immunoglobulins and deficiencies in immune responsiveness have been reported to occur in such patients.

Several investigators have reported a generalized increase in the immunoglobulins in both acute and chronic stages of schizophrenia, although not all investigators have been able to confirm this. There is some evidence that antibrain antibodies which could selectively destroy specific types of brain cells have been detected in schizophrenic patients. Some years ago, a factor was isolated from the serum of schizophrenic patients that produced catatonia and an abnormal electroencephalographic pattern when injected intravenously into monkeys or human volunteers; the electroencephalogram changes were similar to those seen in schizophrenic patients. The serum protein causing these abnormalities was termed taraxein. These findings were confimed by some researchers but not by those who used a more reliable radioimmunoassay method. However, in an extensive study of antibrain antibodies in 69 schizophrenics and 58 controls, it has been shown that if antibrain antibodies play any role in psychiatric disorders they are non-specific and only present in a small percentage of patients.

Allergic reactions entail disordered immune functioning, and controversy exists regarding allergies to various food substances and the incidence of schizophrenia. Some studies have suggested that schizophrenics have an increased incidence of allergies in childhood, especially involving an intolerance to wheat gluten. However, there are few adequately controlled studies to show that food allergies play any role in the aetiology of schizophrenia and, to date, there is little unequivocal evidence to support the view that allergies play a causal role in this illness.

There is evidence to suggest that there are at least two genetically determined components in those at risk from schizophrenia. One of these components facilitates a decrease in suppressor cells, while the other promotes the accumulation of antithymic immunoglobulins. The conse-quences of the resultant imbalance between the helper and suppressor mechanism which arises from these immune malfunctions are the occurrence of specific antitissue antibodies, the formation of which is normally controlled by a balance between helper and suppressor T cell mechanisms.

There have been several suggestions whereby the negative symptoms of schizophrenia could represent an autoimmune encephalitis-like syndrome in which a viral infection, for example, could initiate an autoimmune response against dopaminergic pathways. One possibility is that dopamine receptor stimulating antibodies could be produced as part of the pathological processes that have a high affinity for the dopamine autoreceptors and thereby decrease the release of the neurotransmitter in specific dopaminergic pathways. However, it must be emphasized that the clinical data upon which many of these speculations are based have been obtained from patients on prolonged treatment with neuroleptics. These drugs are known to modify the immune system which could increase the subsequent vulnerability of the patient to viral infections.

It may be speculated that an inherited primary defect in the immune system could initiate schizophrenia by stimulating the production of antibrain antibodies or by increasing the vulnerability of the patient to a viral infection. Alternatively, a primary defect in central neurotransmitter metabolism, possibly involving dopamine, may cause the immune abnormalities which have been described. In this case it may be argued that the immune changes are an epiphenomenon of the disease and not necessarily the primary cause.

Although there has been considerable interest in investigating the changes in the immune system of patients with depression, it is only more recently that researchers have turned their attention to the possible involvement of the immune system in the pathogenesis of schizophrenia. As has already been mentioned, antibrain antibodies have been detected in the CSF of chronic schizophrenic patients while the presence of an increase in the concentration of immunoglobulin G in the CSF, which correlates with the presence of negative symptoms, is a further suggestion that an inflammatory process is operational in the brain of the schizophrenic patient. With regard to the pro-inflammatory cytokines, IL-6 is increased in both the CSF and serum from medicated and unmedicated patients; this is reduced by effective antipsychotic drug treatment. Studies in children with schizophrenia have shown that interferon alpha is raised in the CSF and that this cytokine correlates both with the severity of the symptoms and in their refractoriness to drug treatment. It is of interest to note that the secretion of interferon is an important component of the antiviral immune response that may provide further evidence in favour of the viral hypothesis of schizophrenia. Unlike depression, IL-2 concentrations have been found to increase in the CSF of schizophrenic patients. As there is some evidence that this cytokine can increase the release of dopamine from central neurons, it is possible that IL-2 could contribute to the hyperdopaminergic state which characterizes the acute form of the disease. Support for a central inflammatory process being involved in the pathology of schizophrenia comes from the recent report that cyclo-oxygenase 2 inhibitors, such as celecoxib, potentiate the action of atypical antipsychotics such as clozapine in schizophrenic patients who appear to be resistant to the therapeutic effects of atypical antipsychotics.

In CONCLUSION, it seems probable that some disturbances in immune function do occur in mental illness and are not artefacts of medication or the effects of institutionalization. The known effects of the neuroendocrine system on the immune response and the recent evidence that receptor sites for neurotransmitters and neuroendocrine factor occur on lymphocytes and macrophages, support the hypothesis that immunological abnormalities may assist in precipitating the symptoms of anxiety, depression and schizophrenia. Nevertheless, the nature of specific immunological disturbances which underlie these diseases remains elusive.

19 Endocoids and their Importance in Psychopharmacology

Introduction

Natural products have been known to contain pharmacologically active substances that have been exploited by man since antiquity. In addition to the natural products that have been used to treat the physical symptoms of disease, such as atropine derivatives to reduce gastrointestinal spasm and aspirin derivatives to treat pyrexia, several plant extracts have been used specifically for their psychotropic actions. Reference has already been made in Chapter 15 to the opioids, cocaine and the natural psychostimulants, and to the cannabinoids as drugs of abuse. However the purpose of this chapter is to summarize the evidence implicating naturally occurring substances which occur within the mammalian brain and which appear to produce their psychotropic effects by activating specific receptors within the brain. Such substances are termed endocoids and they include the enkephalins and endorphins, which activate specific opioid receptors, the anandamide related compounds, which activate cannabinoid receptors, the endopsychosins and related compounds that activate sigma receptors and natural agonists and antagonists that show an affinity for the benzodiazepine receptors. These different types of endocoids will be discussed in terms of their possible physiological effects. The abuse potential of such substances has already been referred to in Chapter 15.

Endogenous cannabinoids and cannabinoid receptors

The Chinese emperor Shen Nung is believed to have produced the first written account of the medicinal properties of cannabis over 2000 years ago and various formulations of herbal cannabis have been used over the centuries to treat seizures, neuralgia, dysmenorrhoea, insomnia and even gonorrhoea. The hemp plant, *Cannabis sativa*, from which cannabis and

Fundamentals of Psychopharmacology. Third Edition. By Brian E. Leonard
2003 John Wiley & Sons, Ltd. ISBN 0 471 52178 7

many of the related compounds are obtained, has a long history in medicine. Thus over the centuries the cannabinoids have been used for the treatment of pain, asthma, dysentery, as sedatives, for the suppression of nausea and vomiting and as anticonvulsants. Although the clinical uses of the cannabinoids declined in the 20th century there has been a renewed interest in these natural compounds in recent years for the control of spasticity associated with multiple sclerosis and in the treatment of chronic pain. Such renewed interest coincided with greater attention being paid by the medical profession and society at large to herbal remedies.

Understanding the mechanism of action of the cannabinoids has been advanced by the identification and cloning of specific cannabinoid receptors in the mammalian brain and spleen and the identification of endogenous substances which bind to these receptors. Thus the cannabinoid receptors in the brain are primarily of the CB1 type. These receptors are widely distributed in areas concerned with motor activity (basal ganglia and cerebellum), memory and cognition (cerebral cortex and hippocampus), emotion (amygdala and hippocampus), sensory perception (thalamus) and with endocrine function (hypothalamus and pons). The distribution of radio-labelled tetrahydrocannabinol, the main active ingredient of *Cannabis sativa*, is similar to the distribution of the CB1 receptors and there is good evidence that the cannabinoids exact their action through these receptors. In addition to the CB1 receptors, CB2 receptors have been identified on macrophages in the spleen where they probably mediate the immunological effects of the cannabinoids. CB1 receptors have also been detected in peripheral tissues.

The discovery of cannabinoid receptors has raised the possibility that therapeutic agents could be developed that may combine the therapeutic uses of the cannabinoids with lack of abuse and drug dependency. The first endogenous substances to be shown to have a high affinity for the cannabinoid receptors were the anandamides, named after the Sanskrit word for "bliss"=ananda. Structurally the endogenous ligands for the cannabinoid receptors are unlike those of plant origin (see Figure 19.1). The endogenous parent compound is a derivative of the endogenous fatty acid arachidonic acid, arachidonyl ethanolamide. More recently, two other endogenous unsaturated fatty acid ethanolamides with a high affinity for cannabinoid receptors have been identified in brain tissue. These are homo-gamma-linolenylethanolamide and docotetraenylethanolamide. These substances are agonists at central cannabinoid receptors and their structures are shown in Figure 19.1. The system comprising the cannabinoid receptors and endogenous anandamide-related compounds is referred to as the anandamide system. However, it must be borne in mind that endogenous ligands for cannabinoid receptors may exist with properties that differ from those of the anandamide series of compounds.

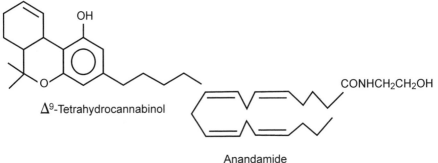

Δ^9-Tetrahydrocannabinol

CONHCH$_2$CH$_2$OH

Anandamide
(Arachidonyl ethanolamide)

Figure 19.1. Chemical structure of main active ingredient of *Cannabis sativa*, Δ^9-tetrahydrocannabinol (THC) and the naturally occurring ligand for cannabinoid receptors anandamide (arachidonyl ethanolamide).

While there is convincing evidence that endogenous compounds exist in the mammalian brain that have properties which resemble those of tetrahydrocannabinol, the most potent cannabinoid from a plant source, the question arises regarding the need to postulate the existence of specific receptors for these natural ligands. After all, although opioid peptides have been isolated from brain extracts, the search for other receptor ligands, including those which bind to the benzodiazepine and sigma receptors, has not been nearly as successful. Nevertheless, due to the special nature of receptors which are coupled to G proteins, it is highly probable that there are natural ligands for all such receptors. This is because G proteins are single molecules that do not contain allosteric binding sites, unlike the benzodiazepine–GABA receptor where the benzodiazepine binding site is an allosteric regulatory site for GABA. For all G protein-coupled receptors, every receptor has an endogenous ligand associated with its binding site. Thus it is reasonable to conclude that the binding sites for the anandamide system in the mammalian brain are true receptor sites through which the physiological changes initiated by the cannabinoids are expressed.

Despite the recent advances in molecular biology, the mechanisms of action and the physiological functions of the anandamide system remain obscure. It would appear that the cannabinoid receptors and the anandamides reside within the neurons. Thus unlike the classical neurotransmitters noradrenaline and serotonin, the anandamides are not released into the synaptic cleft and are not involved in interneuronal communication. Instead the anandamides modulate the excitability and inhibitory responsiveness of neurons by acting on cannabinoid hetero-ceptors located on inhibitory and excitatory terminals. In this way, the cannabinoid receptors reduce the activity of these neurons by decreasing the influx of calcium through the calcium channels and increasing the efflux of potassium ions through the potassium channels located on the neuronal membrane. In some regions such as the cerebellum, there is a convergence of the G protein-linked receptors such as the GABA-B, adenosine A1, cannabinoid and kappa opioid receptors that inhibit the activity of adenylate cyclase thereby leading to a reduction in the release of glutamate. Thus it seems possible that the anandamide system modulates the activity of the major neurotransmitter systems including the opioid, prostenoid and glucocorticoid systems.

Sites of action of the cannabinoids

CB1 receptors are present in a high density in the hippocampus and cerebral cortex and the effects of cannabinoids on cognition and memory are undoubtedly related to their activation of the receptors in this brain region. These regions also mediate the effects of the cannabinoids on perception of time, sound, colour and taste. With regard to the motor effects, and effects on posture, of the cannabinoids it would appear that this is related to their agonist action on CB1 receptors located in the basal ganglia and cerebellum. Other central actions of the anandamide system include the hypothalamus (effect on body temperature), the spinal cord (antinociception) and the brain stem (suppression of nausea and vomiting).

The discovery that cells of the immune system contain both cannabinoid binding sites and cannabinoid receptor mRNA suggests that the immunosuppressive actions of the naturally occurring cannabinoids are receptor mediated. There is now evidence that cannabinoid receptors occur on spleen cells in rodents and man and in human thymus cells and monocytes, but the receptor density is lower than that occurring in the brain. The B-lymphocytes have been shown to contain the highest quantity of cannabinoid receptor mRNA. The specific binding of cannabinoids to the small intestine and testis has also been reported to occur in different mammalian species. As the peripheral cannabinoid receptor appears to be of the CB2 type which appears to be absent from the brain, there have been attempts to develop selective agonists which would lack psychotropic properties but which would be of therapeutic value as immunosuppressants and in the control of such autoimmune diseases as rheumatoid arthritis. Conversely, CB2 receptor antagonists may act as drugs to enhance immune function. To date, no compounds have reached clinical application despite showing promising pharmacological profiles in the preclinical stages of their development. There is hope that a new approach in which analogues of the anandamides are developed will be

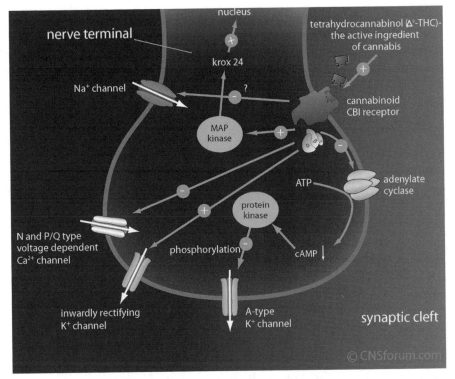

Figure 19.2. Intracellular changes that occur following the activation of the cannabinoid-1 (CB1) receptor by cannabinoids.

more fruitful. A summary of the intracellular changes that occur in response to the stimulation of the CB1 receptor is shown in Figure 19.2.

Physiological processes in that endogenous cannabinoids may act as mediators

The possible physiological importance of the endogenous cannabinoids has largely been based on an extrapolation from the pharmacological properties of the THC-like compounds that are known for their psychotropic effects. Such drugs may differ in action from the endogenous cannabinoids because of their broad range of activity that follows the activation of both the CB1 and CB2 receptors, but also their ability to inhibit membrane bound enzymes and to cause a disruption of the normal function of the phospholipid compounds of neuronal and other membranes. Thus it would be anticipated that endogenous cannabinoids would show more selective actions both in the brain and periphery.

Tolerance is known to develop rapidly to many of the effects of the psychotropic cannabinoids but little is known regarding the mechanisms responsible for the development of tolerance to these drugs. One possibility to account for the development of tolerance is that compensatory decreases in the sensitivity or density of cannabinoid receptors occurs following the prolonged stimulation of these receptors, perhaps by inducing changes in the genetic expression of the receptor protein. This could occur as a result of a decrease in the signal transduction mechanism or in the affinity of the receptor sites for the cannabinoids. There are several *in vitro* and *in vivo* experimental studies in support of such mechanisms, but it is presently unproven whether such mechanisms apply to the components of the anandamide system.

In SUMMARY, there is abundant evidence that endogenous cannabinoids are components of the anandamide system and that they share many of the properties known to occur following the administration of the cannabinoids of plant origin. Thus the endogenous cannabinoids have been shown to induce sleep and thermoregulation. Whether they also cause other changes which are associated with the cannabinoids of plant origin (such as disturbances in cognition, memory, mood, coordination, perception and appetite) at physiologically relevant concentrations is presently unclear. Nevertheless, the anandamide system is of importance because of the therapeutic potential that drugs acting on specific CB1 or CB2 receptors may have. This is an area of psychopharmacology that may hold important therapeutic prospects for the future.

Endozepines as endogenous anxiolytic and anxiogenic agents

It has been postulated that, at the cellular level, the symptoms of anxiety can arise because:

1. There is inadequate activity of an endogenous anxiolytic ligand.
2. There is excessive activity of an endogenous inverse agonist at the benzodiazepine receptor site (see p. 232 for a detailed discussion).
3. There is a dysfunctional GABA-A receptor causing a shift in the GABA-A complex towards inverse agonist activity.

It is uncertain which of these three possibilities apply to patients with anxiety disorders. There is evidence that the binding of the benzodiazepine receptor antagonist, flumazenil, is lower than normal in patients with panic disorder and that it increases the panic attack frequency in these patients but not in normal subjects. This has been interpreted as a slight shift in the benzodiazepine receptor towards the inverse agonist state.

Another possibility that may account for an increase or decrease in the anxiety state relates to the presence of endogenous ligands that act on the benzodiazepine receptors. These ligands have been called endozepines and although a number of compounds have been isolated from mammalian brain it is uncertain whether the endogenous concentration is sufficiently high for them to modulate GABA-A receptor or benzodiazepine receptor function.

Three types of endozapines have been isolated. It is known that the beta-carbolines can be synthesized in the mammalian brain and that, *in vitro*, they act as inverse agonists at benzodiazepine receptor sites. Theoretically such compounds could induce anxiety. However, none of these compounds has been isolated *in vivo* and the original detection of a beta-carboline in the urine of anxious patients was later found to be an artifact, possibly caused by bacterial contamination.

A diazepam binding inhibitor has been isolated from mammalian brain and found to be a mixture of two peptides (an octodecaneuropeptide and a trikontatetra neuropeptide) which stimulates neurosteroid synthesis by acting on peripheral benzodiazepine receptors. There are two main neurosteroids present in the mammalian brain which are antagonists of GABA-A receptors, namely dehydroepiandrosterone and its sulphate form (DHEA and DHEAS). These neurosteroids are also synthesized in the adrenal glands. These neurosteroids are known to have multiple effects of brain function by affecting mood, cognition and sleep; they also enhance neuronal plasticity and are neuroprotective.

The third group of compounds are the naturally occurring benzodiazepines. Desmethyldiazepam has been isolated from human brains which were stored frozen in the 1930s, at least two decades before the benzodiazepines were developed. While there is no evidence that the benzodiazepine structure can be synthesized enzymatically in the mammalian brain, several other compounds of this type have since been isolated from cattle brain and from human breast milk. One possibility is that gastrointestinal flora can partially synthesize the benzodiazepine molecule and it is also known that plants such as wheat and potatoes are a potential source of diazepam, desmethyldiazepam and lormetazepam. If it is eventually shown that the local brain concentration of these benzodiazepines is sufficiently high to activate the benzodiazepine receptors then the possibility arises that anxiety disorders could result from a lack of these endozepines.

Several species of plant also contain compounds that have been shown to act as agonists on benzodiazepine receptors. These include: *Valeriana officinalis* which contains hydroxypinoresinol, *Matricaria recutita* which contains 5,7,4'-trihydroxyflavone, *Passiflora coeruleus* which contains chrysin and Karmelitter Geist which contains amentoflavin. *Hypericum perforatum* (St John's Wort) also contains unknown compounds which have affinity for these receptors. Extracts of these drugs are commonly recommended by herbalists for the treatment of insomnia and anxiety.

Endogenous sleep factors

Early in the 20th century, Pierin in Paris infused the CSF of sleep-deprived dogs into normal dogs and showed that the CSF contained a sleep-inducing (somnogenic) factor. This was thought to be a muramyl peptide but later suggested to be the result of bacterial contamination as these peptides cannot be synthesized by the mammalian brain.

Pro-inflammatory cytokines (see p. 432 et seq.) can also induce sleep, the effect depending on the concentration of the cytokine and the time of day. The effect on the sleep profile (increased non-REM and decreased REM sleep) appears to depend on the increased synthesis of prostaglandin D_2 and nitric oxide which then alter the circadian rhythm. It is also known that some pro-inflammatory cytokines can affect the reuptake of 5-HT which plays an important role in regulating the sleep–wake profile. The endogenous fatty acid, oleamide, can cause sedation and induce sleep by activating cannabinoid receptors but also by potentiating the action of benzodiazepines on their receptor sites. Whether such action is of physiological relevance is presently unknown.

In SUMMARY, the naturally occurring ligands for the benzodiazepine and/or GABA-A receptor sites that act as sedative-hypnotics or anxiolytics all directly or indirectly augment GABA-A receptors and thereby depress neuronal activity. In this respect they act in a similar way to the various classes of drugs used to treat anxiety and insomnia. Such compounds do not induce natural sleep. They all increase slow-wave sleep but reduce REM sleep.

Function and therapeutic effects of sigma receptors

The sigma opiate receptor was originally proposed by the American neuropharmacologist William R. Martin as the site that mediates the psychotomimetic and stimulatory effects of cyclazocine, pentazocine, N-allyl normetazocine (SKF 10047) and related opiates in humans and dogs. However, there is now considerable evidence to suggest that these effects are not mediated by opioid receptors. Many of the opiates that have psychotomimetic properties also bind with a high affinity to phencyclidine (PCP) receptor sites situated in the channel of the N-methyl-D-aspartate (NMDA) receptor. It now appears from electrophysiological, biochemical, anatomical and molecular studies that there are two distinct sites that bind opioid analgesics that have an affinity for sigma receptors. One site is on the PCP receptor situated in the NMDA receptor. The other sigma site is defined as non-opioid, non-dopaminergic and shows a high affinity for haloperidol and N-allyl normetazocine. Using a highly selective ligand for sigma receptors such as ditolyguanidine (DTG), it has now been possible to separate sigma receptors into two major types. Sigma-1 receptors are the main neuronal type and exhibit a high affinity for centrally acting antitussive and anticonvulsant drugs. The other site has a low affinity for most sigma ligands except DTG and haloperidol. This site is found in the red nucleus and cerebellum (as well as many other brain regions) where it may mediate the motor (dystonic) effects of different types of sigma ligand. Biochemically the sigma-1 and sigma-2 receptors may also be distinguished by the nature of the second messenger to which they are attached. Thus the sigma-1 receptors appear to be linked to guanylyl nucleotide binding proteins (G proteins) whereas the sigma-2 sites are not and may bring about their physiological effects by modulating K^+ channels.

Sigma receptors and psychosis

Some 20 years ago, Martin and coworkers proposed that the psychoto-mimetic effects of pentazocine and related opiate analgesics was due to their effect on sigma receptors. It is now known that the sigma receptors are quite distinct from PCP, opioid, serotonin and dopamine receptors. However, many psychotropic drugs that bind to dopamine, serotonin and PCP receptors also have a high affinity for sigma receptors. For example, haloperidol and the novel benzamide neuroleptic remoxipride bind with high affinity for both D_2 and sigma receptors. Nevertheless, there are many potent neuroleptics that have a negligible affinity for sigma receptors and conversely, many sigma ligands that do not apparently have any neuroleptic activity, but it remains a possibility that there could be an involvement of sigma receptors in the pathology of schizophrenia. Thus receptor autoradiographic studies of post-mortem schizophrenic brain have demonstrated a significant reduction of sigma binding sites in the frontal cortex, amygdala and hippocampus without any significant change in the density of PCP binding sites. Therefore, the evidence linking a malfunc-tional sigma receptor system to schizophrenia, or the use of selective sigma receptor ligands as putative neuroleptics, is inconclusive.

Sigma receptors and the immune and endocrine systems

Experimental evidence suggests that sigma receptors play an important role in regulating and integrating both immune and endocrine functions. In experimental studies, it has been shown that the selective sigma ligand N-allyl-normetazocine stimulates the hypothalamic–pituitary–adrenal axis but suppresses luteinizing hormone and prolactin secretion. A high density of sigma receptors has been identified on human leucocytes and in the rat spleen, testis, ovary and adrenal gland. In human leucocytes it has also been shown that sigma receptors are involved in the second signalling mechanisms that are essential for cellular activation. In addition, sigma receptors have been identified on human and rat T and B cells. There is experimental evidence to show that the suppression of T cell replication, and enhanced activity of monocyte phagocytosis, that occurs in some rodent models of depression, can be effectively reversed by the chronic administration of selective sigma ligands such as igmesine. This suggests that such compounds may be of benefit in correcting the diverse immune and possibly endocrine defects that characterize depression.

Clinical implications

Schizophrenia

Following the discovery that some antipsychotic drugs bind to sigma receptors, the suggestion arose that sigma receptors may be involved in schizophrenia and in the mode of action of antipsychotic drugs. Support for this hypothesis arose from the observation that the density of sigma receptors was dramatically reduced in several brain regions of post-mortem brains from schizophrenic patients. Such changes appeared to be restricted to the sigma receptor and did not involve the NMDA receptor or the PCP receptor. Whether such findings implicate alterations in sigma receptor function in schizophrenia is uncertain as it is possible that the changes in the density of these receptors is a function of the duration of treatment with neuroleptics. Support for the possible involvement of sigma receptors in schizophrenia, and in the action of antipsychotic drugs comes from the observation that haloperidol had a high affinity for these receptors in rat brain. Furthermore rimcazole, a putative neuroleptic, was found to have a high affinity for sigma receptors with little action on dopamine receptors. Several other sigma-selective ligands were also developed as possible neuroleptics. Unfortunately, despite convincing pre-clinical data showing that many of the sigma-selective ligands were active in animal models predictive of antipsychotic activity, none proved to have efficacy in clinical trials. It would therefore seem that the sigma ligands so far developed are unlikely to become the novel neuroleptics of the future.

Movement disorders

The most common symptomatic dystonias result from the administration of neuroleptics and occur as acute dystonic reactions or as tardive dyskinesia.

The dystonias are disorders that involve sustained, involuntary muscle contractions and abnormal posture which interferes with normal motor function. Dystonias can be focal, as in the case of torticollis in which the neck involuntarily rotates, or they may be progressive and generalized as in torsion dystonia in which the body slowly becomes contorted. Torsian dystonia is familial and recent studies have identified a defective gene which may be responsible.

Acute dystonic reactions occurring following the administration of potent neuroleptics are reported primarily in young men and usually develop shortly after the start of therapy. By contrast, tardive dystonia occurs following chronic neuroleptic treatments; as with tardive dyskinesia, symptoms often begin after the abrupt withdrawal of the neuroleptic. Although less severe than acute dystonic reactions, tardive dystonia is frequently permanent and difficult to treat.

Until recently, the cause of dystonia has been assumed to involve a dysfunction of the basal ganglia. However, it is now known that most patients with lesions of the basal ganglia show no evidence of dystonia while those patients with dystonia exhibit little biochemical or anatomical change in basal ganglia function. More recently, there is clinical evidence that dystonia is associated with lesions of the brainstem and the cerebellum. The cerebellum is closely linked to the red nucleus which contains a high density of sigma receptors but few dopamine, serotonin or glutamate receptors. The brainstem region is also implicated in the hereditary mutant mouse model of dystonia in which the symptoms are known to be associated with both brainstem and cerebellar lesions.

The presence of sigma receptors in anatomical structures that control movement and posture provides indirect evidence for the link between sigma receptors and dystonia. Further support for the involvement of these receptors is provided by the effects induced by the direct administration of sigma ligands into the red nucleus of rats; the degree of dystonia produced is directly proportional to the affinity of the drug for the sigma receptors. Additional experimental support for the involvement of sigma receptors in idiopathic dystonias comes from studies on a strain of rats which can develop a lethal dystonia but which are free of any identifiable anatomical lesions. It would appear that the density of sigma receptors is dramatically reduced compared to their non-affected litter-mates.

Regarding neuroleptic-induced dystonias, it is well known that typical neuroleptics cause catalepsy in rats and movement disorders in man. By contrast, the atypical neuroleptics clozapine and sulpiride have a low propensity to cause movement disorders in man even though they have established antipsychotic effects. These atypical neuroleptics, unlike many of the typical neuroleptics, have a low affinity for sigma receptors which lends support to the hypothesis that the dystonias produced by typical neuroleptics are related to their affinity for sigma receptors in the brainstem–cerebellar region.

Neurodegenerative disorders

So far all the evidence implicating the neuroprotective action of sigma ligands has been based on animal models of stroke or neurodegeneration. Several sigma ligands such as igmesine (JO 1784), NPC 26377, ifenprodil and eliprodil have been shown to protect gerbils against ischaemic insult resulting from the bilateral occlusion of the carotid arteries; this is a popular experimental model of stroke. Similarly, ifenprodil and eliprodil, which have high affinity for sigma receptors in rat brain, are effective in protecting the mouse against focal cerebral ischaemia when administered after the induction of ischaemia. It would appear that the neuroprotective action is due to modulation of the polyamine site on the NMDA-glutamate receptor. However, as sigma ligands such as DTG, 3-PPP and BM4 14802 (which lack affinity for the NMDA glutamate receptor) have no neuroprotective action in the mouse model of focal cerebral ischaemia, it is uncertain whether highly selective sigma ligands would be effective in focal ischaemia in man.

In other experimental studies, the potent sigma ligand igmesine has been shown to potentiate the potassium-evoked release of acetylcholine from rat hippocampal slices *in vitro*, an effect which is blocked by haloperidol. This suggests that igmesine may act as a sigma-1 agonist and may facilitate memory formation. Further evidence for this possibility is provided by the anti-amnestic action of igmesine in scopolamine-treated rats. These experimental studies suggest that sigma ligands, particularly sigma-1 agonists, may have therapeutic potential in the treatment of stroke and possibly in facilitating memory formation in the aged brain. Only double-blind clinical trials of drugs such as igmesine, which appear to be relatively devoid of peripheral organ toxicity, will determine whether the various animal models of memory deficit and neurodegeneration are really predictive of potential therapeutic activity.

Anxiety and depression

There is experimental evidence to show that representative drugs for most classes of antidepressants have a modest affinity for sigma-1 receptors *in vitro*. Some antidepressants, such as sertraline and the monoamine oxidase-A inhibitor clorgyline, are moderately potent ligands for their receptor site. However, more recent studies have indicated that the most important final common pathway for the action of antidepressants involves the modulation of the NMDA-glutamate receptor possibly via the sigma receptor. It therefore seems uncertain that potent and selective sigma ligands will form the basis of a new group of antidepressants. However, there is more convincing experimental evidence to suggest that sigma ligands could have anxiolytic or anti-stress activity. Thus igmesine and DTG have been shown to block environmentally induced stress or corticotrophin-releasing factor induced colonic activity in the rat. Recently there has been renewed interest in the clinical development of igmesine as an antidepressant. Other experimental studies have shown that selective sigma ligands such as Lu 28-178 are potent anxiolytics in rodent models of anxiety.

The future of sigma receptor ligands

Besides the obvious need to develop highly potent and selective drugs for the sigma-1 and sigma-2 receptor sites, knowledge of the precise structures of the sigma receptors is required in order to establish firmly their identity. The presence of sigma receptors in the brain, in the gastrointestinal tract and endocrine and immune systems suggests that there must be endogenous factors that act as agonists and antagonists for these receptors. To date the nature of these endogenous factors is unknown but there is experimental evidence to implicate some neuropeptides (such as neuropeptides-Y and PYY) and steroids such as progesterone and deoxycorticosterone as putative ligands. In addition to the need for more detailed experimental studies to characterize the cellular mechanism of action of the different types of sigma receptors it is also essential to broaden the clinical profile of these drugs. So far, attention has been almost exclusively directed at the action of relatively non-selective sigma ligands in the treatment of psychotic disorders. The experimental findings that sigma compounds may have putative neuroprotective and anxiolytic/anti-stress effects will hopefully encourage the further development of the highly selective sigma compounds for their therapeutic application.

Appendix 1: Some Important Psychotropic Drug Interactions

Antidepressants and lithium

Tricyclic antidepressants + fluoxetine, paroxetine or sertraline → increased pharmacological and toxicological effects of the tricyclic due to decreased hepatic metabolism. This is a potentially hazardous combination.

Tricyclic antidepressants + MAOIs → stroke, hyperpyrexia and convulsions can occur. Potentially a hazardous combination.

Tricyclic antidepressants + directly acting sympathomimetic amines (e.g. noradrenaline, adrenaline) → hypertension and arrhythmias due to enhancement of the sympathomimetic effects.

Tricyclic antidepressants + phenothiazines → additive anticholinergic effects that can cause psychosis and agitation.

Tricyclic antidepressants + phenytoin → reduction in phenytoin metabolism can increase phenytoin toxicity.

Tricyclic antidepressants + warfarin → increased bleeding due to reduced metabolism of warfarin.

Tricyclic antidepressants + barbiturates, carbamazepine → increased metabolism of the tricyclic due to enzyme induction leading to a reduced antidepressant effect.

Irreversible MAOIs + tricyclic antidepressants → as above, plus hypertension.

Irreversible MAOIs + SSRIs → serotonin syndrome (see p. 171).

Irreversible MAOIs + sympathomimetic amines, tyramine-containing foods ("cheese effect") and buspirone → hypertension, possibly leading to stroke.

Irreversible MAOIs + pethidine → severe excitation, hypertension and coma that can lead to death. This is a very hazardous combination.

Irreversible MAOIs + oral hypoglycaemic drugs → increased hypoglycaemic effect.

Lithium + diuretics → reduced lithium clearance and raised plasma lithium concentration thereby enhancing toxicity.

Lithium + non-steroidal anti-inflammatory drugs → decreased lithium clearance and raised plasma lithium concentration thereby enhancing toxicity.

Fundamentals of Psychopharmacology. Third Edition. By Brian E. Leonard
© 2003 John Wiley & Sons, Ltd. ISBN 0 471 52178 7

Lithium + typical neuroleptics → increased extrapyramidal side effects and possibly increased neurotoxicity.

Lithium + antiarrhythmic drugs → potentiation of the cardiac conduction effects of the antiarrhythmic drugs.

Lithium + carbamazepine, valproate → enhanced therapeutic effects of lithium.

Lithium + tetracycline antibiotics → enhanced toxicity of lithium due to increased lithium absorption and impaired excretion.

Lithium + succinylcholine → prolonged muscle paralysis; synergic effect of the drugs at the neuromuscular junction.

Second-generation antidepressants

Venlafaxine + cimetidine → increased plasma venlafaxine concentration due to impaired metabolism. ?Increased side effects.

Venlafaxine + MAOIs → serotonin syndrome likely.

Mirtazepine + diazepam, alcohol → increased sedation and possible cognitive impairment.

Nefazodone + triazolam → increased effect of triazolam due to impaired hepatic metabolism.

Nefazodone + digoxin → increased plasma digoxin concentration due to impaired metabolism.

Nefazodone + morphine → increased analgesic effect of morphine due to impaired metabolism.

Trazodone + CNS depressants → enhanced sedation.

Trazodone + SSRIs, buspirone, MAOIs → serotonin syndrome possible due to additive serotonergic effects.

Bupropion + MAOIs → hypertensive crisis.

Bupropion + L-dopa → enhanced therapeutic and toxic effects of L-dopa; can cause hallucinations, confusion and dyskinesias. Changes due to additive dopaminergic effects.

Bupropion + fluoxetine (?other SSRIs) → delirium and possible grand-mal seizures.

Bupropion + lithium → seizures can occur.

Bupropion + valproate → increased plasma valproate concentrations.

Anxiolytics

Benzodiazepines + cimetidine, disulfiram → inhibition of benzodiazepine metabolism causing increased sedation.

Benzodiazepines + antacids → reduced absorption of benzodiazepines leading to reduced therapeutic effects.

Benzodiazepines + digoxin → reduced metabolism of digoxin leading to prolonged action and increased toxicity.

Benzodiazepines + smoking, rifampicin → due to enzyme induction, plasma concentration of the benzodiazepine is reduced.

Buspirone + MAOIs → hypertension due to increased serotonergic effect.

Buspirone + haloperidol → elevated plasma haloperidol concentration leading to increased side effects.

Buspirone + cyclosporin A → elevated cyclosporin concentrations leading to renal toxicity.

Anticonvulsants and sedatives

Carbamazepine + phenytoin, tricyclic antidepressants, typical neuroleptics, valproate, clonazepam, warfarin, nefazodone and propoxyphene → reduced plasma concentration of carbamazepine due to increased metabolism.

Carbamazepine + antiarrhythmic drugs → additive effect on cardiac conduction time can cause increased cardiotoxicity.

Carbamazepine + erythromycin → increased toxicity of carbamazepine due to reduced metabolism.

Carbamazepine + oral contraceptives → reduced contraceptive efficacy due to enhanced hepatic metabolism.

Phenytoin + oral anticoagulants → decreased anticoagulant effect due to increased hepatic metabolism.

Barbiturates + phenytoin → decreased anticonvulsant effect due to hepatic enzyme induction; enhanced phenytoin toxicity on abruptly stopping barbiturate.

Barbiturates + oral anticoagulants → decreased anticoagulant effects due to hepatic enzyme induction.

Antipsychotics

All antipsychotics + L-dopa → decreased therapeutic effect of L-dopa due to dopamine receptor blockade.

All antipsychotics + anticholinergic drugs → decreased absorption resulting in decreased plasma concentrations.

Phenothiazine neuroleptics (e.g. chlorpromazine, thioridazine) + vasodilators and antihypertensive drugs → increased hypotensive effects due to increased peripheral vasodilation.

Atypical antipsychotics: interactions with the cytochrome P450 system (see p. 89).

Cyt 1A2 metabolizes clozapine: common substrates – amitriptyline, clomipramine, propranolol, theophylline, warfarin, caffeine. Common inhibitors – fluvoxamine, paroxetine.

Cyt 2D6 metabolizes haloperidol, risperidone, thioridazine, sertindole, olanzapine and clozapine: common substrates – fluoxetine, paroxetine, sertraline, venlafaxine, amitriptyline, clomipramine, desipramine, imipramine, nortriptyline, propranolol, metoprolol, timolol, codeine, encainide, flecanide. Common inhibitors – paroxetine, sertraline, fluoxetine.

Cyt 3A3/4 metabolizes clozapine, sertindole, quetiapine: common substrates – tricyclic antidepressants, nefazodone, sertraline, carbamazepine, ethosuximide, terfenadine, benzodiazepines, diltiazem, nifedipine, verapamil, erythromycin, cyclosporine, lidocaine, quinidine, cisapride, paracetamol. Common inhibitors – nefazodone, fluvoxamine, fluoxetine, ketoconazole.

Summary of some amine-containing foods which could interact with MAOIs, particularly irreversible inhibitors (e.g. phenelzine, isocarboxazid, tranycypromine, selegiline)

Cheeses, particularly any type of ripe cheese
Over-ripe fruit
Broad beans (fava beans)
Sausages, salami
Sauerkraut
Pickled fish
Beef, chicken or other types of liver
Any fermented products, e.g. red wine, beers (including non-alcoholic beers)
Food containing monosodium glutamate

Note: This list is only intended as a brief guideline and is based largely on the types of food commonly available in Europe.

Appendix 2: Glossary of some Common Terms Used in Psychopharmacology

This glossary should be used in conjunction with the index.

Abuse	Use of a legal or illicit substance or medication for non-medical or pleasurable purposes unconnected with medically approved indications.
Abuse liability	Capacity of a drug to produce physiological or psychological dependence and alter the behaviour in a manner detrimental to the individual.
Acetylator status	Refers to ability to acetylate organic compounds in the liver. A rapid acetylator refers to an individual whose N-acetyl transferase is hyperactive. Such individuals are more likely to require larger doses of drugs such as phenelzine. Conversely, slow acetylators have a genetically linked deficit in N-acetyl transferase and therefore require a lower dose of the drug.
Action potential	Wave of electrical impulses that travel down an axon to initiate the release of a neurotransmitter.
Addiction	State in which the individual is dependent on a drug of abuse. Term now replaced by *dependence*.
Adenylate cyclase	The intracellular enzyme associated with some types of receptor that on activation produces the secondary messenger cyclic adenosine monophosphate (cyclic AMP).
Affect	Mood or emotional state.
Affective disorder	Mental illness where the predominant abnormality is a disturbance of affect. Such disorders include depression and mania.
Affinity	The potency of a ligand to bind to a receptor or active site on an enzyme. This may be quantified by the affinity constant (K_m or B_{max}).
Age-associated memory	Disorder alleged to occur in those over 60 years of age in the absence of clinical evidence of dementia.

Fundamentals of Psychopharmacology. Third Edition. By Brian E. Leonard
2003 John Wiley & Sons, Ltd. ISBN 0 471 52178 7

Agitation   Defined in DSM-IV as the inability to sit still, pacing, fidgeting, continuous movement of the legs or fingers, wringing hands. These movements are not limited to isolated periods when an upsetting subject is being discussed.

Agnosia   Loss of the ability to recognize sensory stimuli.

Agonist   A compound that acts on a receptor to produce similar effects to the natural ligand.

Agonist-inverse   Drug that produces effects at a receptor that are qualitatively opposite to those produced by an agonist.

Agonist, partial   Drug that acts as an agonist at a low concentration but which, at higher concentrations, blocks the receptor thereby acting as an antagonist.

Agoraphobia   A phobia characterized by the need to avoid being trapped, usually in a public place.

Agraphia   Impairment of the ability to communicate ideas in writing; usually related to a brain disorder.

Agranulocytosis   Usually an iatrogenic state in which the white blood cell count is less than 2000/cu.mm and the leucocyte count is less than 500/cu.mm.

Akathisia   Term used to describe a patient's restlessness and inability to sit still. Shortly after the introduction of neuroleptics, akathisia was recognized as one of the most common and distressing side effects. Propranolol is often useful in treating such symptoms.

Akinesia   Movement disorder characterized by reduction or loss of ability to initiate voluntary muscle movements. Often associated with side effects of neuroleptics: mask-like facial expression, absent arm swing, low voice.

Alcoholic dementia   An organic brain syndrome associated with prolonged, heavy ingestion of alcohol characterized by impairment of short- and long-term memory, abstract thinking and judgement.

Alcoholic hallucinosis   Persistent auditory and/or visual hallucinations after recovery from delirium tremens.

Alcoholism   (a) Primary chronic disease with genetic, psychological and environmental factors influencing its development and manifestations.
(b) Often progressive and fatal, characterized by impaired control over drinking, preoccupation with alcohol, use of alcohol despite adverse consequences, distortion in thinking – particularly denial.

Alkaloid   Complex nitrogen containing organic base of plant origin (e.g. morphine).

Alkyl group   A radical derived from an open chain hydrocarbon. Often referred to as an aliphatic group (e.g. a methyl or ethyl group).

Allele (allelomorph)   Alternative form of a gene found in the corresponding loci on homologous chromosomes, that determines alternative characteristics in inheritance.

Alogia	Marked poverty of speech or speech content. Alogia is one of the negative symptoms of schizophrenia.
Alpha electroencephalogram	EEG that shows 8–13 Hz waves (alpha waves) in all recording leads from a resting subject with closed eyes.
Amnesia	Loss of memory, inability to recall past experience. *Anterograde* amnesia refers to an inability to recall events after a drug (e.g. a benzodiazepine) or ECT. *Retrograde* amnesia refers to the loss of memory occurring prior to the incident that causes amnesia.
Amyotrophic lateral sclerosis (ALS)	In UK, known as motor neuron disease. A devastating adult onset paralytic disorder caused by degeneration of large motor neurons in the brain and spinal cord.
Analeptic	Stimulant such as caffeine or amphetamine that reverses drug-induced depression of the CNS.
Analysis of covariance (ANCOVA)	Statistical method to determine if two or more related dependent variables exposed to two or more related variables differ significantly from chance.
Analysis of variance (ANOVA)	Statistical test to compare the mean values from two or more groups.
Anhedonia	Inability to derive pleasure from situations that usually induce pleasure. This is a characteristic feature of major depressive disorder.
Anorectic	Drug that reduces appetite; used in weight reduction.
Anorexia nervosa	Heterogeneous, multifactorial eating disorder that occurs most commonly in pre-pubertal adolescents and young women.
Anorexiant	Drug that reduces appetite or induces aversion to food.
Anorgasmia	Failure to achieve orgasm. Usually psychological or interpersonal but can be iatrogenic due to antidepressants (particularly selective serotonin reuptake inhibitors), neuroleptics or benzodiazepines.
Anosmia	Loss of sense of smell.
Antagonist	A compound that blocks a receptor thereby preventing an agonist from eliciting a physiological response. An antagonist should have no biological activity of its own.
Antigen	Substance that can elicit antibody formation by immune-competent cells and react with a specific antibody.
Antinociceptive	Having the action of reducing or abolishing a painful stimulus (e.g. an analgesic).
Antisense oligonucleotide	Short piece of synthetic DNA with a nucleotide sequence that is the reverse of, and complementary to, part of the messenger RNA (mRNA)
Aphrodisiac	Substance that positively enhances sexual arousal.
Apoptosis	Programmed cell death characterized by cellular DNA fragmentation and specific cellular changes.

APUD cell   Amine precursor, uptake and decarboxylation cell from which the platelet is derived.

Arousal   Abrupt change from a deeper state of non-rapid eye movement (non-REM) sleep to a lighter stage, or from REM sleep to wakefulness.

Arteriosclerosis   The thickening, hardening and loss of elasticity of arteries.

Aryl   Chemical group that is derived from, or related to, an aromatic hydrocarbon (e.g. a benzene-like molecule).

Ataxia   Loss of muscle co-ordination.

Attention deficit hyperactivity disorder (ADHD)   Heterogeneous group of behavioural disorders of unknown aetiology usually first evident in childhood.

Augmentation   The addition of a second drug to enhance the response to the first drug.

Autopsy   Post-mortem.

Autoreceptor   A receptor situated on the presynaptic nerve ending which responds to the transmitter released from the same nerve ending. Also termed a presynaptic receptor.

Autosome   Chromosome not determinant of sexual differentiation.

Aversive conditioning   Behavioural method whereby a sensory stimulus is paired with a painful, distasteful or unpleasant reinforcement. In behavioural therapy this method is used to produce an association between a negative experience and undesirable behaviour.

Axon   Part of the neuron consisting of a single fibre down which the action potential is transmitted to the nerve terminal.

Basal ganglia   A collection of nuclei in the brain concerned primarily with the initiation and control of movement consisting of the corpus striatum (globus pallidus and the putamen) and the substantia nigra.

Behavioural dyscontrol (inhibition)   Increase in hostility and aggressiveness provoked by alcohol and sedative/anxiolytics such as the benzodiazepines.

Behavioural sensitization   Process whereby intermittent stimulant exposure produces a time-dependent, enduring and progressively more enhanced behavioural response.

Behavioural toxicity   Impairment of psychomotor and cognitive abilities by psychotropic drugs.

Benefit–risk ratio   Balance of the therapeutic efficacy of a drug with its liability to cause side effects.

Binding site   Domain on receptor surface that has a characteristic arrangement of functional groups that recognize and bind specific ligands. Also sometimes called a recognition site.

Bimodal distribution   Distribution with two peaks at which the frequency is greater than at either side of these points.

Binomial distribution   Probability distribution that describes the number of successes observed in independent trials, each with the same probability of occurrences.

Bioassay	Quantitative assessment of the potency of a drug's effect on an isolated tissue, cell, animal or man.
Bioinformatics	Computer-based science of logging and comparing DNA sequences.
Bipolar	Affective illness characterized by mood swings between mania and depression.
Blood dyscrasia	Abnormality ranging from a reduction in the white blood cells (leucopenia, agranulocytosis) to haemolytic anaemia.
Bolus	Rapid intravenous infusion of a drug.
Borna virus disease (BVD)	A neurotropic, enveloped and negative single-stranded RNA virus that persistently infects domestic animals (e.g. horses) causing behavioural and cognitive dysfunction.
Bovine spongiform encephalopathy (BSE)	Transmissible prion disease of cattle; variation of Creutzfeldt–Jakob disease.
Bradykinesia	Extrapyramidal disorder characterized by reduction in velocity of normal movements, paucity of movements and inability to initiate normal movements. Cardinal sign of Parkinson's disease.
Brain stimulation reward	Experimental procedure whereby an animal learns to receive brief, low intensity electrical stimuli to subcortical regions of the brain that elicit a reward.
Bulimia	Eating disorder that may be either a symptom or a syndrome. Manifested by insatiable hunger resulting in compulsive binge eating.
Candidate gene	Cloned human gene that is functionally related to the disease of interest (e.g. a gene for a specific receptor or ion channel).
Cannabinoid	Derivative or preparation from *Cannabis sativa*. This contains several dozen that are chemically related to cannabinol.
Carcinoid syndrome	Disease in which symptoms are due to a 5-hydroxytryptamine secreting tumour, usually located in the gastrointestinal tract.
Catalepsy	A state of rigidity with either resistance to alteration or ready adoption of a newly imposed posture.
Catatonia	A clinical symptom which is associated either with a marked reduction or increase in mobility or alternation between the two states. This term may also be used to describe automatism or stereotyped movements.
Catechol	A 1,2-dihydrobenzene structure, exemplified by the catecholamine transmitters noradrenaline and dopamine.
CD4 cell	T helper (Th) lymphocyte, a subset of lymphocytes identified by their differential function and specific cell surface markers.
cDNA library	Clones containing a single independent DNA molecule.

Cerebral insufficiency	State in the elderly characterized by difficulties in concentration and memory.
Cerebrospinal fluid (CSF)	Physiological fluid that bathes the brain and spinal cord and may be monitored by removing the fluid from the lumbar region of the spinal cord or occasionally from the lateral ventricles.
c-fos	Immediate early gene that serves as a transcription factor for the expression of other genes.
Chelating agent	Compound that sequesters a metallic ion, thereby inactivating it (e.g. EDTA).
Chemokines	Chemoattractant cytokines; soluble factors that induce chemotaxis of lymphocytes.
Chorea	Repetitive involuntary jerky movements.
Chronic fatigue syndrome (CFS)	Symptom complex of extreme fatigue in combination with signs of an impaired immune and endocrine state. Frequently occurs after an acute, viral infection.
Chronopharmacology	Study of the influence of biological rhythms on the pharmacokinetics, pharmacodynamics and toxicity of drugs.
Circling	Behaviour initiated in animals by dopamine agonists following a unilateral lesion of the nigrostriatal pathway.
Classical benzodiazepines	1,4-Benzodiazepines that are structurally related to diazepam and that have qualitatively similar pharmacological profiles (e.g anxiolytic, anticonvulsant, muscle relaxant and sedative).
Clearance	The rate of elimination of a drug from the body.
Cloning	Process that involves removing the nucleus from an adult cell, transferring it to an unfertilized oocyte, destroying the genome of the oocyte and allowing the resulting cloned cell to develop.
Clonus	Movement characterized by involuntary, alternating rapid muscle contractions and relaxations.
Codon	Triplet of three bases in a DNA or RNA molecule that encodes a specific amino acid according to the genetic code.
Coefficient of variation	Standard deviation as a percentage of the mean.
Cofactor	A compound or ion that, while not being directly involved in a chemical reaction, facilitates an enzyme-catalysed reaction.
Comorbidity	Occurrence of more than one disease at the same time in the same patient (e.g. anxiety and depression).
Compartments	Areas of the body in which a drug or neurotransmitter has different kinetic characteristics.
Competitive inhibition	Inhibition of an enzyme or receptor that is dependent on the relative concentration of the inhibitor, substrate or agonist.
Complement	Plasma proteins that, when activated, bind to a target antigen or pathogen.
Concordance	In genetics, similarity in a twin pair with respect to the presence or absence of a disease or trait.

Confidence interval (CI)	Measurement of the range of values within which the true population value probably lies.
Corpus striatum	Part of the basal ganglia containing the caudate nucleus and the putamen.
Co-transmission	Release of two or more neurotransmitters from the same neuron.
Cytochromes	Part of the family of hepatic microsomal drug metabolizing enzymes. Two isozymes (P450 2D6 and 3A4) responsible for biotransformation of 90% of drugs used clinically.
Cytotoxic T cell	T-cell that, on activation by a specific antigen, targets and attacks cells bearing that type of antigen. Also called natural killer cell (NKC)
Dale's law	Principle that each neuron contains only one neurotransmitter (now no longer true!)
Delirium	Transient organic mental syndrome characterized by global impairment of cognition, including memory and perception.
Delirium tremens (DTs)	Acute, sometimes lethal, brain disorder precipitated by total or partial withdrawal from excessive alcohol intake. Shown by confusion, disorientation, fluctuating or clouded consciousness, agitation and insomnia.
Delusion	A belief held without any supportive evidence.
Dementia	An acquired global impairment of intellect, memory and personality but without global impairment of consciousness.
Dependence	(a) A behavioural syndrome that implies compulsive use of a drug. (b) Physical dependence, or change in brain function in tolerance and withdrawal, when a chronically administered drug is abruptly discontinued.
Depersonalization	Subjective experience that the body is unreal.
Depolarization	The inside of a nerve cell becoming less negatively charged relative to the outside of the nerve membrane.
Depression, major/chronic	Unremitting major depression that persists for at least 2 years.
Desensitization	Reduction in the sensitivity of a receptor in response to excessive stimulation. Also termed *down-regulation*. Such changes may be associated with a decrease in the number of receptors and/or their functional responsiveness. Desensitization is also a term used to describe the reduction in anxiety and panic states caused by controlled exposure to a specific anxiety-provoking stimulus.
Designer drug	Illegally manufactured drug with similarity in structure or effect to a drug already registered as a drug of abuse.
Diencephalon	Anterior region of the brain that includes the thalamus, hypothalamus and pituitary gland.

Discordance Dissimilarity in a twin pair with respect to the presence or absence of a disease or trait.

Dissociation constant Term used to describe quantitatively the separation of a ligand from a receptor. In ligand binding studies it may be expressed as the reciprocal of the affinity constant.

Dizygotic In genetic studies this refers to twins who have developed from two ova and therefore have different genetic characteristics.

Double depression Major depression superimposed on underlying dysthymia (chronic minor depression).

Down-regulation Reduction in response following the exposure of a receptor to a higher than normal concentration of an agonist.

Drug abuse Use of any drug in a manner which is at variance with the approved use in that culture.

Drug dependence Syndrome in which an individual continues to take a drug for its pleasurable effect despite the adverse medical and social consequences. The individual then continues to take the drug for his or her well-being.

Dyskinesia Impairment of voluntary movements.

Dysphasia Impairment of language.

Dysphoria Acute, transient changes in mood (e.g. feelings of sadness, sorrow, anguish).

Dyspraxia Impairment of ability to perform co-ordinated movement.

Dystonia Neurological condition characterized by slow, tonic sustained muscle contractions often of the tongue, jaw, eyes, neck and occasionally the whole body.

Effect size The clinically meaningful result required to detect a specific result or end-point; related to the probability of declaring a true positive.

Electrolytic lesion Destruction of a specific nerve pathway by the passage of a current between electrodes inserted into the brain region which is innervated by the nerve pathway.

Endocoids Unspecified endogenous compounds that may modulate synaptic neurotransmission.

Enteroviruses Small ribonucleic acid (RNA) containing viruses. For example, polio viruses, which destroy the anterior horn cells leading to lower motor neuron paralysis, are of this type.

Entorhinal cortex Critical area of the brain linking limbic structures to the cerebral cortex. The hippocampus receives its major input from the entorhinal cortex via the perforant pathway.

Entrainment Synchronization of a biological rhythm by a stimulus such as an environmental time cue (zeitgeber).

Enzyme induction Increase in enzyme activity in response to an increase in the amount of substrate available. For example, barbiturates increase the activity of the hepatic microsomal enzyme system following their repeated administration.

Eosinophilia myalgia syndrome (EMS)
Toxic, potentially fatal disorder attributed to a contaminant of tryptophan.

Evoked potential (EP)
Electrophysiological measurement in which a sensory (flight flash, tone) or cognitive signal stimulates a response that is detected from the scalp or cortex.

Exon
Part of a gene that encodes information present in messenger RNA.

Extrapyramidal
Motor control that does not involve the pyramidal tracts. It originates in the basal ganglia.

Extrapyramidal system
Polysynaptic neuronal pathways involving the basal ganglia and related subcortical nuclei that influence motor behaviour.

Fatal toxicity index
Number of deaths due to poisoning per million National Health Service prescriptions.

Fatigue
The patient tires abnormally early during prolonged mental or physical activity or cannot sustain the same level of activity as normal.

Fibromyalgia
Form of non-articular rheumatism characterized by a syndrome of chronic, diffuse musculoskeletal pain and stiffness, chronic fatigue and sleep disturbance.

Flashback
Spontaneous occurrence of previously experienced drug effects (e.g. hallucinations, delusions, depersonalization) or distressing emotions originally associated with trauma. Generally associated with LSD-like drugs and occasionally cannabis.

Flicker fusion threshold
Measure of CNS drug effects that assesses temporal information processing in the visual system; the threshold for flicker detection at high frequencies ($>30\,Hz$).

Flight of ideas
Rapid succession of thoughts without logical connections.

Foetal alcohol syndrome
Specific, recognizable pattern of malformation (brain, skull, heart) in offspring of alcoholic mothers.

Gangliosides
Group of complex sphingolipids containing sphingosine linked to a fatty acid and a branched chain polysaccharide molecule.

Gas chromatography
Method whereby volatile compounds are separated by injecting them into a stream of inert gas which percolates over a solid or liquid stationary phase. The separated compounds are then detected and quantified by means of an electrochemical or fluorescent probe. GC-MS is a method whereby the gas chromatograph is linked to a mass spectrograph, thereby allowing very small quantities of the compound to be quantified.

Gene, candidate
A gene that may be associated with a disease phenotype.

Gene, family   A family of related genes that control a similar biological process.

Gene, penetrance   The proportion of subjects with the genotype who manifest the disease.

Gene, polymorphism   Variations in DNA sequences that do not affect the corresponding gene product.

Glia   Supporting cells within the brain that act as a physical and metabolic buffer around nerve cells.

G proteins   Family of proteins within neurons that link receptors to ion channels or secondary messengers.

Grand mal   Major seizure disorder characterized by tonic and clonic muscular movements and loss of consciousness.

Guanylate cyclase   The intracellular enzyme associated with some types of receptor that on activation produces the secondary messenger cyclic guanylate monophosphate (cyclic GMP).

Guillain–Barré syndrome Acute idiopathic polyneuritis characterized by muscular weakness and paraesthesia.

Half-life   The time taken for the concentration of a compound in a tissue to decrease by 50%.

Hallucinations   Sensory perception that is not based on a real stimulus.

Hebephrenia   Chronic form of schizophrenia, usually starting before the age of 20 years, characterized by marked disorder in thinking, shallow and inappropriate affect, severe emotional disturbance, hallucinations and delusions.

Helper T-cell   T-cell that activates B-cells to produce antibodies and secretes interleukin-2 to facilitate natural killer cell proliferation and activity.

Hepatic encephalopathy A progressive metabolic liver disorder that results in altered intellectual function and emotion.

Heteroceptor   Presynaptic receptor that is activated by a neurotransmitter from an adjacent neuron; the type of neurotransmitter activating the heteroceptor differs from that released from the axon.

5-HIAA   5-Hydroxyindoleacetic acid, the main metabolite of 5-hydroxytryptamine (serotonin) formed by monoamine oxidase.

High performance liquid chromatography (HPLC)   Form of chromatography in which mobile solvent passes through a column packed with a non-polar solid phase. The organic molecules are then detected fluorimetrically or electrochemically. Commonly used to determine trace concentrations of biogenic amines.

Hippocampus   Region of the temporal lobe that is thought to play a role in learning and memory.

HVA   Homovanillic acid, one of the main metabolites of dopamine formed by the actions of monoamine oxidase and catechol-*O*-methyltransferase.

Hyperbaric	Raised pressure.
Hyperkinetic	Increased movements or activity.
Hypertension	Raised blood pressure.
Hypnotic	Sleep inducing.
Hypochondriasis	Over-concern about health.
Hypofrontality	Hypofunction of prefrontal cortex as shown by positron emission tomography imaging or cerebral blood flow determinations. Hypofrontality occurs in both medicated and unmedicated schizophrenics.
Hypophysis	The pituitary gland. Hypophysectomy is removal of the pituitary gland.
Hypotension	Lowered blood pressure.
Hypothalamus	Region at the base of the brain concerned with the regulation of autonomic activity and some aspects of behaviour.
Hypothermia	Low body temperature.
Iatrogenic	Complications of drug treatment; unwise use of drugs producing adverse effects; drug-induced disorder.
Ideas of reference	Ideas that normal events have specific reference to the individual or are commenting on the individual.
Idiosynchratic drug reaction	Unpredictable side effects of a drug, including hypersensitivity reactions, that usually develop suddenly. Such reactions are often genetically determined and not related to the pharmacological properties of the drug.
Illusion	Perceptual distortion of a genuine stimulus; visual and auditory distortions most common.
Immunofluorescence	Fluorescence histochemistry using antibodies to identify the compounds under investigation.
Indoles	Compounds with a 2,3-benzpyrrole structure. The indoleamines, e.g. 5-hydroxytryptamine, are compounds containing the indole structure.
Infarct	An area of dead tissue caused by a reduced blood supply.
Interneuron	One of the four major fundamental types of neurons that establish inter-relationships between sensory afferents and motor efferents.
Intrinsic activity	The inherent ability of a ligand to elicit a biological response once it is bound to a receptor.
Inverse agonist	A substance that produces effects at a receptor that are the opposite to those produced by the usual agonist. Thus the inverse agonists at benzodiazepine receptors have anxiogenic, proconvulsant and promnestic properties.
Ion channel	Pore on the nerve membrane through which sodium, potassium and other metal and non-metal ions (e.g. chloride) pass to produce changes in the electrical activity of the nerve membrane. These channels are controlled by receptors located in the nerve membrane.

Iontophoresis   Administration of compounds through micropipettes which are released by an electric current.

Isomerism   The existence of a molecule that possesses two or more structural forms. *Stereo-isomerism* refers to the existence of two or more compounds possessing the same molecular and structural formulae but having different spatial configurations.

Isozyme   Multiple molecular forms of an enzyme within the same individual.

Kindling   Consequences of repeated subthreshold electrical or chemical stimuli that progressively increase convulsive or behavioural responses, eventually resulting in a seizure. Subsequent application of a single subthreshold stimulus will also evoke a seizure.

Korsakoff's psychosis   An organic brain syndrome associated with prolonged, heavy ingestion of alcohol. It is characterized by amnesia for recent events and an inability to memorize new information.

LD_{50}; ED_{50}   Dose of a compound which is lethal (LD_{50}) or effective (ED_{50}) in 50% of the test population.

Learned helplessness   Behavioural phenomenon consisting of passivity and withdrawal after exposure to an uncontrollable adverse event.

Leptin   The gene product of the obesity (ob) gene.

Lewy body dementia   Cortical dementia characterized by diffuse Lewy bodies with neuronal degeneration, mild parkinsonism and slowing of the electroencephalogram.

Life events   Experiences which are part of normal life but which are stressful and thought to trigger a psychiatric disorder in a vulnerable individual.

Lifetime prevalence   Number of individuals who may have a disease any time during their lifetime.

Ligand   Compound which specifically binds to a receptor.

Ligase chain reaction (LCR) Recently developed amplification method used to detect a gene mutation. The method uses the coupling of two adjacent synthetic oligonucleotides aligned on the template of the target deoxyribonucleic acid (DNA).

Limbic system   Area of the brain associated with small, involuntary functions, emotions and behaviour. Comprises the hypothalamus, parahippocampus, olfactory lobe, dentate gyrus, amygdala, anterior thalamus, fornix and stria terminalis.

Linkage analysis   Analysis of genetic markers linked to genes (e.g. genetic traits or phenotype markers such as enzyme deficiencies occurring in patients with mood disorders).

Liver enzyme induction   Increased liver enzyme activity due to chronic use of drugs such as barbiturates.

Lumbar puncture   The sampling of cerebrospinal fluid by insertion of a needle through the lumbar region of the spine into the space surrounding the spinal cord.

Malignant hyperthermia	Rare, familial hyperthermia (41 °C) associated with inhalation anaesthetics, muscle relaxants, tricyclic antidepressants, phenothiazine neuroleptics (particularly chlorpromazine) monoamine oxidase inhibitors and haloperidol.
Mass fragmentography	Quantitative analysis of compounds by measurement of specific fragments using mass spectrometry.
Mass spectrometry	Analysis of the chemical structure of a compound by measurement of the molecular weight of fragments formed by bombardment of the molecule by ions.
Medulla oblongata	Area of the brain lying below the pons.
Mesencephalon	Area of the brain also called the midbrain, which contains the tegmentum and the substantia nigra.
Mesocortical system	Part of the dopaminergic system with the cell bodies mainly in the ventral tegmental area which project to the prefrontal cortex, accumbens, septum and olfactory tubercles.
Mesolimbic system	Area of the brain containing the nucleus accumbens, olfactory tubercle and projections to the cortex.
Messenger RNA (mRNA)	RNA that carries genetic information for a specific polypeptide from the nuclear gene to the cytoplasm where it combines with transfer RNA (tRNA) to initiate protein synthesis.
Meta-analysis	Statistical overview of randomized, controlled trials that reduce random errors and may detect small treatment effects that are not apparent in a single study.
MHPG	3-Methoxy-4-hydroxyphenylglycol, the main brain metabolite or noradrenaline formed by the actions of monoamine oxidase and catechol-O-methyltransferase.
Microglia	Cells in the CNS that modify their behaviour in response to diverse signals from other cells; these cells represent the immune system in the CNS.
Microsatellite	A variable number of tandem repeats of a relatively short oligonucleotide sequence.
Microsomal ethanol oxidizing system	An enzyme complex in the liver that metabolizes alcohols and other compounds.
Microsomes	Subcellular particles occurring in most types of cell and involved in the metabolism of drugs as well as natural substances.
Migraine	A syndrome thought to involve 5-HT characterized by localized headache and often accompanied by nausea, vomiting and sensory disturbances.
Mitochondria	Rod-shaped subcellular particles involved in energy production (e.g. ATP) and metabolism.
Mitogen	Substance foreign to the body that induces lymphocytes to proliferate.
Monoamine	General name for catecholamine and indoleamine neurotransmitters.

Monozygotic	In genetic studies this refers to twins who are derived from a single ovum and therefore have identical genetic characteristics.
Narcolepsy	Rare, disabling sleep disorder of unknown origin. Characterized by sudden attacks of flaccid paralysis (cataplexy), extensive daytime sleepiness, sleep paralysis, hypnagogic hallucinations and rapid onset of rapid eye movement (REM) phase of sleep.
Natural killer cell (NKC)	Any class of white blood cells that can spontaneously recognize and kill tumour or virus infected cells without previous exposure to an antigen. NKC cytotoxicity decreased in depression and in alcoholism.
Nerve growth factor (NGF)	Member of a class of proteins, the neurotrophins, that regulate neuronal cell death during development, aiding neural recovery from injury and ageing.
Neuritic plaques	Found in high density throughout the hippocampus and neocortex of patients with Alzheimer's disease. Density of plaques correlated with degree of cognitive impairment.
Neuroendocrine challenge test	Any of a variety of tests used to examine the functional integrity of the monoamine pathways that control the secretion of pituitary hormones.
Neurofibrillary tangle (NFT)	One of the principal histopathological changes observed in Alzheimer's disease.
Neuromodulator	A substance that modifies the function or effects of a neurotransmitter, e.g. peptides.
Neuron	A nerve cell.
Neuroregulator	A compound that has not been shown to fulfil the criteria of a neurotransmitter.
Neurosis	Behaviour showing undue adherence to an unrealistic idea of things and showing an inability to take a rationally objective view of life.
Neurotransmitter	A chemical messenger released by a neuron to excite or inhibit adjacent neurons.
Nigrostriatal pathway	The neural projection from cell bodies in the substantia nigra to the striatum.
NMDA	N-Methyl-D-aspartate, a synthetic amino acid that activates a subclass of excitatory amino acid (glutamate) receptors.
Nociceptive	Impulses that give rise to pain.
Novel anxiolytics	Drugs chemically unrelated to diazepam that produce their anxiolytic effects by facilitating inhibitory transmission through mechanisms other than the GABA-benzodiazepine receptor complex (e.g. buspirone).
Nuclear schizophrenia	The core symptoms of schizophrenia rather than the associated or social factors.
Nutraceuticals	Plants used for food but also for health benefits, including disease prevention and treatment.

Nystagmus	Oscillatory movements of the eyes.
Obsessive–compulsive disorder (OCD)	State characterized by recurrent, intrusive thoughts and compulsive stereotyped, repetitive behaviour or cognitions.
Oedema	Swelling due to the presence of excess fluid in the intercellular spaces of the body.
Oligodendroglia	One of the three types of glia cells responsible for creating the myelin sheath surrounding neurons in the CNS.
Oligonucleotide	Short (less than 30 nucleotides) piece of DNA.
Oncogene	Gene involved in development and differentiation that causes cancer when mutated.
"On-off" phenomenon	Occurs in patients with Parkinson's disease. The "on" phase (choreoathetotic dyskinesia) occurs at peak dose effect. In the "off" phase (akinesia), patients suddenly "freeze".
Operant conditioning	Response to a stimulus that increases the probability that the behavioural response to the stimulus will be repeated.
Palpitations	An unduly rapid heart beat which is noticed by the subject.
Panic attack	Sudden attack of fear or anxiety associated with one or more of 12 autonomic symptoms (e.g. shortness of breath, dizziness, palpitations, sweating).
Paper chromatography	Separation of a mixture of compounds on filter paper according to their relative solubility in organic solvents that diffuse through the paper by capillary action.
Paranoia	The occurrence of delusions that are frequently of a persecutory nature.
Para suicide	Deliberately non-fatal self-poisoning or injury.
Particulate fraction	Usually applied to a fraction of a tissue homogenate which contains subcellular particles.
Passivity	A feeling of being under the control or will of an outside agency.
Penetrance	Genetic term referring to the degree to which an inherited characteristic is expressed.
Phobia	A persistent and unreasonable fear of some situation or object.
Phosphatidylinositol system (PI system)	G protein linked secondary messenger system which, by controlling the concentration of intracellular calcium, modulates the actions of some transmitters. The action of lithium may be mediated via the PI system.
Phospholipid	A phosphorus-containing lipid that comprises about 50% of the cell membrane.
Physical dependence	Phenomenon in which abnormal behavioural and autonomic symptoms occur following the abrupt withdrawal of a drug of dependence or when the effect of the drug is terminated by means of a specific antagonist.

Plasma	Blood from which the cells have been removed but without the blood being allowed to clot.
Platelet	Small blood constituents formed from APUD cells which are involved in blood clotting. Platelets are also called *thrombocytes*.
Polydipsia	Excessive drinking.
Polymerase chain reaction (PCR)	Technique using enzymes and specific primers to generate multiple copies of the original (usually viral) nucleic acid, thereby increasing its numbers so that it may more easily be detected.
Polymorphism	Occurrence of two or more gene structures in the same population.
Polypeptide	Protein-like molecule consisting of a chain of amino acids.
Polyuria	Voiding of excessive amounts of urine.
Pons	Area of the hindbrain under the cerebellum.
Postsynaptic	Part of the membrane lying adjacent to the nerve terminal that contains the postsynaptic receptors.
Post-traumatic stress	Anxiety disorder attributed to a severe, adverse life experience (e.g. threat to life) that is experienced again without the stimulus of the adverse experience.
Precursor	Usually used in reference to compounds which are metabolized in neurotransmitters (e.g. tryptophan is the precursor of 5-hydroxytryptamine).
Prepulse inhibition (PPI)	Partially automatic response involving an inhibitory process in which the normal startle reflex is reduced when the startling stimulus is preceded 30–50 msec earlier by a weak prepulse. This provides an operational measure of sensory motor gating.
Presynaptic	Events or structures occurring proximal to the synapse.
Prion disease	Transmissible spongiform encephalopathy is an example, together with Creutzfeldt–Jakob disease and bovine spongiform encephalopathy. Caused by abnormal proteins.
Protein kinases	A group of enzymes that transfer charged phosphate groups on proteins, thereby regulating intracellular processes in response to extracellular signals (see *PI system*).
Psychological dependence	Dysphoria and craving which arise following the abrupt withdrawal of a drug of abuse.
Psychosis	A psychiatric condition in which contact with reality and insight are lost.
Psychotropic drug	A drug acting on the brain to cause a change in mood or behaviour.
Purinergic	Neurons in the brain and heart that secrete purine neurotransmitters such as adenosine.
Putamen	Area of the brain within the corpus striatum.
QT interval	Electrocardiographic measure that estimates an entire cycle of electrical depolarization and repolarization and which varies with age, gender and heart rate.

Radioimmunoassay Assay technique in which an antibody against a specific compound is used to measure the concentration of that compound.

Radiolabelled compound Compound synthesized to contain one or more radioactive atoms (usually ^{3}H or ^{14}C).

Randomization Chance allocation of study subjects to either the control or experimental group.

Rank Arrangement by order of magnitude of components in a series.

Rank order Set of markers ranked from the lowest to the highest, or vice versa.

Raphé nuclei These are serotonin containing neurons that project from the brainstem throughout the brain and act as filters for sensory impulses.

Rapid eye movement (REM) sleep Stage of sleep associated with high frequency, low voltage waves on the electroencephalogram. It is linked with dreaming, rapid movement of the eyes and pronounced changes in blood pressure and respiration.

Rating scale Instrument to record and quantify the extended magnitude of a trait.

Rebound Recurrence of symptoms of the original disorder after discontinuation of the drug; the symptoms are of equal or greater intensity to those occurring before the start of the drug treatment.

Receptor A protein-containing site in the neuronal cell wall to which a natural or synthetic ligand may bind to produce a physiological or pharmacological effect.

Recombinant DNA Technique to manipulate and clone DNA molecules. This type of DNA consists of a vector for propagation of the nucleotide sequence and an insertor site.

Regulatory sequence Region of DNA responsible for regulating the transcription of the gene.

Reinforcement The process by which a specific stimulus appears to increase the probability that a particular behaviour will occur.

Relapse Re-emergence of symptoms that improved spontaneously or following treatment.

Restriction enzyme Enzyme that recognizes short stretches (4–8 base pairs) in a sequence-specific manner and cleaves the DNA at specific points.

Restriction fragment length polymorphism (RFLP) Genetic tool from the direct analysis of the human genome to detect new genes that predispose to genetic disease.

Reticular formation Brainstem region consisting of the tegmental part of the medulla, pons and midbrain; plays a major role in sleep and wakefulness.

Reverse transcriptase Enzyme that forms complementary DNA (cDNA).

Saccade Abrupt, high velocity eye movement produced by a precisely timed pattern of activity in the motor neurons innervating the extraocular muscles.

Scatchard plot

Relationship between the applied concentration (in molar units) and the ratio of bound to free drug following the binding of a hormone, drug or neurotransmitter to a receptor.

Seasonal affective disorder (SAD)

Seasonal subtype of major depressive disorder characterized by an annual pattern of symptoms (e.g. depression occurring in the autumn or spring).

Secondary messenger

A molecule such as cyclic AMP, cyclic GMP or phosphatidylinositol that regulates intracellular processes in response to an extracellular signal.

Seizure

Uncontrolled or paroxysmal brain activity that is usually expressed through the motor system.

Selective 5-HT reuptake inhibitors

Antidepressants such as fluoxetine and fluvoxamine that show specificity in inhibiting the uptake of 5-hydroxytryptamine into platelets or brain tissue *in vitro* and *in vivo*.

Single photon emission computed tomography (SPECT)

Neuroimaging technique for measuring cerebral blood flow, cerebral blood volume, metabolic rate, oxygen utilization and the oxygen extraction volume.

Sleep apnoea

Disorder characterized by respiratory cessations during sleep.

Standard deviation (SD)

Measure of the dispersion or spread of points clustered around the mean value; SD=square root of the variance.

Standard error of the mean (SEM)

Measure of the variability of the mean value from one sample to another (e.g. control versus experimental sample).

Startle reflex

Jerky movements produced by a loud sound or stimulus.

Stereoisomerism

Two or more compounds with the same molecular and structural formulae but having different spatial configurations.

Stereotaxic surgery

A method for accurately placing lesions in the brain by electrocoagulation, selective neurotoxins or radioactive pellets.

Stereotypy

The persistent repetition of body movements.

Subcaudate tractotomy

A neurosurgical procedure used for the treatment of therapy-resistant depression.

Subsensitivity

The decreased response of a receptor to a fixed concentration of an agonist, shown as a shift in the dose–response curve to the right. In behaviour, subsensitivity represents a decreased response to a fixed dose of a drug. *Supersensitivity* is the opposite of subsensitivity and the dose–response curve is shifted to the left.

Suprachiasmatic nucleus (SCN)

Collection of cells in the anterior hypothalamus acting as a biological clock or oscillator that maintains the circadian rhythm of the sleep–wake cycle.

Synapse

The gap separating adjacent neurons.

Synaptosomes	The pinched off and resealed nerve endings formed following the homogenization and high speed centrifugation of brain tissue in an isotonic medium.
Tachycardia	Rapid heart beat.
Tardive dyskinesia (TD)	Potentially irreversible, late onset, extrapyramidal hyperkinetic movement disorder often associated with the long-term administration of neuroleptics. Abnormal movements generally involve the mouth, lips and tongue.
Tau	A microtubule associated protein that is a major component of the neurofibrillary tangles found in the Alzheimer brain.
T-cell suppressor	T-cell that specifically inhibits antibody formation in beta cells as well as other cytotoxic T-cells.
Teratogenesis	Physical malformation of foetal organs that can be caused by exposure to psychotropic drugs (e.g. thalidomide) during the first trimester of pregnancy in females.
Therapeutic index	The ratio between the dose of a drug needed to produce a therapeutic effect (assumed to be unity) and the toxic dose.
Thymoleptic	Drug affecting mood state; formerly used to describe antidepressants.
Tolerance	Reduced effect of an agonist or antagonist following its prolonged administration resulting from the increased metabolism (called *metabolic tolerance*) or decreased receptor sensitivity (termed *pharmaco-* or *tissue tolerance*).
Trait marker	A variable factor that is specific for a particular disease and remains stable over time, as distinct from a STATE marker which only appears when the disease symptoms are present.
Transcranial magnetic stimulation (TMS)	Procedure that involves rapidly passing an electric current through a coil thereby creating a powerful, localized and transient magnetic field. This field depolarizes superficial cortical neurons.
Transcription factor	Regulatory protein that controls the transcription of specific genes; transcription is the first step from DNA to RNA by RNA polymerase.
TRAP	Acronym for the major symptoms of Parkinson's disease (T=tremor, R=rigidity, A=akinesia, P=postural disturbance).
Tuberoinfundibular system	The system connecting the hypothalamus with the pituitary gland.
Up-regulation	An increase in the number and/or sensitivity of receptors to compensate for the decreased effect of an agonist.
Vagus nerve stimulation	Chronic stimulation of vagus as a non-drug treatment for epilepsy and depression.
Vasoconstriction	Reduction in the diameter of blood vessels by contraction of the circular muscles in the vessel wall.

Ventral tegmental area
  (VTA)

Area of the midbrain dorsal to the substantia nigra.

Ventricles

Cavities within the brain containing the CSF.

Voltage-sensitive calcium
  channels

Ion channels for calcium uptake whose regulation is controlled by nerve impulses.

Volume of distribution

The apparent volume of the body in which a drug would be distributed if it was present throughout the body at the same concentration as that occurring in plasma.

Appendix 3: Generic and Proprietary Names of Some Common Psychotropic Drugs

This list of drugs is not intended to be entirely comprehensive and in most cases only the most frequently used proprietary names are given. For detailed coverage of the area the reader is referred to a local pharmacopoeia. Our best efforts to ensure accuracy have been made. The publisher bears no responsibility for inaccuracy.

Approved name	European (mainly Irish/ UK) trade name	USA trade name
Acetazolamide	Diamox	Diamox
Alprazolam	Xanax	Xanax
Amantadine	Symmetrel	Symmetrel
Amisulpride	Solian	—
Amitriptyline	Tryptizol; Lentizol	Elaril; Endep
Amoxapine	Asendin	Asendin
Amphetamine	Benzedrine	Benzedrine
Antipyrine (phenazone)	—	Auralgan
Baclofen	Lioresal	Lioresal
Benperidol	Anquil; Frenactil; Concilium	—
Benserazide	Madopar (with L-dopa)	Madopar (with L-dopa)
Benzhexol	Artane	Artane
Benztropine	Cogentin	Cogentin
Biperiden	Akineton	Akineton
Bromazepam	Lexotan	Lexomil
Bromocriptine	Parlodel	Parlodel
Brotizolam	Ladormin; Lendorm	—
Buprenorphine	Temgesic	—
Bupropion	Zyban	Wellbutrin
Buspirone	Buspar	Buspar
Butorphanol	Torbutrol; Torate; Torbutesic	—

Fundamentals of Psychopharmacology. Third Edition. By Brian E. Leonard
2003 John Wiley & Sons, Ltd. ISBN 0 471 52178 7

Approved name	European (mainly Irish/ UK) trade name	USA trade name
Cabergoline	Cabaser; Dostinex	Dostinex
Captopril	Capoten; Capozide; Acepril	Capoten; Capozide
Carbamazepine	Tegretol	Tegretol
Carbidopa	Sinemet (with L-dopa)	Sinemet (with L-dopa)
Chlordiazepoxide	Librium	Librium; Limbitrol
Chlormethiazole	Heminevrin	—
Chlorpromazine	Largactil	Thorazine
Cisapride	Prepulsid	Propulsid
Citalopram	Cipramil	Celexa; Lexapro
Clobazam	Frisium	—
Clomipramine	Anafranil	—
Clonazepam	Rivotril	Klonopin
Clonidine	Catapres; Dixarit	Catapres; Dixarit
Clopenthixol	Clopixol	—
Clorazepate	Tranxene	Tranxene
Clozapine	Leponex; Lepotex; Clozaril	Leponex; Lepotex; Clozaril
Co-dergocrine	Hydergine	Hydergine
Corticotrophin	Acthar gel	Acthar
Cyproheptadine	Periactin	Periactin
Cyproterone acetate	Androcur	—
Debrisoquine	Declinax	—
Desferrioxamine mesylate	Desferal	Desferal
Desipramine	Pertofran	Pertofran; Norpramin
Dexamethasone	Decadron	Decadron; Nexadrol
Dexamphetamine	Dexedrine	Dexedrine; Desoxyn
Dextromethorphan	Benylin; Robitussin	Benylin DM; Delsym
Dextropropoxyphene	Distalgesic	Darvon; Darvocet; Propacet
Diazepam	Valium	Valium
Diethylpropion	Tenuate	Tenuate; Tepanil
Digoxin	Lanoxin	Lanoxin
Dihydrocodeine	DF 118; DHC Continus	—
Diphenylhydantoin – see Phenytoin		
Disulfiram	Antabuse	Antabuse
L-Dopa (levodopa)	Larodopa	Larodopa
Dothiepin	Prothiaden	—
Doxepin	Sinequan; Xepin	Sinequan; Zonalon
Ergometrine	Syntometrine	—
Ergotamine	Migril	Ergomar; Ergostat
Ethchlorvynol	Avinol; Serenesil; Normoson	Placidyl
Ethosuximide	Zarontin; Emeside	Zarontin
Ethytoin (ethotoin)	—	Peganone
Fenfluramine	Ponderax	Pondimin
Fentanyl	Durogesic	Sublimaze

Approved name	European (mainly Irish/UK) trade name	USA trade name
Flumazenil	Anexate	Romazicon
Flunitrazepam	Rohypnol	Rohypnol
Fluoxetine	Affex; Prozac; Prozamel	Prozac
Flupenthixol	Depixol; Fluanxol	—
Fluphenazine	Modecate	Prolixin; Permitil
Flurazepam	Dalmane	Dalmane
Fluvoxamine	Faverin	—
Gabapentin	Neurontin	Neurontin
Galantamine	Reminyl	Reminyl
Haloperidol	Serenace; Haldol	Haldol
Heroin (diacetylmorphine)	Diamorphine	Diamorphine
Hydrocodone	—	Codinal; Codan
Hydromorphine	Palladone	Dilaudid
Imipramine	Tofranil	Tofranil
Iproniazid	Marsilid	Marsilid
Isocarboxazid	Marplan	Marplan
Ketamine	Ketalar	—
Ketanserin	Serefrex; Sufrexal	—
Lamotrigine	Lamical	Lamictal
Levadopa	Madopar; Sinemet	Dopar; Larodopa
Levallorphan	Naloxiphan; Naloxifan	—
Levorphanol	Dromoran	Levo-Dromoran
Lithium	Priadel; Phasal; Camcolit	Lithonate; Lithane; Eskalith
Lofepramine	Gamanil	—
Loprazolam	Dormonoct	—
Lorazepam	Ativan	Ativan
Lormetazepam	Loramet	Noctamid
Loxapine	Cloxazepam; Oxilapine	Loxitane
Maprotiline	Ludiomil	—
Medazolam	Nobrium	—
Melperone	Buronil; Eunerpan	—
Meprobamate	Miltown; Equanil	Miltown; Equanil
Mesoridazine	Lidanar; Lidanil	Serentil
Methadone	Physeptone	Dolophrine
Methylphenidate	Ritalin	Ritalin
Metoclopromide	Antimet; Gastrobid; Maxolon; Paramax	Reglan
Metyrapone	Metopirone	Metopirone
Mianserin	Tolvon; Bolvidon	—
Midazolam	Hypnovel	—
Mirtazepine	Zispin; Remeron	—
Moclobemide	Mannerix	—

Approved name	European (mainly Irish/ UK) trade name	USA trade name
Molindone	Lidone; Moban	—
Morphine	Duromorph; MST-Continus	Duromorph; Roxanol
Nabilone	Cesamet	Cesamet
Nalorphine	Allorphine; Anarcon	—
Naloxone	Narcan	Narcan
Nefazodone	Dutonin	Serzone
Nitrazepam	Mogadon	Mogadon
Nomifensine	Merital	Merital
Nortriptyline	Aventyl	Aventyl
Olanzapine	Zyprexa	Zyprexa
Ondansetron	Zofran	Zofran
Oxazepam	Serenid	Serax
Oxcarbamazepine	Trieptal	Trileptal
Oxycodone	Oxycontin	—
Pargyline	Eutonyl	—
Paroxetine	Seroxat; Paxil	Paxil
Pemoline	Volital	Cylert
Penfluridol	Flupidol; Oraleptin	—
Pentazocine	Fortral; Fortagesic	Talwin; Talacem
Pentobarbitone	Nembutal	Nembutal
Pentoxifylline	Trental	Trental
Pergolide	Celance	Permax
Perphenazine	Fentazin	—
Pethidine (meperidine in USA)	Pethilorfan (with leval-lorphan); Pamergan	Demerol
Phenazocine	Narphen	—
Phenelzine	Nardil	Nardil
Phenmetrazine	—	Adipost; Bontril
Phenobarbitone	Luminal	Luminal
Phentermine	Ionamine; Duromine	—
Phenytoin	Epanutin	Dilantin
Physostigmine	Eserine	Antilirium
Pimozide	Orap	Orap
Pindolol	Vistaldix	Visken
Piribedil	Trivastal	—
Pramipexole	Mirapexin	Mirapex; Sifrol
Prazepam	Contrax	Centrax
Primidone	Mysoline	Mysoline
Prochlorperazine	Stemetil	Compazine
Promazine	Sparine	Sparine
Propranolol	Inderal	Inderal
Quetiapine	Serequal	Seoquel

Approved name	European (mainly Irish/UK) trade name	USA trade name
Reboxetine	Edronax	—
Reserpine	Serpasil	Serpasil
Risperidone	Risperdal	Risperdol
Rivastigmine	Exelon	—
Selegiline	Eldepryl	Eldepryl
Sertraline	Lustral	Zoloft
Sodium valproate (valproic acid)	Epilim	Depakene
Spiroperidol (spiperone)	Spiropitan	—
Sulpiride	Dogmatil; Sulpital	—
Sulthiame	Ospolat; Elisal; Trolone	—
Tacrine (THA)	Cognex	Cognex
Temazepam	Euhypnos; Normison	Levanxol; Cerepax
Thioridazine	Melleril	Melleri
Tiagabine	Gabitril	Gabitril
Topiramate	Topamax	Topamax
Tramadol	Tramex; Xymel; Zydol	Ultram
Tranylcypromine	Parnate	Parnate
Trazodone	Molipaxin	Desyrel
Triazolam	Halcion	Halcion
Triclofos	Tricloryl	—
Trifluoperazine	Stelazine	Stelazine
Trimethadione (troxidone)	Tridione	Tridione
Trimipramine	Surmontil	—
Venlafaxine	Efexor	Effexon
Verapamil	Cordilox; Securon; Univer	Calan; Isoptin
Vigabatrin	Sabril	—
Viloxazine	Vivalan	—
Yohimbine	Aphrodine; Corynine	Actibine; Aphrodyne
Zimelidine	Zelmid; Zelmidine	—
Zolpidem	Stinoct	Ambien
Zopiclone	Zimovane; Imovane	—
Zuclopenthixol	Clopixol	—

Appendix 4: Key References for Further Reading

No attempt will be made to give details of the experimental and clinical studies which have been surveyed in this text. I trust that the authors of these studies will forgive me for this deliberate omission, but my intention has been to create a readable text, not a detailed monograph, in which the flavour and excitement of the advances in psychopharmacology will encourage those interested to read further. With this in mind, a list of key monographs, review articles and textbooks is included merely as a guide for the reader. The choice of texts may seem idiosyncratic to some readers, but they include those which have appealed to the author because of their clarity, comprehensive nature or contribution to the advances in psychopharmacology.

General reading

Bazier, S. *Psychotropic Drugs Directory*. Salisbury: Quay Books, 2001.

Davis, K. L., Charney, D., Coyle, J. T. and Nemeroff, C. B. (Eds) *Neuropsychopharmacology – The Fifth Generation of Progress*. New York: Raven Press, 2002.

D'haenen, H. A. H., den Boer, J. A. and Willner, P. (Eds) *Biological Psychiatry*, Vols 1 and 2. Chichester: John Wiley & Sons, 2002.

Feldman, R. S., Meyer, J. S. and Quenzer, L. F. *Principles of Neuropsychopharmacology*. Sunderland, MA: Sinauer Associates Inc., 1997.

Janicak P. G., Davis, J. M., Preskorn, S. H. and Ayd, F. J. *Principles and Practice of Psychopharmacology* (Third Edition). Philadelphia: Lippincott, Williams and Wilkins, 2001.

Kasper, S., den Boer, J. A. and Sitsen, A. J. M. (Eds). *Handbook of Depression and Anxiety* (Second Edition). New York: Marcel Dekker, 2003.

King, D. J. *Seminars in Clinical Psychopharmacology* (Second Edition). London: Gaskell, 2003.

Lopez-Ibor, J. J., Goebel, W., Maj, M. and Sartorius, N. *Psychiatry as a Neuroscience*. Chichester: John Wiley & Sons, 2002.

Schatzberg, A. F. and Nemeroff, C. B. *Textbook of Psychopharmacology*. Washington, DC: American Psychiatric Press, 1998.

Webster, R. A. (Ed.) *Neurotransmitters, Drugs and Brain Function*. Chichester: John Wiley & Sons, 2001.

Fundamentals of Psychopharmacology. Third Edition. By Brian E. Leonard
© 2003 John Wiley & Sons, Ltd. ISBN 0 471 52178 7

Chapter 1 – Functional Neuroanatomy of the Brain

Fitzgerald, M. J. T. and Folan-Curran, J. *Clinical Neuroanatomy* (Fourth Edition). Edinburgh: W. B. Saunders, 2002.

Chapter 2 – Basic Aspects of Neurotransmitter Function

Barbour, B. and Hausser, M. Intersynaptic diffusion of neurotransmitters. *TINS* 20 (1997): 377–384.

Conn, P. T. and Pin, J.-P. Pharmacology and functions of metabotropic glutamate receptors. *Ann. Rev. Pharmacol.* 37 (1997): 205–232.

Dingledine, R. The glutamate receptor ion channel. *Pharmacol. Rev.* 51 (1999): 7–61.

Kandel, E. R., Schwartz, J. H. and Jessell, T. M. *Principles of Neural Science* (Fourth Edition). Englewood Cliffs, NJ: Prentice-Hall, 2000.

Kerr, D. I. and Ong, J. GABA-B receptor. *Pharmacol. Ther.* 67 (1995): 187–246.

Langer, S. Z. 25 Years since the discovery of presynaptic receptors: present knowledge and future prospects. *TIPS* 18 (1997): 95–99.

Lindstrom, J. M. Nicotinic acetylcholine receptors in health and disease. *Mol. Neurol.* 15 (1997): 193–222.

Moss, S. T. and Smart, T. G. Constructing inhibitory synapses. *Nat. Rev. Neurosci.* 2 (2001): 240–250.

Nicoll, R. A. The coupling of neurotransmitter receptors to ion channels in the brain. *Science* 241 (1988): 545–551.

Povlock, S. L. and Amara, S. G. The structure and function of noradrenaline, dopamine and 5-hydroxytryptamine transporters. In: *Neurotransmitter Transporters.* Totowa, NJ: Humana Press, 1999, pp. 1–28.

Sautel, M. and Milligan, G. Molecular manipulation of G-protein coupled receptors: a new avenue into drug discovery. *Curr. Opin. Med. Chem.* 7 (2000): 889–894.

Shepherd, G. M. and Erulkar, S. D. Centenary of the synapse: from Sherrington to the molecular biology of the synapse and beyond. *TINS* 20 (1997): 385–392.

Soellner, T. and Rothman, J. E. Neurotransmission: harnessing fusion machinery at the synapse. *TINS* 17 (1994): 344–348.

Stanford, S. C. and Salman, P. Beta-adrenoceptors and resistance to stress: old problems and new possibilities. *J. Psychopharmacol.* 6 (1992): 15–19.

Wess, K. A. and Neve, R. L. (Eds) *The Dopamine Receptors.* Totowa, NJ: Humana Press, 1997.

Chapter 3 – Pharmacokinetic Aspects of Psychopharmacology

Bertilson, L. and Dahl, M. L. Polymorphic drug oxidation: relevance to the treatment of psychiatric disorders. *CNS Drugs* 5 (1996): 200–212.

Brosen, K. Are pharmacokinetic drug interactions with SSRIs an issue? *Int. J. Psychopharmacol.* 11 (Suppl. 1) (1996): 23–27.

Catterson, M. O. and Preskorn, S. H. Pharmacokinetics of selective serotonin reuptake inhibitors: clinical relevance. *Pharmacol. Toxicol.* 78 (1996): 203–228.

Fugh-Berman, A. Herb drug interactions. *Lancet* 355 (2000): 134–138.

Fuhr, U. Drug interactions with grapefruit juice: extent, probable mechanism and clinical relevance. *Drug Safety* 18 (1998): 251–272.

Horsmans, Y. Major cytochrome P450 families: implications in health and liver disease. *Acta Gastro-Enterol. Belg.* 15 (1997): 2–10.

Nemeroff, C. B., De Vane, C. L. and Pollock, B. G. Newer antidepressants and the cytochrome P450 system. *Am J. Psychiat.* 153 (1996): 311–320.

Stockley, I. H. *Drug Interactions: A source book of adverse interactions, their mechanisms, clinical importance and management* (Fifth Edition). London: Pharmaceutical Press, 1999.

Chapter 4 – Clinical Trials and their Importance in Assessing the Efficacy and Safety of Psychotropic Drugs

Healy, D. and Doogan, D. P. (Eds) *Psychotropic Drug Development*. London: Chapman and Hall Medical, 1996.

Jick, H. Adverse drug reactions: the magnitude of the problem. *J. Allergy Clin. Immunol.* 74 (1984): 555–557.

Kaitin, K. I., Richard, B. W. and Lasagna, L. Trends in drug development. *J. Clin. Pharmacol.* 27 (1987): 542–548.

McDevitt, D. G. and MacDonald, T. M. Post-marketing drug surveillance – how far have we got? *Quart. J. Med.* 78 (1991): 1–3.

Passamani, E. Clinical trials – are they ethical? *N. Engl. J. Med.* 324 (1991): 1589–1592.

Temple, R. Trends in pharmaceutical development. *Drug Inf. J.* 27 (1993): 355–366.

Chapter 5 – Molecular Genetics and Psychopharmacology

Heilig, M. Antisense technology: prospects for treatment in neuropsychiatric disorders. *CNS Drugs* 1 (1994): 405–420.

Lerer, B. (Ed.) *Pharmacogenetics of Psychotropic Drugs*. Cambridge: Cambridge University Press, 2002.

Mallet, J. Catecholamines: from gene regulation to neuropsychiatric disorders. *TIPS* 17 (1996): 129–135.

Mueller, R. F. and Young, I. D. *Emery's Elements of Medical Genetics* (Seventh Edition). Edinburgh: Churchill Livingstone, 2001.

Stahl, S. M. New drug discovery in the post genomic era: from genomes to proteomics. *J. Clin. Psychiat.* 61 (2000): 894–895.

Wagner-Savill, K. and Kay, S. A. Circadian rhythm genetics: from flies to mice and humans. *Nat. Genet.* 26 (2000): 23–27.

Watson, S. T., Meng, F., Thompson, R. C. and Abil, H. The "chip" as a specific genetic tool. *Biol. Psychiat.* 48 (2000): 1147–1156.

Chapter 6 – Psychotropic Drugs that Modify the Serotonergic System

Aghajanian, G. K. and Marck, G. J. Serotonin and hallucinogens. *Neuropsychopharmacol.* 21 (1999): 16S–23S.

Barnes, N. M. and Sharp, T. A review of central serotonin receptors and their function. *Neuropsychopharmacol.* 13 (1999): 983–1152.

Baumgarten, H. G. and Goethert, M. (Eds) Serotoninergic neurons and 5-hydroxytryptamine receptors in the CNS. *Handbook of Experimental Pharmacology*, Vol. 129. Berlin: Springer-Verlag, 1997.

Gillman, P. K. The serotonin syndrome and its treatment. *J. Psychopharmacol.* 13 (1999): 100–109.

Heils, A., Mossner, R. and Lesch, K. P. The human serotonin transporter gene polymorphism – basic research and clinical implications. *J. Neural. Trans.* 104 (1997): 1005–1014.

Hoyer, D., Clarke, D. E. and Fozard, J. R. International Union of Pharmacology classification of receptors for 5-hydroxytryptamine (serotonin). *Pharmacol. Rev.* 46 (1994): 157–164.

Jacobs, B. L. and Fornal, C. A. Activation of serotonergic neurons in behaving animals. *Neuropsychopharmacol.* 21 (1999): 95–158.

Marshall, S. E., Bird, T. G. and Hart, K. Unified approach to the analysis of genetic variation in serotonergic pathways. *Am. J. Med. Genet.* 88 (1999): 621–627.

Naughton, M., Mulrooney, J. B. and Leonard, B. E. A review of the role of serotonin receptors in psychiatric disorders. *Hum. Psychopharmacol.* 15 (2000): 397–415.

Pinegro, G. and Blier, P. Autoregulation of serotonin neurons: role in antidepresant drug action. *Pharmacol. Rev.* 51 (1999): 533–591.

Uphouse, L. Multiple serotonin receptors: too many, not enough or just the right number. *Neurosci. Biobehav. Rev.* 21 (1997): 679–698.

Chapter 7 – Drug Treatment of Depression

Artigas, F., Perez, V. and Alvarez, E. Pindolol induces a rapid improvement of depressed patients treated with serotonin reuptake inhibitors. *Arch. Gen. Psychiat.* 51 (1994): 248–251.

Asberg, M., Traskman, L. and Thoren, P. 5HIAA in the CSF: a biological chemical suicide predictor. *Arch. Gen. Psychiat.* 33 (1976): 1193–1197.

Benedetti, F. Polymorphism within the promoter of the serotonin transporter gene and antidepressant efficiency of fluvoxamine. *Mol. Psychiat.* 3 (1998): 508–511.

Cassidy, S. L. and Henry, J. A. Fatal toxicity of antidepressant drugs in overdose. *Br. Med. J.* 295 (1987): 1021–1024.

Davis, L. L., Yonkers, K. A., Trivedi, M., Kramwer, G. L. and Petty, F. The mechanism of action of SSRIs: a new hypothesis. In: *Selective Serotonin Reuptake Inhibitors: Past, Present and Future*, Stanford, S. C. (Ed.). Austin, TX: R. G. Lander, 1999, pp. 171–185.

Farmer, R. D. T. Suicide and poisons. *Hum. Psychopharmacol.* 9 (Suppl. 1) (1994): S11–S18.

Grasby, P. M. Imaging strategies in depression. *J. Psychopharmacol.* 13 (1999): 346–351.

Kasper, S., den Boer, J. A. and Sitsen, A. J. M. (Eds) *Handbook of Depression and Anxiety* (Second Edition). New York: Marcel Dekker, 2003.

Ordway, G. A. Pathophysiology of the locus caeruleus in suicide. *Ann. NY Acad. Sci.* 836 (1997): 233–252.

Schildkraut, J. J. The catecholamine hypothesis of affective disorders: review of the supporting evidence. *Am. J. Psychiat.* 122 (1965): 509–522.

Spina, E. and Perucca, E. Newer and older antidepressants: a comparative review of their drug interactions. *CNS Drugs* 2 (1994): 479–490.

Yamada, M. and Higuchi, T. Functional genomics and depression research: beyond the monoamine hypothesis. *Eur. Neuropsychopharmacol.* 12 (2002): 235–244.

Chapter 8 – Drug Treatment of Mania

Belmaker, R. H. How does lithium work in manic depression? Clinical and psychological correlates of the inositol theory. *Ann. Rev. Med.* 47 (1996): 47–60.

Finley, P. R. Clinical relevance of drug interactions with lithium. *Clin. Pharmacokinetics* 29 (1995): 172–187.

Guscott, R. and Taylor, L. Lithium prophylaxis in recurrent affective illness; efficacy, effectiveness and efficiency. *Br. J. Psychiat.* 164 (1994): 741–750.

Keck, P. E. and McElroy, S. L. Outcome of the pharmacological treatment of bipolar disorder. *J. Clin. Psychopharmacol.* 16 (Suppl.) (1996): 15–23.

Manji, H. K., Moore, G. J. and Chen, G. Lithium at 50: have the neuroprotective effects of this unique cation been overlooked? *Biol. Psychiat.* 46 (1999): 929–940.

McElroy, S. L. and Keck, P. E. Pharmacological agents for the treatment of acute bipolar mania. *Biol. Psychiat.* 48 (2000): 539–557.

Chapter 9 – Anxiolytics and the Treatment of Anxiety Disorders

Barbaccia, M. L., Berkovich, A., Guarneri, P. and Slobodyansky, E. Diazepam binding inhibitor: the precursor of a family of endogenous modulators of GABA-A receptor function. History, perspectives and clinical implications. *Neurochem. Res.* 15 (1990): 160–173.

Charney, D. S. and Bremner, J. D. The neurobiology of anxiety disorders. In: *Neurobiology of Mental Illness.* Charney, D. S., Nestler, E. J. and Bunney, B. S. (Eds). Oxford: Oxford University Press, 1999, pp. 494–517.

Davis, M. Neurobiology of fear responses; the role of amygdala. *J. Neuropsychiat. Clin. Neurosci.* 9 (1999): 382–402.

Den Boer, J. A. and Westenberg, H. G. M. Serotonergic compounds in panic disorder, obsessive compulsive disorder and anxious depression. *Hum. Psychopharmacol.* 10 (Suppl. 3) (1995): S173–184.

Dupont, R. L., Rice, D. P., Miller, L. S. and Shiraki, S. S. Economic cost of anxiety disorders. *Depress. Anxiety* 2 (1996): 167–172.

Haefely, W. The GABA–benzodiazepine interaction fifteen years later. *Neurochem. Res.* 15 (1990): 169–182.

Uhde, T. W. Genetics and brain function: implications for the treatment of anxiety. *Biol. Psychiat.* 48 (2000): 1142–1143.

Wolff, M., Alsobrook, J. P. and Pauls, D. L. Genetic aspects of OCD. *Psychiat. Clin. North Am.* 23 (2000): 535–544.

Woods, J. H. Current benzodiazepine issues. *Psychopharmacol.* 118 (1995): 107–120.

Yehuda, R. Are glucocorticosteroids responsible for putative hippocampal damage in PTSD? How and when to decide. *Hippocampus* 11 (2001): 85–89.

Zohar, J., Mueller, E. A., Insel, T. R., Zohar-Kadouch, R. C. and Murphy, D. L. Serotonergic responsivity in OCD: comparison of patients with healthy controls. *Arch. Gen. Psychiat.* 44 (1987): 946–951.

Chapter 10 – Drug Treatment of Insomnia

Garcia-Garcia, F. and Drucker-Colin, R. Endogenous and exogenous factors on sleep–wake cycle regulation. *Prog. Neurobiol.* 58 (1999): 297–314.

Hartmann, P. M. Drug treatment of insomnia: indications and newer agents. *Am. Fam. Physician* 51 (1995): 191–200.

Holbrook, A. M., Crowther, R. and Lotter, A. Meta-analysis of benzodiazepine use in the treatment of insomnia. *CMAT* 162 (2000): 225–233.

Lancel, M. Role of GABA-A receptors in sleep regulation: differential effects of muscimol and midazolam on sleep in rats. *Neuropsychopharmacol.* 15 (1996): 63–74.

Tecott, L. H. Genes and anti-anxiety drugs. *Nature Neurosci.* 3 (2000): 529–530.

Tzischinisky, O. and Lavie, P. Melatonin possesses time-dependent hypnotic effects. *Sleep* 17 (1994): 638–645.

Walsh, T. K. and Schweitzer, P. K. Ten-year trends in the pharmacological treatment of insomnia. *Sleep* 22 (1999): 371–375.

Zammit, G. K., Werner, J. and Damato, N. Quality of life in people with insomnia. *Sleep* 22 (1999): S379–S385.

Chapter 11 – Drug Treatment of Schizophrenia and the Psychoses

Brunello, N. New insights into the biology of schizophrenia through the mechanism of action of clozapine. *Neuropsychopharmacol.* 13 (1995): 177–188.

Conley, R. R., Tamminga, C. A. and Beasley, C. Olanzapine versus chlorpromazine in therapy-refractory schizophrenia. *Schizophren. Res.* 24 (1997): 190–202.

Coyle, J. T. The glutamatergic dysfunction hypothesis of schizophrenia. *Harvard Rev. Psychiat.* 3 (1996): 241–250.

Kane, J. M. Management strategies for the treatment of schizophrenia. *J. Clin. Psychiat.* 60 (Suppl. 12) (1999): 13–17.

Kinan, B. J. and Lieberman, J. A. Mechanism of action of atypical and antipsychotic drugs – a critical analysis. *Psychopharmacol.* 124 (1996): 2–12.

Lawrie, S. M. and Abukineil, S. S. Brain abnormality in schizophrenia. A systematic and quantitative review of volumetric magnetic resonance imaging studies. *Br. J. Psychiat.* 172 (1998): 110–120.

Liddle, P. F. Functional imaging in schizophrenia. *Br. Med. Bull.* 52 (1996): 486–494.

Meltzer, H. Y. The role of serotonin in antipsychotic drug action. *Neuropsychopharmacol.* 21 (Suppl. 2) (1999): 106S–115S.

Sartorius, N. (Ed.) The usefulness and use of second generation antipsychotic medication: review of evidence and recommendations by a task force of the World Psychiatric Association. *Curr. Opin. Psychiat.* 15 (Suppl. 1) (2002).

Sartorius, N. (Ed.) The usefulness and use of second generation antipsychotic medication – an update. *Curr. Opin. Psychiat.* 16 (Suppl. 2) (2003).

Chapter 12 – Drug Treatment of the Epilepsies

Albini, F. Carbamazepine: clinical pharmacology – a review. *Pharmacopsychiat.* 28 (1995): 235–245.

Baulac, A., Arzimanoglu, A., Semah, F. and Cavalcanti, D. Therapeutic opinions provided by new anti-epileptic drugs. *Rev. Neurol.* 155 (1997): 21–33.
Chadwick, D. General review of the efficacy and tolerance of new anti-epileptics. *Epilepsia* 38 (Suppl. 1) (1996): S59–S62.
Feely, M. Drug treatment in epilepsy. *Br. Med. J.* 318 (1999): 106–109.
Joffe, R. T. and Calabrese, J. R. *Anticonvulsants in Mood Disorders.* New York: Marcel Dekker, 1994.
Loiseau, P. Tolerability of newer and older anticonvulsants: a comparative review. *CNS Drugs* 6 (1995): 148–166.
Meldrum, B. S. Update of the mechanisms of action of antiepileptic drugs. *Epilepsia* 37 (Suppl. 6) (1996): 4–11.
Sander, T. and Was, B. New drugs for epilepsy. *Curr. Opin. Neurol.* (11) (1998): 141–148.
Shorvan, S. D. *Handbook of Epilepsy Treatment.* Oxford: Blackwell Science, 2000.
Vermeulen, J. and Aldenkamp, A. P. Cognitive side effects of chronic antiepileptic drug treatment: a review of 25 years' research. *Epilepsy Res.* 22 (1995): 65–80.

Chapter 13 – Drug Treatment of Parkinson's Disease

Calne, D. W. Treatment of Parkinson's disease. *N. Engl. J. Med.* 329 (1997): 1021–1027.
Hirsh, E. C. and Hunot, S. Nitric oxide, glial cells and neural degeneration in Parkinson's disease. *TIPS* 21 (2000): 163–165.
Hogan, J. J., Middlemas, D. N., Scharpe, P. C. and Poste, G. H. Parkinson's disease: prospects for improved therapy. *TIPS* 18 (1997): 156–163.
Le Witt, P. and Oertel, W. *Parkinson's Disease: The Treatment Options.* London: Martin Dunitz, 1999.
Quinn, N. Drug treatment in Parkinson's disease. *Br. Med. J.* 310 (1995): 575–580.
Reddy, H. P., Williams, M. and Tagle, D. A. Recent advances in understanding the pathogenesis of Huntington's disease. *TINS* 22 (1999): 248–255.

Chapter 14 – Alzheimer's Disease and Stroke: Possible Biochemical Causes and Treatment Strategies

Adams, M. P. Treating ischaemic stroke as an emergency. *Arch. Neurol.* 55 (1998): 457–461.
Allen, N. H. P. The treatment of Alzheimer's disease. *J. Psychopharmacol.* 9 (1995): 43–50.
Auld, D. S., Kar, S. and Quiron, R. Beta amyloid peptides as direct cholinergic neuromodulators: a missing link? *TINS* 21 (1958): 43–49.
Barinaga, M. Finding new drugs to treat stroke. *Science* 272 (1996): 664–666.
Brioni, J. D. and Decker, M. W. (Eds) *Pharmacological Treatment of Alzheimer's Disease.* New York: John Wiley & Sons, 1997.
Daniel, S. E., Lees, A. J. and Cruz-Sanchez, F. F. *Dementia in Parkinsonism.* Vienna: Springer-Verlag, 1997.
Eagger, S. A. Tacrine and older anticholinesterase drugs in dementia. *Curr. Opin. Psychiat.* 8 (1995): 264–270.
Hardy, J. Amyloid, the presenilins and Alzheimer's disease. *TINS* 20 (1997): 154–159.
Kumar, V. Advances in pharmacotherapy for decline in memory and cognition in patients with Alzheimer's disease. *Psychiat. Serv.* 47 (1996): 249–259.

Neve, R. L. and Robakis, N. K. Amyloid disease: a re-examination of the amyloid hypothesis. *TINS* 21 (1998): 15–19.

Selkoe, D. J. Translating cell biology into therapeutic advances in Alzheimer's disease. *Nature* 399 (Suppl.) (1999): A23–A31.

Smith, M. A. Alzheimer's disease. *Int. Rev. Neurobiol.* 42 (1998): 1–44.

Chapter 15 – Psychopharmacology of Drugs of Abuse

British Medical Association. *The Therapeutic Uses of Cannabis*. London: Harwood Academic, 1997.

Burgess, C., O'Donohoe, A. and Gill, M. Agony and ecstasy: a review of MDMA effects and toxicity. *Eur. Psychiat.* 15 (2000): 287–294.

Chick, J. and Cantwell, R. *Seminars in Alcohol and Drug Misuse*. London: Gaskell, 1994.

Daws, L. C. and White, J. M. Regulation of opioid receptors by opioid antagonists: implications for rapid opioid detoxification. *Addiction Biol.* 4 (1999): 391–397.

Maldonado, R. (Ed.) *Molecular Biology of Drug Addiction*. Totowa, NJ: Humana Press, 2003.

Nestler, E. J. and Aghajanian, G. Molecular and cellular basis of addiction. *Science* 278 (1997): 58–63.

Robbins, T. W. and Everitt, B. Drug addiction: bad habits add up. *Nature* 398 (1999): 567–571.

Simonata, M. The neurochemistry of morphine addiction in the neocortex. *TIPS* 17 (1996): 410–415.

Spangel, R. and Weiss, F. The dopamine hypothesis of reward: past and current status. *TINS* 22 (1999): 521–527.

Spangel, R. and Ziegansberger, W. Anti-craving compounds for ethanol: new pharmacological tools to study addictive processes. *TIPS* 18 (1997): 54–58.

Zernig, G., Saria, A., Kurz, M. and O'Malley, S. S. (Eds) *Handbook of Alcoholism*. Boca Raton, FL: CRC Press, 2001.

Chapter 16 – Paediatric Psychopharmacology

Battino, D., Estienne, M. and Aanzini, G. Clinical pharmacokinetics of anti-epileptic drugs in pediatric patients. *Clin. Pharmacokinetics* 29 (1995): 341–369.

Brown, C. S. and Cooke, S. C. Attention deficit hyperactivity disorder – clinical features and drug treatment options. *CNS Drugs* 1 (1994): 95–109.

Campbell, M. and Cueva, J. E. Psychopharmacology in child and adolescent psychiatry: a review of the past seven years. *J. Am. Acad. Child. Adolesc. Psychiat.* 34 (1995): 1124–1130.

Posey, D. J. and McDougle, C. J. The pharmacology of target symptoms associated with autistic disorder and other pervasive developmental disorders. *Harvard Rev. Psychiat.* 8 (2000): 45–63.

Chapter 17 – Geriatric Psychopharmacology

Altamura, A. C., De Novalis, F., Guercetti, G. *et al.* Fluoxetine compared with amitriptyline in elderly depression: a controlled clinical trial. *Int. J. Clin. Pharmacol. Res.* 9 (1989): 391–396.

Ashtari, M., Greenwald, B. S. and Kramer-Ginsberg, E. Hippocampal/amygdala volumes in geriatric depression. *Psychol. Med.* 29 (1999): 629–638.

Ganguli, M., Reynolds, C. F. and Gilby, J. E. Prevalence and persistence of sleep complaints in a rural elderly community sample: the MOVIES project. *J. Am. Ger. Soc.* 44 (1996): 778–784.

George, C. F., Woodhouse, K. W., Denham, M. J. and MacLennon, W. T. (Eds) *Drug Therapy in Old Age*. Chichester: John Wiley & Sons, 1998.

Livingston, G., Blizard, B. and Mann, A. Does sleep disturbance predict depression in elderly people? A study in inner London. *Br. J. Gen. Pract.* 43 (1993): 445–448.

Robertson, D. R. Drug therapy for Parkinson's disease in the elderly. *Br. Med. Bull.* 46 (1998): 124–136.

Zaleon, C. R. and Guthrie, S. K. Antipsychotic drug use in older adults. *Am. J. Hosp. Pharm.* 51 (1994): 2917–2925.

Chapter 18 – The Inter-relationship Between Psychopharmacology and Psychoneuroimmunology

Ader, R., Felten, D. L. and Cohen, N. (Eds) *Psychoneuroimmunology* (Third Edition). San Diego: Academic Press, 2001.

Blalock, J. E. (Ed.) *Neuroimmunoendocrinology*. Basel: Karger, 1997.

Dantzer, R., Wollman, E. E. and Yirmiya, R. *Cytokines, Stress and Depression*. New York: Kluwer Academic/Plenum Publishers, 1999.

Leonard, B. E. Brain cytokines and the psychopathology of depression. In: *Antidepressants*, Leonard, B. E. (Ed.). Basel: Birkhäuser-Verlag, 2000, pp. 109–122.

Leonard, B. E. and Miller, K. (Eds) *Stress, the Immune System and Psychiatry*. Chichester: John Wiley & Sons, 1995.

Merrill, J. E. and Beneviste, E. N. Cytokines in inflammatory brain lesions: helpful and harmful. *TINS* 19 (1996): 331–336.

Rabin, B. S. *Stress, Immune Function and Health*. New York: Wiley-Liss, 1999.

Smith, R. S. The macrophage theory of depression. *Med. Hypoth.* 35 (1991): 298–306.

Song, C. and Leonard, B. E. *Fundamentals of Psychoneuroimmunology*. Chichester: John Wiley & Sons, 2000.

Chapter 19 – Endocoids and their Importance in Psychopharmacology

Apfel, S. C. (Ed.) *Clinical Applications of Neurotrophic Factors*. Philadelphia: Lippincott-Raven Press, 1997.

Itzhak, Y. (Ed.) *Sigma Receptors*. San Diego: Academic Press, 1994.

Izquierdo, I. and Medina, J. (Eds) *Naturally Occurring Benzodiazepines*. New York: Ellis Horwood, 1993.

Leonard, B. E. The potential contribution of sigma receptors to the action of antidepressant drugs. In: *Antidepressants – New Pharmacological Strategies*, Skolnick, P. (Ed.). Totowa, NJ: Humana Press, 1997, pp. 159–172.

Index

Notes. Page numbers in italics refer to figures in tables. Abbreviations used in subheadings are: AD=Alzheimer's disease; ADHD=attention deficit/hyperactivity disorder; ECT=electroconvulsive shock treatment; MAOIs=monoamine oxidase inhibitors; OCD=obsessive–compulsive disorder; PTSD=post traumatic stress disorder; SNRIs=selective serotonin and noradrenaline reuptake inhibitors; SSRIs= selective serotonin reuptake inhibitors; TCAs=tricyclic antidepressants.

α receptors *see* adrenergic receptors, α receptors
abercarnil, insomnia, 252–3
acamprosate, 386–7, 388
acetazolamide, *303*, 304, *305*, 308
acetylcholine/cholinergic system, *18*
   AD, 38–9, 61–2, 350, 351, 352–3, 361–4
   and co-transmitters, 27–8
   epilepsies, 301
   functional neuroanatomy, 11–12, 18
   and lithium, 203–4
   mania, 194, 196–7, 204
   metabolism, 62–5
   Parkinson's disease, 324, 326, 332–5
   psychoneuroimmunology, 434
   receptors, *18*, 22, 37–42, *42*
      AD, 38–9, 61–2, 350, 351, 352–3, 361–4
      ADHD, 420
      alcohol, 386
      anatomical distribution, *64*, 65
      depression, 157, *161*, 162, 184
      drugs of abuse, 386, 398
      ECT, 184
      nicotine, 398
      Parkinson's disease, 332–5
     sleep, 243
     synthesis, 61–2
action potentials, 16–18, 24–5
addiction, definition, 377
adenosine
   anxiolysis, 218

Parkinson's disease, 328
adenosine triphosphate (ATP), 25, *26*, 43
adenylate cyclase, 25, *26*, 27
   adrenergic receptors, 25, *43*
   antidepressant mechanisms, 165
   dopaminergic receptors, 44–5, 264
   5-HT receptors, 47, 136, *141*
   and lithium, 203, 204
   opioid receptors, 394
adolescents *see* paediatric psychopharmacology
adrenaline, 65, 70
adrenergic receptors, 42–3
   α receptors, *18*, 22–3, 42–4
      antidepressants, 177, 178
      buspirone, 237–8
      depression, 156, *159*
      mania, 208
      Parkinson's disease, 325
      schizophrenia, 279, 281–2
      antipsychotic action, 279
   β receptors, *18*, 25, 27, 44
      antidepressant mechanisms, 163
      anxiety disorders, 236
      depression, 44, 156–7, *159*, 163
      lithium, 204
      mania, 202
      Parkinson's disease, 325
      psychoneuroimmunology, 435
   depression, 44, 156–7, *159*, 161–2, 163
   Parkinson's disease, 325

Fundamentals of Psychopharmacology. Third Edition. By Brian E. Leonard
  2003 John Wiley & Sons, Ltd. ISBN 0 471 52178 7

adrenergic receptors (*cont'd*)
  presynaptic mechanisms, 22–3
  psychoneuroimmunology, 435
  PTSD, 227
  second messenger systems, 24, 26,
    42–4
adrenergic system *see* noradrenaline/
    adrenergic system
adrenoceptors *see* adrenergic receptors
adrenocorticotrophic hormone (ACTH),
    434, 435–6, 437–8
affective disorders, 193–4
  amine theory, 155–60, 192, 194, 196
  psychoneuroimmunology, 431, 439–
    42
  see also bipolar disorder; depression;
    mania
agonists, 37
  adrenergic receptors, 23, 44, 156, 208,
    227, 421
  benzodiazepine receptors, 53–4
    AD, 368
    anxiety disorders, 231–2, 233–4
    endozepines, 451–2
    insomnia, 252–3
  cannabinoid, 413–14, 446, *447*, 448
  cholinergic receptors, 38, 39, 40, 363–4
  dopamine receptors, 44, 45–6
    Parkinson's disease, 331–2, *333*
    schizophrenia, 264, 265, 266
  GABA receptors, 52, 53–4, 229, 280–1
  glutamate receptors
    AD, 355–6
    antipsychotic action, 279–80
    cannabis, 413–14
  5-HT receptors
    depression, 50–1, *137*, 138, *143*, 144–
      5, 147–8, 173
    mania, 196
    OCD, 225
  inverse, 53–4, 232, 368
  mania, 196, 208
  partial, 53, 54, 231–2, 252–3
  receptor down-regulation, 26, 234
  sigma receptors, 456
agoraphobia, genetics, 123–4
alcohol(s), 64–5, 145, 229, 246–7, *376*,
    381–8
  drug interactions, 386, 460
  hypnotic use, 251, 429
allergies, schizophrenia, 443

alpha receptors *see* adrenergic receptors,
    α receptors
alprazolam, *212*, 223, 228, 429
Alzheimer's disease (AD), 341–71
  functional neuroanatomy, 5, *6*, 9, 10
  genetics, 118–19, 346, 348, 370
  Hirano bodies, 341–2
  immune function, 358–61, 367
  neurochemical changes, 350–61
    cholinergic, 38–9, 61, 350, 351, 352–
      3, 361–4
    dopaminergic, 352
    excitotoxins, 354–8
    glutamatergic, 57, 59, 353–6, 369
    inflammatory, 358–61, 364–5
    noradrenergic, 352
    peptides, 351, *352*, 369, 370
    serotonergic, 352
    treatment strategies, 38–9, 361–
      70
  neuropathological change, 345–8
    environmental excitotoxins, 356
    future research, 370
    gross changes, 342–3, *344*, 345
    inflammatory, 358–61
    neuritic plaques, 341, *342*, 345–6,
      348, *350*, 359
    neurofibrillary tangles, 341, *343*,
      345–6, 348, *349*, *350*
  treatment, 361–70
    ampakines, 369
    anti-inflammatories, 364–5, *368*
    antioxidants, 365, *368*, 369
    benzodiazepine inverse agonists,
      368
    chelating agents, 365–6, *368*
    cholinergic function, 38–9, 353, 361–
      4, *368*
    oestrogens, 366, *368*, 369
    secretase inhibitors, 366–7
    vaccines, 367
amantadine, 332, *334*
amine theory, affective disorders, 155–
    60, 192, 194, 196
amino acid neurotransmitters *see* aspar-
    tate; GABA; glutamate; glycine
gamma-aminobutyric acid *see* GABA
amisulpride, 273, 275
amitriptyline, 236
AMPA receptors
  AD, 354–5, 369

antipsychotic action, 280
Parkinson's disease, 328
ampakines, 369
amperozide, *137*, 275
amphetamines
  ADHD, 420
  as drugs of abuse, 399–400, 402–3
amygdala, *2, 4, 5*
  anxiety, 219, 221
amyloid beta peptide (Ab), 346, 366–7,
  369
amyloid precursor protein (APP), 346,
  347, 348, 366
analgesics
  enantiomers, 96–7
  opioid, 96–7, 145, *376*, 381, 389–97
anandamide system, 446–9
angel dust *see* phencyclidine (PCP)
angiotensin peptides, anxiolysis, 218
animal models
  epilepsies, 297–300
  pre-clinical tests, 102–3
  transgenic mice, 102–3, 117, 128–9
anoxia, *6*
antagonists, 36–7
  adenosine receptors, 328
  adrenergic receptors, 22–3, 42, *43*, 177,
    178
    as antipsychotics, 279
    anxiety disorders, 236, 237–8
    schizophrenia, 279, 281–2
  benzodiazepine receptor ligands, 231–
    2
  cannabinoid, 413, 414, 448–9
  cholinergic receptors, 38–9, 40
    AD, 38–9
    Parkinson's disease, 332–5
  dopamine receptors, 46, 47
    cannabis, 414
    schizophrenia, 264, 265, 266, 269,
      275–6, 282
  GABA receptors, 52, 53, 217–18, 451
  glutamate receptors, 59, 164
    AD, 353, 354–5
    epilepsies, 357
    hypoxia, 357–8
    Parkinson's disease, 328
    stroke, 373, 409
  5-HT receptors, 49, *137*, 138, *143*, 144–
    5, 146–8, 151–2
    as antipsychotics, 146–7, 278–9

down-regulation, 163
  schizophrenia, 271, 272, 273–4,
    275–6
  tetracyclic antidepressants, 177
  Parkinson's disease, 328, 332–5
  sigma receptors, 280, 453
anticholinergics
  drug interactions, 461
  nocturnal enuresis, 422
  Parkinson's disease, 332–5
anticholinesterases, 62–4
  AD, 38, 39, 362–3, *368*
  mania, 197
anticoagulants, stroke, 374
anticonvulsants *see* antiepileptics
antidementia drugs, 38–9, 361–8
antidepressants
  as anxiolytics, 147–9, 175, 223, 224–5,
    227, 228, 236
  atypical, 164, *174*, 177–80, *186*, 228,
    251, 427
  bipolar disorder, 209
  children
    depression, 422
    emotional disorders, 421
    nocturnal enuresis, 422
  and circadian rhythm, 160
  classification, *174*
  dopaminergic system, 159–60, 163–4
  drug–drug interactions, 88, 89, 94
    MAOIs, 170, 171, 187, 188–9, 191,
      459, 460
    SSRIs, 171, 189, 191, 459, 460
    TCAs, 87, 88, 94, 187, 188, 189, 191,
      459, 461
  drug–protein interactions, 99
  ECT, 182–5, 427
  elderly people, 173–5, 185, 189, 190,
    425, 427
  genetic polymorphism, 88, 89
  glutamate receptors, 164, 456
  herbal, 180, 451–2
  historical development, 154–5
  5-HT, *137, 143*
    anxiolysis, 147–9, 175, 223, 224–5
    chronic administration, *150–1*
    mechanism, 163–4
    sites of action, *50*
    SSRIs, 47–9, 171, 173, 175, 223
    TCAs, 177
  for insomnia, 251

antidepressants (cont'd)
  mechanisms of action, 161–9, 192
    cholinergic function, 161, 162
    dopaminergic system, 163–4
    endocrine function, 167–8
    glucocorticoid receptors, 165–7
    glutamatergic system, 164
    immune function, 167–8, 441–2
    intracellular changes, 165
    neuronal structure, 168–9
    noradrenergic system, 163
    response delay, 161–2
    serotonergic system, 163–4
  noradrenergic activity, 42, 159, 161–2,
    163
  pain, 180
  pharmacogenomics, 130, 131
  pharmacokinetics, 82–5
    drug–drug interactions, 88, 89, 94
    drug–protein interactions, 99
    enantiomers, 98–9
    SSRIs, 88, 94, 98, 99, 172–5
  pharmacological properties, 169–80
  psychoneuroimmunology, 441–2
  side effects, 169, 170–1, 175, 185–90,
    427
  sigma receptors, 456–7
  sites of action, 150–1, 181
  sleep, 247
  treatment decisions, 181, 209
  treatment-resistant depression, 190–1,
    203
antiemetics
  cannabis, 416
  5-HT receptor antagonism, 49, 137,
    140
antiepileptics, 303, 308–18
  action on neurotransmitters, 51, 52,
    57, 59, 304–6, 318
    benzodiazepines, 304–5, 306, 311
    carbamazepine, 207, 304, 306, 309
    excitotoxins, 357
    felbamate, 312
    gabapentin, 313
    imaging, 35–6
    lamotrigine, 314
    tiagabine, 315
    topiramate, 316
    valproate, 281, 305–6, 316
    vigabactin, 317
  antipsychotic action, 281

conduct disorders, 420
generic formulations, 301
imaging, 35–6
intractable epilepsy, 303
ionic effects, 306
major groups, 304
mania, 205–7, 208
membrane effects, 306
pharmacokinetics, 301–3, 306–7, 310
serum concentration monitoring, 301–
  3
summary of, 303, 308, 317–18
therapeutic range, 302
treatment-resistant depression, 191
antihistamines, anxiolysis, 236
anti-inflammatory drugs
  AD, 364–5, 368, 369
  drug interactions, 459
  stroke, 374
antimigraine drugs, 47, 50
antioxidants, AD, 365, 368, 369
antipsychotics see neuroleptics
antispastic drugs
  cannabis, 414
  GABA receptors, 54
anxiety disorders
  children, 423
  elderly people, 428–9
  genetics, 123–4
  and MDMA, 404–5
  neurobiology of, 213–18
    benzodiazepines, 147, 214, 215–18,
      234
    endozepines, 450–2
    integrated theory, 219, 220
    OCD, 148, 224–5, 226
    panic disorder, 148, 219, 221–4
    peptides, 218, 223–4
    PTSD, 227–8
    social phobia, 224, 225, 227
  neurotransmitters, 18, 70, 74, 147–9,
    214–18, 220
    endozepines, 451
    GABA, 217–18, 234
    OCD, 148, 224–5, 226
    panic, 148, 221, 223–4
    PTSD, 227–8
    social phobia, 227
  sigma receptors, 456–7
  SSRIs, 148–9, 175, 224–5

treatment *see* anxiolytics; benzodiazepines, anxiolytic
anxiolytics, 211–39
  azaspirodecanedione, 237–9
    5-HT receptors, 47, *50*, *137*, 147, 148,
     149, 238, 239
    pharmacokinetics, 88
    treatment-resistant depression, 191
  benzodiazepines *see* benzodiazepines,
    anxiolytic
  dependence, 235–6, *376*, 388–9
  elderly people, 235, 426, 428, 429
  endogenous, 450–2
  GABA receptors, 51, 54, *55*, 56, 217–
    18, 228–9, 230–1, 234–5
  genetic polymorphism, *89*
  5-HT, *137*, *143*
    antidepressants, 147–9, 175, 223,
     224–5
    benzodiazepines, 147, 215, 217
    buspirone, 47, *50*, 147, 148, 149, 238,
     239
    OCD, 224–5
    panic disorder, 148, 223–4
    social phobia, 227
  non-benzodiazepines, 236–9
    antidepressants, 147–9, 175, 223,
     224–5, 227, 228, 236
    azaspirodecanedione *see above*
  OCD, 148, 224–5, 228, 423
  panic disorder, 148, 221, 223–4, 228
  partial agonists, 54–5, 231–2
  pathogenesis of anxiety, 214–18
  pharmacokinetics, 86–8, *89*, 212
  pharmacological properties, 212–13
  PTSD, 227, 228
  side effects, 235–6
  sigma receptors, 456–7
  social phobia, 225, 227, 228
  tolerance, 235
  treatment decision summary, 228
  treatment-resistant depression, 191
  withdrawal, 236
apolipoprotein E_4 (ApoE$_4$), 348, *350*
apomorphine, 331–2, *333*
arginine vasopressin (AVP), 438
aspartate, *18*, 57, 74, 75
association studies, 119–20, 121, 122–3
astrocytes, 10
attention deficit/hyperactivity disorder
  (ADHD), 124–6, 419–20

autoinhibition, 22–3
autoradiography, 33
azaspirodecanedione anxiolytics, 147,
  237–9
  5-HT receptors, 47, *50*, *137*, 147, 148,
   149
  pharmacokinetics, 88
  treatment-resistant depression, 191

β carbolines *see* carbolines
β receptors *see* adrenergic receptors, *β*
  receptors
B lymphocytes, 432–3, 435, 448
baclofen, 54
barbiturates, 211, 236
  dependence, 388
  drug interactions, 461
  GABA receptors, 55, 229
  insomnia, 241, 251
  NMDA receptors, 355
  see also phenobarbitone; primidone
basal ganglia, 3
  cannabinoid receptors, 448
  dystonia, 455
  Parkinson's disease, 324, 326–8
bed wetting, 421–2
benserazide, 67
benzhexol, 333
benzodiazepine receptor ligands, 54–5,
  231–2, 251–3
  see also zopiclone
benzodiazepines
  aetiology of anxiety
    GABA, 217–18, 234
    5-HT, 147, 215, 217
    noradrenaline, 214
  antiepileptics, 87, *303*, 304–5, 308–9,
   311
  antipsychotic action, 281
  anxiolytic, 211–12
    buspirone compared, 238, 239
    chronic administration, 234–5
    dependence, 235–6, *376*, 388–9
    drug interactions, 235, 460–1
    elderly people, 235, 426, 428, 429
    inverse agonism, 54–5, 232
    metabolic pathways, *213*
    OCD, 228
    panic disorder, 228
    pharmacological properties, 212–13
    PTSD, 227

benzodiazepines (*cont'd*)
  anxiolytic (*cont'd*)
    receptors, 228–35, 451
    side effects, 235–6
    tolerance, 235
    withdrawal, 236
  chemical structures, *214, 305*
  children, 421
  drug interactions, 235, 460–1
  elderly people, 235, 426, 428, 429
  genetic polymorphism, *89*
  hypnotic, 241–2, 246, 248–51, 429
  inverse agonism, 54–5, 232, 368, 450
  mania, 208
  naturally occurring, 451
  pharmacokinetics, 86–7, *89, 212*
  receptors, 228–35
    drugs acting on, 231–2, 251–3
    endozepines, 451–2
    and GABA, 51, 54, *55*, 56, 218, 228–
      9, 230–1, 234–5, 304–5
    natural ligands, 56, 232–4
    sensitivity, 234–5
    types, 230–1
  side effects, 235–6, 311
  tolerance, 235, 311
  withdrawal, 236, 250, 378, 388
benztropine, 332–3, *334*
beta adrenoceptors *see* adrenergic
    receptors, β receptors
beta carbolines *see* carbolines
biperiden, 332–3, *334*
bipolar disorder, 193
  genetics, 118, 119, 120, 131, 193–4, *195*
  incidence, 193–4
  maintenance treatments, 208–9
  mania biochemistry, 194–7
  mania treatment, 198–208
  pharmacogenomics, 131
  treatment decisions, 209
  see also depression
B lymphocytes, 432–3, 435, 448
blood–brain barrier, 6–7
brain
  functional neuroanatomy, 1–13
    blood–brain barrier, 6–7
    cellular, 7–13, 16
    structural subdivisions, 1–6
  imaging methods, 33–7
  and immune system *see* psycho-
    neuroimmunology

neurotransmitters *see* neurotransmit-
    ters
brain infarction, 371–4
brain stem, 1
  dystonia, 455
brain tissue, pre-clinical drug tests, 103–
  4
brain transplants, 337
bretazenil, 252, 253
bromocriptine, 332, *333*
brotizolam, 248, *249*, 250
buproprion, 176, *178*, 181, 189–90, 399,
  460
buspirone, 237
  anxiolytic action, 237–9
  drug interactions, 461
  5-HT receptors, 47, *49*, *137*, 147, 148,
    149, 238, 239
  pharmacokinetics, 88
  treatment-resistant depression, 191
butyrophenones, 288, *289*
  see also haloperidol

calcium, AD, 353–4, 369
calcium channel antagonists
  AD, 369
  mania, 207
  stroke, 374, 409
  see also lamotrigine
cannabinoids
  abuse, *376*, 410–16
  endogenous, 445–50
cannabis, abuse, *376*, 410–16
carbamazepine, 309
  action on neurotransmitters, 207, 304,
    306, 309
  chemical structure, *305*
  conduct disorders, 420
  drug interactions, 94, 309, 459, 460,
    461
  indications, *303*, 308, 318
  kindled seizures, 206
  mania, 206–7, 209
  mode of action, 309
  pharmacokinetics, 307
  PTSD, 227
  side effects, 94, 309, 318
  therapeutic range, *302*
carbidopa, 65, 67
β carbolines, 56, 231, 232, 252–3, 451
carbon monoxide (CO), 61

cardiotoxicity
  amphetamines, 402
  antidepressants
    MAOIs, 171, 191
    SNRIs, 176
    TCAs, 169, 170, 186, 191, 427
  cocaine, 400–1
  neuroleptics, 293
  thioridazine enantiomers, 97
cardiovascular system
  and 5-HT, *143*
  see also cardiotoxicity
catecholamines *see* dopamine; noradrenaline
cellular structure, brain, 7–13, 16
  psychoneuroimmunology, 435
  see also neurons
cerebellum, 2
  dystonia, 455
cerebrospinal fluid, 7
cerebrum, 3
  see also basal ganglia; cortex
charas, 411
chelating agents, 67, 365–6, *368*
children *see* paediatric psychopharmacology
China white, 403
chiral structures, 95–6
chiral switching, 96
chloral hydrate, 251, 429
chlordiazepoxide, *212, 213*, 241, 429
chlormethiazole, 251
chlorpromazine
  anxiety disorders, 236
  conduct disorders, 420
  drug interactions, 461
  elderly people, 428
  and functional neuroanatomy, 13
  schizophrenia, 255–6, 269, 284, 286
cholecystokinin, 218, 223–4
choline uptake, 62, *63*
cholinergic system *see* acetylcholine/cholinergic system
cholinomimetic drugs
  AD, 39, 40, 361, 363–4, *368*
  mania, 197
  receptor sequestration, 39–40
cigarettes
  cannabis, 411, 412, 415–16
  drug interactions, 461
  nicotine, 398–9

circadian rhythm
  neurotransmitters, 160–1, 243–4
  sleep, 242–4
citalopram, 171, 172, 173
  chemical structure, *173*
  elderly people, 427
  enantiomers, 98, 175
  side effects, 189
clinical trials, 101, 104–11
  confidence intervals, 105–6
  costs of treatment, 109
  double-blind, 106
  error types, 106
  evaluation, 105–6
  informed consent, 107–8
  interim analyses, 108
  limitations, 110
  meta-analyses, 108
  null hypotheses, 105
  numbers of patients in, 108
  open, 106–7
  placebos, 107–8, 110
  pre-clinical drug tests, 101–4, 109–10
  prescribing decisions, 110–11
  purpose, 104–5
  statistical significance, 105, 106, 108
  types, 106–7
clobazam, 87, *303, 304, 305*, 308–9, 311
clomipramine
  children, 421, 423
  OCD, 224, 225, 423
clonazepam, *303, 304, 305*, 308
clonidine
  childhood tic disorders, 421
  depression, 156
  mania, 208
  PTSD, 227
cloning, 126–8
clozapine, 270–1, 275
  chemical structure, *274*
  drug interactions, 94
  5-HT receptor activity, 49, *50*, 146
  in vitro receptor binding, *271*
  sigma receptors, 455–6
cocaine abuse, *376*, 380–1, 399, 400–2, 403
computed tomography, SPECT, 34
conduct disorders, 420
confidence intervals, 105–6
contraceptive pill, 71
corpus callosum, 1, 3

cortex, 2, 3, 4–5
  cannabinoid receptors, 448
  drug dependence, 381
corticotrophin releasing factor (CRF)
  anxiolysis, 218
  psychoneuroimmunology, 434, 437–8
cortisol, 434, 437–8, 439–40
costs of treatment, 109
co-transmitters see peptide co-transmitters/neurotransmitters
crystal see phencyclidine (PCP)
cyclic adenosine monophosphate
  (cAMP), 24–5, 26, 27, 38, 43, 380
cytochrome P450 isoenzymes
  classification, 92
  drugs metabolized by, 93
  genetic polymorphism, 88–9
  oxidative reactions, 90–1
  pharmacogenomics, 130
cytokines
  AD, 358–9
  antidepressant mechanisms, 167, 168,
    441
  psychoneuroimmunology, 432, 433–4,
    436, 441, 444
  schizophrenia, 444
  sleep, 433–4, 452
  stroke, 374
cytoskeleton, 9, 165
cytosol, 9

Dale's Law, 11, 19
delusional states, 428
dementias, 426
  genetics, 118–19
  neurotransmitters, 18
  see also Alzheimer's disease; Parkinson's syndromes
dendrites, 8, 11, 12, 16
deoxyribonucleic acid (DNA), 7, 113–14,
  115
  cloning, 127–8
  complementary (cDNA), 103–4, 115–
    17
    antidepressants, 130
    libraries, 115, 127
  gene manipulation, 115–17
  microarray technology, 103–4, 120,
    127, 130
dependence, 376–81, 382, 383
  specific drugs see drugs of abuse

deprenyl (selegiline)
  AD, 365, 369
  Parkinson's disease, 330–1
  psychoneuroimmunology, 435
depression
  children, 422
  classification, 153–4
  and contraceptive pill, 70
  definition, 153
  or dementia, 426
  ECT, 182–5, 427
  elderly people, 426, 427
  genetics, 123–4, 130, 131
  neurotransmitters, 18, 191–2
    adrenergic receptors, 44, 156–7, 159,
      161–2, 163
    cholinergic, 157, 161, 162, 184
    circadian changes, 160–1
    dopamine, 159–60, 161–2, 163–4
    ECT, 183–5
    GABA, 36, 162, 184
    glutamate, 36, 164
    5-HT, 70, 71, 143, 149–52, 157–9,
      160–2, 163–4
    macrophage hypothesis, 441
    noradrenaline, 42, 155–7, 159, 161–
      2, 163, 192
    and prostaglandins, 167–8
    psychoneuroimmunology, 439–42
    TMS treatment, 37
  pharmacogenomics, 130, 131
  physical pain, 180
  psychoneuroimmunology, 431, 439–
    42
  sigma receptors, 454, 456–7
  sleep, 245–6, 247
  treatment see antidepressants
  treatment-resistant, 190–1, 203
designer drugs, abuse of, 403–5
desmethyldiazepam, 451
desmopressin, 422
development of drugs
  clinical trials, 101, 104–11
  pre-clinical testing, 101–4, 109–10
dexamethasone, 191, 434
diazepam
  antiepileptic use, 308
  chemical structure, 214, 305
  chronic administration, 234–5
  drug interactions, 460
  elderly people, 428, 429

genetic polymorphism, *89*
half-life, *212*
metabolic pathway, *213*
pharmacokinetics, 87
receptors, 228–9
diazepam-binding inhibitor (DBI), 232–3
diencephalon, 1, 2
diphenylbutylpiperidines, 288, *289*
  see also pimozide
diphenylhydantoin (phenytoin), 310
  action on neurotransmitters, 304
  chemical structure, *305*
  drug interactions, 459, 461
  indications, *303*, 308, 318
  pharmacokinetics, 307, 310
  side effects, 310
  therapeutic range, *302*
discontinuation of drugs *see* withdrawal
  of drugs
discovery of drugs, 101–4, 109–10
disulfiram, 67, 386
ditolyguanidine (DTG), 453, 456, 457
divalproex sodium, mania, 208–9
DNA *see* deoxyribonucleic acid
donepezil, 362, 363
L-dopa *see* levodopa
dopamine/dopaminergic system, *18*,
  65
  AD, *352*
  ADHD, 125, 419–20
  anatomical distribution, 68–70, 264–8
  anatomical divisions, 262, *264*
  chemical structure, *333*
  and co-transmitters, 27–8
  depression, 159–60, 161–2, 163–4, 183
  drugs of abuse, 379–81
    alcohol, 387
    amphetamines, 400, 402, 403
    cannabis, 414
    cocaine, 400
    nicotine, 398
    phencyclidine, 410
  end product inhibition, 67
  functional neuroanatomy, 12
  mania, 194, 196, 197, *198*, 202
  metabolism, 65–8
  OCD, 225, *226*
  β-oxidase (β-hydroxylase) inhibitors,
    65–7, 386
  Parkinson's syndromes, 46, 322, 323–
    5, 326–7, 328, 336, 337

receptors, *18*, 44–7
  ADHD, 125
  chronic drug treatment, 45–6
  down-regulation, 46, 234
  drug dependence, 380
  lithium, 202, 203
  measuring in brain, 31–2
  mechanisms, 22, 24
  neuroleptics, 44–5, 46, 47, 146, 256,
    262–76, 281–2, 283–4
  Parkinson's syndromes, 46, 322,
    324, 326–7, 328, 331–2, 336
  subsensitivity, 46, 234
  supersensitivity, 234
  types, 46–7, 264
  up-regulation, 234
  schizophrenia, 46, 47, 146, 256–7, 258–
    76, 281–2, 283–4, 443–4
  sleep, 244
  synthesis, 65–7
dorsal raphé, 2
drug abuse, definition, 375–6
  see also drugs of abuse
drug addiction, 377
drug dependence, 376–81
  diagnostic criteria, 382, *383*
  specific drugs *see* drugs of abuse
drug discontinuation *see* withdrawal of
  drugs
drug–drug interactions, 459–62
  alcohol, 386, 460
  anticonvulsants, 94, 309, 459, 460, 461
  antidepressants, 88, 89, 94, 459–60
    MAOIs, 170, 171, 187, 188–9, 191,
      459, 460
    SSRIs, 171, 189, 191, 459, 460
    TCAs, 87, 88, 94, 187, 188, 189, 191,
      459, 461
  benzodiazepines, 235, 460–1
  biochemistry of, 90–4
  genetic polymorphism, 88–9
  lithium, 205, 459–60
  neuroleptics, 89, 94, 205, 460, 461–2
  pharmacodynamic, 92–4
  pharmacokinetic, 92, 93–4
  valproate, 206, 311, 460
drug–food interactions, MAOIs, 170,
  188, 459, 462
drug-induced psychosis, 427
drug names, 483–7
drug–protein interactions, 99

drug tolerance *see* tolerance
drug trials *see* clinical trials
drug withdrawal *see* withdrawal of drugs
drugs of abuse, 375–416
    alcohol, 67, 145, 246–7, *376*, 381–8
    amphetamines, 399–400, 402–3, 404–5
    anxiolytics, *376*, 388–9
    cannabis and cannabinoids, *376*, 410–
        16
    cocaine, *376*, 380–1, 399, 400–2, 403
    definitions, 375–7
    designer drugs, 403–5
    hallucinogens, 58, *143*, 144–5, *376*,
        405–8
    5-HT antagonists, 145
    neuronal mechanisms, 379–81
    nicotine, 145, *376*, 398–9
    opioid analgesics, 96–7, 145, *376*, 381,
        389–97
    phencyclidine, 408–10
    psychostimulants, *376*, 380–1, 399–403
    sedatives, *376*, 388–9
duloxetine, 176
dystonias, sigma receptors, 454–6

Ecstasy (MDMA), 404–5
efficacy of drugs, trials, 101–11
elderly people *see* geriatric psychophar-
    macology
electroconvulsive shock treatment
    (ECT), 182–5
    elderly people, 427
    mania, 208
eliprodil (SL 820715), 280, 456
emotional disorders, 421
enantiomers, 95–9
endocoids, 445–57
    cannabinoid abuse, *376*, 410–16
    endogenous cannabinoids, 445–50
    endozepines, 450–2
    sigma receptors, 452–7
    sleep factors, 452
endocrine function
    antidepressant mechanisms, 167–8
    and neuroleptics, 291–2
    psychoneuroimmunology, 434, 435–8,
        442
    sigma receptors, 453–4
endoplasmic reticulum, 7, *8*
endozepines, 450–2
enuresis, nocturnal, 421–2

ependymal cells, 10
epilepsies, *6*, 295–318
    classification, 295–6
    and cocaine, 401
    definition, 295
    kindled seizures, 206, 300
    neurotransmitters, *18*, 300–1, 304–6
        and ECT, 184
        excitotoxins, 357
        GABA, 35–6, 72, 184, 301, 304–6, 318
        imaging, 35–6
        see also antiepileptics, action on
            neurotransmitters
    pathological basis, 296–301
    treatment
        drugs used in, 303, 308–18, 357
        GABA transmission, 304–6, 318
        intractable epilepsy, 303
        ionic effects, 306
        major drug groups, 304
        membrane effects, 306
        pharmacokinetics, 301–3, 306–7, 310
        see also antiepileptics, action on
            neurotransmitters
ergolines, 332, *333*
escitalopram, 98, 175
ethchlorvynol, 251
ethosuximide, 309–10
    action on neurotransmitters, 304
    chemical structure, *305*
    indications, *303*, 308, 318
    pharmacokinetics, 307
    therapeutic range, *302*
Eve (MDA), 404–5
evidence-based prescribing, 110–11
excitatory amino acid neurotransmitters
    see aspartate; glutamate
excitotoxins, 354–8, 371–2

family studies, 122, 123
fananserin, 278–9
fatty acids
    schizophrenia, 281
    sleep, 452
feeding behaviour, and 5-HT, *143*
felbamate, *302*, *303*, 312–13
fenfluramine, 400, *401*
fentanyl derivatives, 403, *405*
flunitrazepam, *214*, 249
fluoxetine, 171, 173
    anxiety disorders, 148, 225

chemical structure, *173*
children, 421
drug interactions, 189, 459, 460
enantiomers, 99
genetic polymorphism, *89*
indications, 174–5
side effects, 189
toxicity, *186*
fluphenazine, 284, 285, 287
flurazepam, *214*, 234–5, 249, 429
fluvoxamine, 171, 173
  anxiety disorders, 148, 223
  chemical structure, *173*
  elderly people, 427
  indications, 174
  side effects, 189
  toxicity, *186*
fodrin, 9
food allergies, schizophrenia, 443
food–drug interactions, MAOIs, 170,
  188, 459, 462
free radicals
  AD, 365
  Parkinson's disease, 323
  stroke, 372, 373–4
functional MRI (fMRI), 33–5, 37

G proteins, 25–6, *27*
  antidepressants, *151*
  cannabinoids, 447
  depression, *151*, 158
  5-HT receptors, 141, *151*, 158
  and muscarinic receptors, 38–9
  opioids, 394
  sigma receptors, 453
GABA (gamma-aminobutyric acid), *18*,
  51, 53, 74, 76
  aetiology of anxiety, *216*, 217–18, 234
  alcohol, 229, 384, 385–6
  anatomical distribution, 72, 74, *76*,
    77–8
  benzodiazepines, 53, 55, *56*, 57, 212
    aetiology of anxiety, 217–18, 234
    antiepileptic action, 304–5, 311
    endozepines, 451
    receptors, 228–9, 230–1, 234–5
  depression, 36, 162, 184
  in epilepsies, 35–6, 51, 54, 74, 184, 301,
    304–6, 318
  functional neuroanatomy, 11, 12
  Huntington's disease, 338

imaging, 34, 35–6
mania, 197, *200*, 204, 205, 207, 208
metabolism, *75*
Parkinson's disease, *325*, 326, 328
receptors, 51–7
  aetiology of anxiety, 217–18, 234
  antiepileptics, 51, 52, 304–6, 311,
    312, 313, 314, 315, 316, 318
  antipsychotic action, 280–1
  anxiolytics, 51, 53, *56*, 57, 217–18,
    228–9, 230–1, 234–5
  carbamazepine, 207
  depression, 162, 184
  ECT, 184
  lithium, 204
  mechanisms, 21–2
  types, 54
  valproate, 205
schizophrenia, *263*, 280–1
synthesis, 77, 78
gabapentin, *303*, *312*, 313, 318
galantamine, 362, 363
gamma-aminobutyric acid *see* GABA
generic drug names, 483–7
genetics *see* molecular genetics
gepirone, *137*, 147, 237, 238
geriatric psychopharmacology, 425–30
  anticholinergics, 334–5, 425, 428
  antidepressants, 173–5, 185, 189, 190,
    425, 427
  anxiety disorders, 428–9
  benzodiazepines, 235, 249
  dementia, 426, 428
    see also Alzheimer's disease
  depression, 427
  hypotension, 425–6
  insomnia, 249, 429
  mania, 428
  paranoid disorders, 428
  pseudodementia, 426
  psychosis, 427–8
glial cells, 9–10, 16
gliosis, 10
glucocorticoid receptors
  antidepressant mechanisms, 165–7
  psychoneuroimmunology, 434, 437–8,
    441
  PTSD, 227
glutamate/glutamatergic system, *18*, 49,
  51, 74, 75–6
  anatomical distribution, 72, 74

glutamate/glutamatergic system (*cont'd*)
 anxiolysis, 218
 depression, 36, 164
 epilepsies, 357
 imaging, 34, 35–6
 metabolism, *76*, 78
 receptors, 56–60
  AD, 58, 60, 353, 354–6, 369
  alcohol, 386–7
  antidepressants, 164, 456
  antiepileptics, 58, 60, 309, 312, 314,
   318, 357
  antipsychotic action, 279–80
  cannabis, 413–14
  drugs of abuse, 386–7, 409, 413–14
  gene studies, 128–9
  and glycine, 75
  ketamine, 409
  mechanisms, 21–2
  Parkinson's disease, 328
  phencyclidine, 409
  schizophrenia, 261–2, *263*, 279–80
  sigma receptors, 456
  stroke, 371–2, 373, 409
 schizophrenia, 259–62, *263*, 279–80
 synthesis, 76, *77*
glycine, *18*, 74
 anatomical distribution, 74
 antidepressants, 164
 antipsychotic action, 279–80
 epilepsies, 300–1
 metabolism, *75*
 NMDA receptors, 59, 74, 164, 279–80
 receptor mechanisms, 20–2
Golgi apparatus, 8
grass, 411
grey matter, 3, 34
growth factors
 Parkinson's disease, 337
 schizophrenia, 121

half-life ($t_{1/2}$), 80–1
 drug withdrawal, 111
hallucinogens, 58, *143*, 144–5, *376*, 405–8
haloperidol
 chemical structure, *289*
 childhood tic disorders, 421
 conduct disorders, 420
 and dopamine receptors, 44
 drug interactions, 461
 genetic polymorphism, *89*

in vitro receptor binding, *271*
 mania, 204–5
 schizophrenia, 269, 275, 278, 288
hash, 411
herbal antidepressants, 180, 451–2
heroin-like compounds, 403–4
heteroceptors, 23, *24*
hippocampus, 2, 3–4, 5
 anxiety disorders, 221, 227
 cannabinoid receptors, 448
 drug dependence, 380–1
 schizophrenia, 257–8, 260–1
histamine, sleep, 243–4
homovanillic acid (HVA), 159, 196
human genome, 114, 115, 129–30
Huntington's disease, 118, 338–9, 358
hybridization, molecular genetics, 117
hydantoins *see* diphenylhydantoin
5-hydroxytryptamine (5-HT) *see* seroto-
  nin/serotonergic system
Hypericum officinalis, 180, 451–2
hypnotics, 241–2, 246, 247–54, *376*, 388–9
 elderly people, 426, 429
hypothalamus, 2, 4
 anxiety, 219
hypoxia, excitotoxins, 357–8

ifenprodil, 456
igmesine (JO 1784), 456, 457
imaging methods, 34–7
imipramine
 anti-panic action, 221, 223
 children, 422, 423
 history of development, 154
 toxicity, 185, *186*
 treatment decisions, 181
immune system, 432–4
 AD, 358–61, 367
 antidepressant mechanisms, 167–8,
  441–2
 cannabinoids, 448
 psychoneuroimmunology, 431–44
  affective disorders, 439–42
  endocrine function, 434, 435–8, 442
  immune system structure, 432–4
  nervous system, 435, *436*
  schizophrenia, 442–4
  stress, 435–9
 sigma receptors, 453–4
inflammatory changes
 AD, 358–61, 364–5

psychoneuroimmunology, 441, 444
insomnia, 241–54
  elderly people, 249, 429
  hypnotics, 241–2, 246, 247–54, 429
  physiology of sleep, 242–7
ion channels, 19, 23–4
  AD, 355–6, 369
  adrenergic receptors, 42, *43*
  antiepileptics, 306
  GABA receptors, 55, 229
  glutamate receptors, 57, *58*
    AD, 355–6
    ketamine, 409
    phencyclidine, 409
    stroke, 373, 409
  nicotinic receptors, 38
  stroke, 373, 374, 409
ionotropic receptors, 21–2, 24, 54, 58
  5-HT, 50, 136, *138*
ipsapirone, 50, *137*, 147, 237, 238
ischaemia
  excitotoxins, 357–8, 371–2
  sigma receptors, 456
  stroke, 371–4, 409, 456

ketamine, 408–9
kindling, seizures, 206, 300
"knock-out" mice, 102–3, 117, 128–9
Korsakoff's syndrome, *6*

L-dopa *see* levodopa
lamotrigine, 313–14, 318
  chemical structure, *312*
  indications, *303*
  mania, 208
  therapeutic range, *302*
  treatment-resistant depression, 191
levetiracetam, *303*, 314
levodopa (L-dopa), 67, 324, 328–31, 335–7, 460, 461
ligand receptor binding studies, 29–33
limbic system, 3–4
  anxiety disorders, 219, *220*
  Parkinson's disease, 324
  see also amygdala; hippocampus;
    hypothalamus
linkage analysis studies, 122, 124, 194
lithium
  children, 420, 423
  conduct disorders, 420
  drug–drug interactions, 205, 459–60

elderly people, 428
  mania, 198–204, 208, 209, 423, 428
  pharmacokinetics, 83–4, 428
  PTSD, 227
  side effects, *201*, 203–4
  treatment-resistant depression, 190, 203
locus ceruleus, *2*
lofepramine, 169, 170, *186*, 189, 427
loprazolam, *212*, 249
lorazepam, 208, *212*, 234–5, 308, 428
lormetazepam, *212*, 249
LSD, *143*, 144–5, 406–8
lymphocytes
  cannabinoids, 448
  psychoneuroimmunology, 432–3, 434, 435, 439–41, 443
  sigma receptors, 454
lysergic acid diethylamide *see* LSD
lysosomes, 8

macroglia, 10
magnetic resonance imaging (MRI), 34–5, 36
magnetic resonance spectroscopy (MRS), 34, 35–6
mamillary body, *5*
mania, 193
  biochemistry of, 194–7
  children, 423
  ECT, 208
  elderly people, 428
  genetic factors, 193–4, *195*
  neurotransmitters, *18*, 194–7, 202, 203–4, 205, 206–7
  pharmacological treatment
    benzodiazepines, 208
    calcium channel antagonists, 207
    carbamazepine, 206–7, 209
    children, 423
    clonidine, 208
    lithium, 198–204, 208, 209, 423, 428
    maintenance, 208–9
    neuroleptics, 204–5
    valproate, 205–6, 208
MAOIs *see* monoamine oxidase inhibitors (MAOIs)
marijuana, 411
MDA (Eve), 404–5
MDL 100 907, 278
MDL72222, 145

MDMA (Ecstasy), 404–5
Mendelian inheritance, 118, 119
mescaline, *143*, 145, 406, 407–8
meta-analyses, 108
metabotropic receptors, 22, 25, 51–4, 57–9
    5-HT, 47, 136, *139*
methadone, enantiomers, 96–7
methsuximide, 307, 308, 310
N-methyl-D-aspartate receptors *see*
    NMDA receptors
N-methyl-phenyl-tetrahydropyridine
    (MPTP), 403–4, *405*
metrifonate, 363
mianserin, 177, *186*, 190, 251, 427
microarray technology, 103–4, 120, 127,
    130
microglia, 10
midazolam, 248, *249*, 250
milameline, 364
milnacipran, 176–7, *178*
mirtazepine, 177, *179*, 181, 190, 191, 251
mitochondria, 7, *8*
molecular genetics, 113–31
    AD, 118–19, 346, 348, 370
    ADHD, 124–6, 419
    affective disorders, 118, 119, 120, 194
    cloning, 126–8
    detecting defects, 119–26
    DNA, 103–4, 113–14, 115–17, 120, 127–8
    drug dependence, 380
    drug testing, 103, 104
    gene composition, 113
    gene expression analysis, 103, 104
    gene manipulation, 115–17
    genetic code, 114
    human genome, 114, 115, 129–30
    Huntington's disease, 118, 338
    hybridization, 117
    impact on psychopharmacology, 126–
        32
    "knock-out" mice, 102–3, 117, 128–9
    OCD, 122–3
    panic disorder, 123–4
    Parkinson's disease, 323
    pharmacogenetics, 117–32
    pharmacogenomics, 129–32
    plasmids, 115, 117, 128
    polymorphism, 88–9, 119–22
    regulatory sequences, 114–15
    RNA
        cloning, 127, 128

mRNAs, 113–14, 115, 117
    schizophrenia, 118, 119, 120–2, 257
    theranostics, 130–1
    transfection, 117
    transgenic mice, 117, 128–9
monoamine oxidase
    catecholamine metabolization, 65–8
    5-HT metabolization, 72
    inhibitors *see below*
monoamine oxidase inhibitors
    (MAOIs)
    AD, 365, 369
    anxiety disorders, 224, 227, 228
    chemical structures, *172*
    classification, *174*
    drug interactions, 170, 171, 187, 188–9,
        191, 459, 460
    elderly people, 427
    food interactions, 170, 188, 459, 462
    history of development, 154–5
    5-HT receptors, 48, *49, 150*
    irreversible, 170
    Parkinson's disease, 330–1
    pharmacokinetics, 84–5
    pharmacological properties, 170–1
    psychoneuroimmunology, 435
    reversible (RIMAs), 85, 171, *174*, 228
    selective, 85
    selective irreversible, 170
    see also selegiline (deprenyl)
    side effects, 170–1, *186*, 187–9
    treatment-resistant depression, 191
movement disorders, sigma receptors,
    454–6
MPTP (N-methyl-phenyl-tetrahydro-
    pyridine), 403–4, *405*
muscarinic receptors, *18*, 22, 38–40
    AD, 39–40, 361, 363–4
    alcohol, 386
    anatomical distribution, *64*, 65
    depression, 157, *161*, 162, 184
    Parkinson's disease, 333

nabilone, 416
naltrexone, 387–8
natural killer cells (NKCs), 433, 440–1
nefazodone, *173*, 177–8, 180, 228, 251,
    460
neostigmine, 64
nephentin, 233
nerve cells *see* neurons

neuroanatomy, 1–13
neuroglial cells, 9–10, 16
neuroimaging methods, 33–7
neurokinin (NK), 218
neurolathyrism, 357
neuroleptics, 255–6
  AD, 428
  adrenergic receptors as, 279
  anxiety disorders, 228, 236
  atypical, 270–6, 428, 455–6
  bipolar disorder, 209
  childhood tic disorders, 421
  classification, 269, 285–90
  clinical pharmacology, 283–5
  and cognitive function, 292–3
  conduct disorders, 420
  delusional states, 428
  depot preparations, 284, 285
  drug interactions, 89, 94, 205, 460,
    461–2
  elderly people, 428
  enantiomers, 97–8
  GABAergic receptors as, 280–1
  genetic polymorphism, 89
  glutamate receptors as, 279–80
  high doses, 285, 290
  hormonal changes with, 291–2
  ligand receptor binding studies, 32
  mania, 204–5, 209
  mechanism of action, 256–7, 268–9,
    281–2
  neurotransmitters
    antipsychotic action, 146–7, 278–81
    clinical pharmacology, 283–4
    dopamine receptors, 44–5, 46, 47,
      146, 256, 262–76, 281–2, 283–4
    glutamate receptors, 261–2, 279–80
    5-HT receptors, 51, 146–7, 269, 271,
      272, 273–6, 278–9, 281–2
    and side effects, 46, 47, 266, 275,
      276, 281–2, 283
  omega 3 fatty acids, 281
  pharmacokinetics, 81–2, 89, 94, 97–8
  serotonin receptor antagonists as,
    146–7, 278–9
  side effects, 205
    akathisia, 277–8
    cardiotoxicity, 293
    cognitive function, 292–3
    dystonias, 454–6
    elderly people, 428
  high doses, 290
  hormonal changes, 291–2
  and neurotransmitters, 46, 47, 266,
    275, 276, 281–2, 283
  sigma receptors, 454–6
  tardive dyskinesia, 205, 276–7
  sigma receptors, 278, 280, 453, 454–6
  sites of action, 267
  treatment-resistant depression, 191
  treatment-resistant patients, 290, 444
neuromodulators, 11
  types, 18, 19
  see also prostaglandins
neuronal cell adhesion molecule
    (NCAM), 121
neurons, 7–9, 10–13
  AD, 345–6, 356, 357, 358–61, 364–6,
    370
  antidepressant mechanisms, 165, 166,
    168–9
  effects of drug abuse, 379–81
  neurotransmitters, 11–12, 16–17, 65,
    68–70, 72, 77–8
  Parkinson's disease, 322, 323–7, 336,
    337
  plasticity, 12
  schizophrenic patients, 121, 257–8
  sigma receptors, 456
  stroke, 371–4, 456
neuropeptides see peptide co-transmit-
    ters/neurotransmitters
neurotransmitter receptors
  antidepressant specificity, 162
  gene manipulation, 116–17
  gene studies, 128–9
  heteroceptors, 23, 24
  measuring in brain, 29–33
  mechanisms, 19
  plasticity, 12
  see also under acetylcholine/choliner-
    gic system; dopamine/dopami-
    nergic system; GABA;
    glutamate/glutamatergic system;
    adrenergic receptors; serotonin/
    serotonergic system
  sensitivity, 26–7, 46, 57, 151–2, 202,
    234–5
  types, 21–2, 24, 25, 37–60
neurotransmitters, 15–78
  AD, 350–70
  ADHD, 125, 419–20

neurotransmitters (*cont'd*)
  and anandamide system, 447–8
  anatomical distribution, 64, 67–70, 72,
    74, 77–8, *137*, *140–2*
  in anxiety disorders *see* anxiety dis-
    orders
  anxiolytics, 147–9, 212, 214–18, 223–5,
    227, 238, 239
  circadian rhythm, 160–1, 243–4
  co-transmission, 11, 28, *29*
  criteria for, *19*
  Dale's Law, 11, 19
  in depression *see* depression
  drugs of abuse, 379–81
    alcohol, 67, 145, 384–8
    amphetamines, 400, 402, 403, 404
    cannabis, 413–14
    cocaine, 400, 401
    hallucinogens, *143*, 144–5, 406–7
    ketamine, 409
    MDMA, 404
    nicotine, 398
    opioids, 394
    phencyclidine, 409, 410
  ECT, 182–5
  in epilepsies *see* epilepsies
  functional neuroanatomy, 11–12, 16–
    17
  Huntington's disease, 338, 358
  imaging, 34–7
  mania, 194–7, 202, 203–4, 205, 206–7
  metabolism, 62–78
  molecular genetics, 114, 116–17
  nerve impulse, 16–17
  and neuroleptics *see* neuroleptics
  Parkinson's syndromes, 46, 322, 323–
    8, 336, 337
  peptides *see* peptide co-transmitters/
    neurotransmitters
  psychoneuroimmunology, 434, 435–8,
    439–42
  receptors *see* neurotransmitter recep-
    tors
  in schizophrenia *see* schizophrenia
  sleep, 243–4, 452
  stroke, 371–2, 373–4, 409
  synthesis, 62–78, 114
  types, *18*, 19–20
neurotrophins
  Parkinson's disease, 337
  schizophrenia, 121

nicotine, 145, *376*, 398–9
nicotinic receptors, *18*, 22, 38, 40–1, *42*
  ADHD, 420
  anatomical distribution, *64*, 65
  nicotine as drug of abuse, 398
nitrazepam, *212*, 249
nitric oxide (NO), 60–1, 452
NMDA (N-methyl-D-aspartate) recep-
    tors, 58–60, 75
  AD, 353, 354–6
  antidepressants, 164, 456
  antiepileptics, 58, 60, 309, 312, 318, 357
  antipsychotic action, 279–80
  anxiolysis, 218
  drugs of abuse
    alcohol, 386–7
    ketamine, 409
    phencyclidine, 409
  gene studies, 128–9
  hypoxia, 357–8
  Parkinson's disease, 328
  sigma receptors, 456
  stroke, 373, 409
nocturnal enuresis, 421–2
nomifensine, 176, *186*, 189–90
non-steroidal anti-inflammatories
  AD, 364–5, *368*
  drug interactions, 459
noradrenaline/adrenergic system, *18*, 65
  AD, 352
  ADHD, 419–20
  anatomical distribution, 67, *68*
  anxiety, 214–15, *216*, *217*, *220*, *222*, 223
  depression, 155–7, 159, 161–2, 192
    antidepressant mechanisms, 163,
      177
    ECT, 183
  drugs of abuse
    alcohol, 385
    amphetamines, 402
    cocaine, 401
    opioids, 394
  end product inhibition, 67
  functional neuroanatomy, 11, 17
  mania, 194, 196, *197*, 202
    carbamazepine, 206, 207
    lithium, 202, 204
  metabolism, 67–8
  Parkinson's disease, 325
  psychoneuroimmunology, 434, 435–6
  receptors, *18*, 42–4

antidepressants, 163, 177, 178
antipsychotic action, 279
anxiety disorders, 236
buspirone, 237–8
depression, 44, 156–7, *159*, 161–2,
    163
lithium, 204
mania, 202, 208
Parkinson's disease, 325
presynaptic mechanisms, 22–3
psychoneuroimmunology, 435
PTSD, 227
schizophrenia, 279, 281–2
second messenger systems, 24, 27,
    42–4
sleep, 244
synthesis, 64–7
noradrenaline reuptake inhibitors
    (NARIs)
chemical structure, *178*
classification, *174*
drug interactions, 460
pharmacological properties, 175–6
side effects, 189–90
smoking cessation, 399
treatment decisions, 181
noradrenaline and selective serotonin
    antidepressant (NaSSA) *see* mirta-
    zepine
novel drugs, discovery, 101–4, 109–10
null hypotheses, 105

obsessive–compulsive disorder (OCD),
    224–5
children, 423
genetics, 122–3
5-HT receptors, 148–9
SSRIs, 148, 175, 224–5, 423
treatment decisions, 228
oestrogens, AD, 366, *368*, 369
olanzapine, 271–2
bipolar disorder, 209
chemical structure, *274*
effect on neurotransmitter receptors,
    275
in vitro receptor binding, *271*
mania, 205
oligodendrocytes, 10
omega 3 fatty acids, 281
opioids
abuse of, 96–7, 145, *376*, 381, 389–97

endogenous, 391–2
    alcohol dependence, 387–8
    pain response, 397
    sigma receptors, 452–3
oxazepam, *212*, *213*, 429
oxcarbazepine, *302*, *303*, 309
oxidative stress hypothesis, 323

paediatric psychopharmacology, 417–24
ADHD, 124–6, 419–20
antiepileptics, 317–18
anxiety disorders, 423
conduct disorders, 420
depression, 422
emotional disorders, 421
mania, 423
nocturnal enuresis, 421–2
tic disorders, 421
pain
cannabis, 413
depression, 180
endogenous opioids, 397
panamesine (EMD 57445), 280
panic disorder, 219, 221–4
autonomic nervous system, *215*
genetics, 123–4
and MDMA, 404–5
SSRIs, 148, 175, 228
treatment decisions, 228
paranoid disorders, 428
Parkinson's syndromes, 319–38
aetiology, 323
basal ganglia neuroanatomy, 326–8
brain transplants, 337
causes, 319–20
cholinergic system, 324, 326
dopaminergic system, 45, 322, 323–5,
    326–7, 328, 336, 337
drug treatment, 328–37
elderly people, 428
excitotoxins, 357, 358
GABA, *325*, 326
noradrenergic system, 325
oxidative stress hypothesis, 323
serotonergic system, 325
paroxetine, 171, 173, 175, 189, 459
peptide co-transmitters/neurotransmit-
    ters, 11, 27, *28*
AD, 351, 352, 369, 370
anxiety, 218, 223–4
carbamazepine, 207

peptide co-transmitters/neurotransmitters (*cont'd*)
ECT, 184
Huntington's disease, 338
pharmacogenetics, 117–32
pharmacogenomics, 129–32
pharmacokinetics, 79–99
  alcohol, 382–3
  antidepressants, 82–5, 88, 89, 94, 98–9, 172–5
  antiepileptics, 301–3, 306–7, 310
  anxiolytics, 86–8
  bioavailability, 79
  cannabis, 412
  clearance (Cl), 80
  drug–drug interactions, 88–9, 90–4
  drug–protein interactions, 99
  enantiomers, 95–9
  genetic polymorphism, 88–9
  half-life ($t_{1/2}$), 80–1
  levodopa, 336
  neuroleptics, 81–2, *89*, 94, 97–8
  and pharmacogenomics, 131
  therapeutic window, 81
  volume of distribution (V_d), 79–80
phencyclidine (PCP)
  AD, 355
  as drug of abuse, 408–10
  schizophrenia, 259–60, 453
  sigma receptors, 409, 452, 453, 454
phenobarbitone, 310–11
  action on neurotransmitters, 304, 306
  chemical structure, *305*
  indications, *303*, 308
  pharmacokinetics, 306–7
  therapeutic range, *302*
phenothiazines, 286–7
  drug interactions, 459, 461
  see also chlorpromazine; thioridazine
phenytoin *see* diphenylhydantoin
physical pain *see* pain
physostigmine, 38, 39, 40, 64, 363
pimozide, *137*, 288, *289*, 421
pindolol, *137*, 191
pipamerone, 278
piracetam, 315
placebo controlled trials, 107–8, 110
plasma membrane, 8
plasmids, 115, 117, 128
platelet function, depression, 149, 151, 157–8, 183–4

polyamines, NMDA receptors, 59–60
polyunsaturated fatty acids, schizophrenia, 281
positron emission tomography (PET), 34
post traumatic stress disorder (PTSD), 227–8
pot, 411
pre-clinical drug tests, 101–4, 109–10
pregnancy, antiepileptics, 318
prescribing principles, 111
primidone, 311
  action on neurotransmitters, 304
  chemical structure, *305*
  indications, *303*, 308
  pharmacokinetics, 307
  therapeutic range, *302*
propranolol, *137*, 227, 236
proprietary drug names, 483–7
prostaglandins
  antidepressant action, 167–8
  sleep, 452
protein–drug interactions, 99
proteomics, 104
pseudodementia, 426
psilocybin, 406, 407–8
psychedelics *see* hallucinogens
psychoneuroimmunology, 431–44
  affective disorders, 439–42
  brain–immune system, 435, *436*
  endocrine–immune relation, 434, **435–8**, 442
  immune system structure, 432–4
  schizophrenia, 442–4
  stress–immune system, 435–9
psychosis
  elderly people, 427–8
  schizophrenia *see* schizophrenia
psychostimulant abuse, *376*, 380–1, **399–403**
psychotomimetics *see* hallucinogens

quantitative autoradiography, 33
quetiapine, 271, 272, 273
quinolinic acid, 358

racemic drugs, 95–9
radioligands, 29–33
reboxetine, 175–6, 181
remoxipride, 272–3, *274*, 275
research trials *see* clinical trials
reserpine, 285

resin, cannabis, 411
reversible inhibitors of monoamine oxidase (RIMAs), 85, 171, *174*, 228
ribonucleic acid (RNA), 7
  cloning, 127, 128
  mRNA, 7, 113–14, 115, 117
ribosomes, 7, *8*
risperidone, 272, 275
  bipolar disorder, 209
  chemical structure, *274*
  conduct disorders, 420
  elderly people, 428
  5-HT activity, 146
  in vitro receptor binding, *271*
  mania, 205
ritanserin, *137*, 144, 147
rivastigmine, 362, 363

safety of drugs, trials, 101–11
  see also toxicity
St John's Wort, 180, 451–2
Scatchard plots, *30*, 31
schizophrenia, 255–93
  allergies, 443
  cannabis, 414, 415
  core symptoms, 255, *256*
  drug treatment, 255–6
    adrenergic receptors, 279
    atypical neuroleptics, 270–6
    cardiotoxicity, 293
    cognitive function, 292–3
    effect on neurotransmitters, 262–8, 274–6
    endocrine function, 291–2
    GABAergic receptors, 280–1
    glutamatergic receptors, 279–80
    high doses, 285, 290
    5-HT antagonists, 146–7, 278–9
    mechanisms, 256–7, 268–9, 281–2
    neuroleptic classification, 269, 285–90
    neuroleptic pharmacology, 283–5
    omega 3 fatty acids, 281
    side effects, 266, 275, 276–8, 281–2, 283, 290, 291–3
    sigma receptors, 280, 453, 454
    tardive dyskinesia, 276–7
  genetics, 118, 119, 120–2, 257, 443
  integrated model, *261*
  neuropathology, 257–8
  neurotransmitters, *18*, 122, 256–7, 258–62
    antipsychotic action, 146–7, 278–81
    dopamine receptors, 45, 47, 146, 256–7, 258–76, 281–2, 283–4, 443–4
    effects of neuroleptics on, 262–8, 274–6
    GABA, *263*
    glutamate, 259–62, *263*, 279–80
    5-HT, 146, *263*, 271, 272, 273–6, 278–9, 281–2
    neuroleptic side effects, 266, 275, 276, 281–2, 283
    psychoneuroimmunology, 443–4
    phencyclidine (PCP), 259–60, 453
    psychoneuroimmunology, 442–4
    sigma receptors, 280, 453, 454
school phobia, 423
seasonal affective disorder (SAD), 160–1
secondary messenger systems, 24–7
  adrenergic receptors, 25, 27, 42–4
  antidepressants, 151, 165, *166*
  depression, 151, 158
  dopamine receptors, 264
  5-HT receptors, *48–9*, 50, 135–6, 151, 158
  lithium, 204
  muscarinic receptors, 38–9
secretase, AD, 346
secretase inhibitors, AD, 366–7
sedative hypnotics, 241–2, 246, 247–54, *376*, 388–9
  elderly people, 426, 429
seizures
  cocaine-induced, 401, 403
  ECT-induced, 182, 184
  epileptic *see* epilepsies
selective serotonin and noradrenaline reuptake inhibitors (SNRIs), *174*, 176–7, *178*, 190–1
  see also venlafaxine
selective serotonin reuptake inhibitors (SSRIs)
  anxiety disorders, 148–9, 175, 223, 224–5, 227, 228
  chemical structures, *173*
  children
    ADHD, 420
    depression, 422
    emotional disorders, 421

selective serotonin reuptake inhibitors
    (SSRIs) (cont'd)
  classification, 174
  drug–drug interactions, 459, 460
    genetic polymorphism, 88
    MAOIs, 171, 189, 459
    pharmacodynamic, 94
    pharmacokinetic, 94
    TCAs, 191, 459
  drug–protein interactions, 99
  elderly people, 173–5, 189, 427
  enantiomers, 98, 99, 175
  5-HT receptors, 47–9, 52, 148–9, 150–1,
    163, 164
  indications, 173–5
  mechanisms of action, 163, 164
  pharmacogenomics, 130, 131
  pharmacokinetics, 88, 94, 98, 99, 172–5
  pharmacological properties, 171–5
  side effects, 175, 189
    5-HT receptor activity, 48, 175
    serotonin syndrome, 191
    toxicity, 175, 186
    on withdrawal, 191
  treatment decisions, 181
  treatment-resistant depression, 191
  withdrawal, 191
selegiline (deprenyl)
  AD, 365, 369
  Parkinson's disease, 330–1
  psychoneuroimmunology, 435
separation anxiety, children, 423
septohippocampal system, anxiety, 219,
  221
serotonin/serotonergic system (5-HT),
  18, 70
  AD, 352
  ADHD, 420
  anatomical distribution, 72, 74, 137,
    140–2
  anxiety, 70, 215, 216, 217, 220
    OCD, 148, 224–5, 226
    panic disorder, 148, 222, 223–4
    social phobia, 227
    treatment see anxiolytics, 5-HT
  and co-transmitters, 28
  depression, 70, 71, 149–52, 157–9, 160–
    2, 163–4
    ECT, 183–4
    treatment see antidepressants, 5-HT
  discovery, 15, 133–4

drugs of abuse, 380
  alcohol, 385
  amphetamines, 400, 404
  hallucinogens, 143, 144–5, 406–7
  MDMA, 404
drugs modifying, 133–52
  alcohol, 145
  antidepressants see antidepressants,
    5-HT
  antiemetics, 51, 137, 140
  anxiolytics see anxiolytics, 5-HT
  hallucinogens, 143, 144–5
  lithium, 203
  neuroleptics, 49, 50, 137, 143, 269,
    271, 272, 273–6, 281–2
  sleep, 143–4
main pathways, 74, 135
mania, 194, 196, 197, 199, 203, 206–7
metabolism, 72, 73
Parkinson's disease, 325
psychoneuroimmunology, 434
receptors, 18, 70
  antagonists as antipsychotics, 146–
    7, 278–9
  anxiety, 70, 215, 217, 223
  depression, 149–52, 157–8, 159, 161–
    2, 163, 183–4
  drug dependence, 380
  drugs modifying see above
  ECT, 183–4
  hallucinogens, 143, 144–5, 406–7
  lithium, 203
  mechanisms, 22, 23, 24, 25–6
  second messenger systems, 47–8,
    52, 135–6, 151, 158
  subtypes, 47–8, 52, 134–43
sleep, 143–4, 244
synthesis, 70–2, 73
sertindole, 272, 273, 275, 293
sertraline, 171, 172–4, 189, 459
sexual dysfunction, 143, 292
sigma receptors, 278, 452–7
  antipsychotic action, 280, 453, 454
  anxiety, 456–7
  depression, 454, 456–7
  endocrine function, 453–4
  future, 457
  immune function, 453–4
  movement disorders, 454–6
  neurodegenerative disorders, 456
  phencyclidine, 409, 452, 453, 454

schizophrenia, 280, 453, 454
single photon emission computed
 tomography (SPECT), 34
sleep
 5-HT involvement, 143–4, 244
 insomnia
  hypnotics, 241–2, 246, 247–54
  physiology, 242–7
 psychoneuroimmunology, 433–4
sleep factors, endogenous, 452
smoking
 cannabis, 411, 412, 415–16
 drug interactions, 461
 nicotine, 398–9
social phobia, 224, 225, 227, 228
sodium valproate see valproate
SPECT, 34
spiperone, 137, 289
SSRIs see selective serotonin reuptake
 inhibitors (SSRIs)
statins, AD, 367
stem cells, 104
stress, psychoneuroimmunology, 431,
 435–9
stroke, 6, 371–4, 409, 456
St John's Wort (Hypericum officinalis),
 180, 451–2
substance abuse see drug abuse
succinimides see ethosuximide; methsuximide
sulpiride, 290, 291, 455–6
sumatriptan, 47, 50
synapses, 16, 17, 20–2
synapsins, 23, 122

T lymphocytes, 432–3, 434, 435, 443, 454
tacrine, 362
tardive dyskinesia, 46, 205, 276–7
TCAs see tricyclic antidepressants
 (TCAs)
temazepam, 212, 213, 214, 249, 421, 429
teratogenicity, antiepileptics, 318
tetracyclic antidepressants
 classification, 174
 drug interactions, 460
 insomnia, 251
 pharmacological properties, 177, 179
 side effects, 186, 190
 treatment decisions, 181
 treatment-resistant depression, 190,
  191

thalamus, 2, 4, 5
theranostics, 130–1
thermoregulation, 143
thioridazine, 282, 284, 286
 cardiotoxicity, 293
 drug interactions, 461
 elderly people, 428
 enantiomers, 97–8
thioxanthines, 281–2, 287–8
thrombolysis, stroke, 374
tiagabine, 303, 315
tic disorders, 421
T lymphocytes, 432–3, 434, 435, 443, 454
TMS, 36–7
tolerance, 377
 alcohol, 383, 384–5
 amphetamines, 403
 benzodiazepines, 235, 311
 cannabinoids, 414, 450
 cannabis, 414
 cocaine, 402, 403
 hallucinogens, 407–8
 opioids, 396
 phencyclidine, 410
topiramate, 302, 303, 315–16
Tourette's syndrome, 421
toxicity
 amphetamines, 402
 anticholinesterases, 362
 antidepressants, 185–7
  MAOIs, 171, 186, 187–8, 191
  SNRIs, 176
  SSRIs, 175, 186
  TCAs, 169, 170, 185–6, 191, 427
 antiepileptics, 311, 313, 318
 cocaine, 400–1
 drug-induced psychosis, 427
 lithium, 199–200, 201, 204, 205, 428
 MDA, 404–5
 MDMA, 404–5
 neuroleptics, 205, 293
 thioridazine enantiomers, 97
 valproate, 311
toxicology tests, pre-clinical, 102
transfection, 117
transgenic mice, 102–3, 117, 128–9
tranylcypromine, 189
trazodone, 177–8, 180, 186
 drug interactions, 460
 elderly people, 427
 insomnia, 251

treatment costs, 109
trials *see* clinical trials
triazolam, *212*, *214*, 248, *249*, 250, 460
tribulin, 233
tricyclic antidepressants (TCAs)
  anticholinergic activity, 162
  anxiety disorders, 221, 223, 236, 423
  cardiotoxicity, 169, 170
  children
    anxiety disorders, 423
    depression, 422
    emotional disorders, 421
    nocturnal enuresis, 422
  drug interactions, 187, 459, 461
    genetic polymorphism, 87, 88
    MAOIs, 187, 188, 189, 191, 459
    pharmacodynamic, 94
    pharmacokinetic, 94
    SSRIs, 191, 459
  elderly people, 427, 428
  glutamatergic system, 164
  history of development, 154
  5-HT receptors, *52*, *150–1*
  insomnia, 251
  overdose, 186
  paranoid disorders, 428
  pharmacokinetics, 82–3, 84, 87, 88, 94
  pharmacological properties, 169–70,
    174
  and prostaglandins, 167–8
  side effects, 169, 170, 185–7, 189, 191,
    427
  treatment decisions, 181
  treatment-resistant depression, 191
  withdrawal, 187
tri-iodothyronine (T$_3$), 191
tryptophan, 70–1, *73*, 191
twin studies, 122, 124, 125, 193–4

vaccines, AD, 367
valproate
  action on neurotransmitters, 281, 304,
    305–6, 316

antiepileptic use, *303*, 307, 308, 311,
  316–17
antipsychotic action, 281
chemical structure, *305*
drug interactions, 206, 311, 460
mania, 205–6, 208
side effects, 206, 311
venlafaxine, 176, *178*, 181, 190–1
  drug interactions, 460
  insomnia, 251
  PTSD, 228
verapamil, mania, 207
vigabatrin, 35–6, *303*, *312*, 317, 318
vitamin E, AD, 365, 369

white matter, 3, 34
withdrawal of drugs, 111
  alcohol, 385–6
  amphetamines, 403
  antidepressants, 187, 189, 190–1
  benzodiazepines, 236, 250, 378, 388
  cannabis, 415
  cocaine, 403
  hallucinogens, 408
  hypnotics, 250, 253
  nicotine, 398
  opioids, 396–7
  physical dependence, 377–8
  withdrawal symptoms, 377–8
  withdrawal syndrome, 378–9

xanomeline, 364

zaleplon, *249*, 250
ziprasidone, *271*, 272, 273
ZK 93426, 368
zolpidem, *249*, 250, 252, 253, 429
zopiclone, 55, 231
  chemical structure, *252*
  elderly people, 429
  enantiomers, 97
  insomnia, 251, 252, 253, 429
  pharmacokinetics, 87–8, 97
zotepine, 272, 275